THE PROGRAM:
— PERSONAL EVOLUTION —

A SCIENTIFIC
APPROACH TO
RAPID BODY
RECOMPOSITION

ANDREW WINGE, M.D.

ISBN-10: 0615716644
ISBN-13: 9780615716640

To Russ and Aileen, the most selfless people I know.

TABLE OF CONTENTS

FOREWORD

Daren Korf, MPE-AA, USAW-1

I am thrilled to introduce Andrew Winge, MD, or as I call him Dr. Drew, as an author, and give my testimonial on the life changing effectiveness of The Program: Personal Evolution. For starters, he is highly accomplished in a multitude of fields including medicine, nutrition, strength sports, and martial arts. His direct and honest demeanor makes being a friend, colleague, and former training partner a pleasure. In writing this book, Dr. Drew spent a great deal of time combing through hard science and organizing it into this useful resource. His purpose is clear: help the reader understand how to achieve their personal fitness goals in the most efficient manner possible.

Honored. That's the first thing that came to mind when Dr. Drew, asked me to write the foreword to this book. Our friendship began when we developed respect for each other as hard trainers, and hard studying college students in Eugene, OR, during the early 1990's. Shortly after, he earned a coveted medical school scholarship through the U.S. Air Force while I took advantage of a scholarship to study kinesiology at Boise State. I started a coaching career in collegiate strength and condition, and later shifted my focus to strength sports and physical education. Like Dr. Drew, I appreciate working with athletes from youth to Olympic level athletes, and we share the same joy assisting people in achieving their physical fitness and performance goals.

Dr. Drew has helped people from all walks of life accomplish their fitness goals for over twenty years, myself included. I'm one of the fortunate people who have listened to him, acted on his no-nonsense advice, and enjoyed improving my physique with The Program. At age 39, I used it to go from a soft and round 300lbs to a leaner and athletic 215lbs in less than nine months. What's remarkable is that I did this without being hungry. I enjoyed good food and wine throughout the journey.

Finally, with my lighter body and improved strength I have more fun and do more physically active things now than before. Thanks to The Program, I feel great. Now I am urging you, the reader, to imagine how great you will feel when you get on The Program, and begin your own Personal Evolution.

I urge you to study hard, train hard, and may the next honor be yours.

Sincerely,

Daren Korf, MPEAA, USAW-1

ACKNOWLEDGMENTS

This book has gone through many stages over the years. Many times, it was shelved for years at a time when the demands of work and family life required that it be set aside. If it were not for the following people, and many others whom I haven't mentioned, this book would have remained a scattered collection of Word documents on my hard drive, never having seen the light of day. You have my sincere thanks and appreciation for all you have done.

Daren Korf, MPEAA: The man whose tireless encouragement, fresh perspectives, and countless hours of work behind the scenes made this book possible. No man could ask for a better friend and colleague.

Christopher Alfonzo, MD: His tireless hypomania, creative eye, and unmatched talents transformed this book from simple text to a work of art.

Andrew Henderson: His time and effort going into the stretching images are very appreciated.

The Club Fitness Center for the generous use of their facility and equipment.

There isn't a person anywhere who isn't capable
of doing more than he thinks he can.

—Henry Ford

INTRODUCTION

It is midnight at Balad Air Base, otherwise known as LSA (Logistical Staging Area) Anaconda in Iraq. I have just finished a long shift in the theater hospital emergency department. All day, Blackhawk helicopters brought in a steady stream of casualties, including American soldiers, Iraqi army, and police as well as civilians. Fortunately, my replacement had arrived, and it was time for me to head back to my bunk and try to get some sleep. I quickly reported on the patients still in the emergency room and headed out. Tomorrow would surely be another busy day. Fortunately, this late at night, the temperature had dropped to a very comfortable sixty-five degrees. Walking the four hundred meters or so to my bunk in full body armor during the day when temperatures routinely exceeded 120 degrees was not pleasant. At night though, the cool air actually made the walk enjoyable. I thought about some of the patients my team and I had treated, thought about what I would do at the gym the next morning, and counted how many weeks I had left before I could go home. Despite the late hour, there was activity everywhere. This base never slept. Everywhere, loud gas- and diesel-powered generators roared, vehicles convoyed through the streets, and jets landed and took off. It's a good thing I was a hard sleeper. After a while, you learned to block out the constant droning. I even learned to sleep through it. There was one sound that I never became accustomed to however, one sound that always got my attention. *Thud…Thud…Thud…*

As I strolled home, I was snapped back to reality from my idle daydreaming. Those are incoming mortar rounds. In over four months, there was rarely a day that insurgents did not fire mortar rounds and rockets over the fences and onto the base. I quickly got my bearings and hustled into the nearest concrete bunker. The warning siren blared its all-too-familiar high-pitched tone. "*Alarm red…Alarm red.*" The blasts sounded far off. They were probably over by the airfield a half mile or so away. I didn't feel too threatened, but I wasn't taking my body armor off and I sure as hell wasn't leaving that bunker until the "all-clear" signal was given. Soon, the incoming *thuds* stopped. A few minutes later came a different sound, more high-pitched, and with a more audible "*Whoosh.*" Outgoing rounds. Those I liked to hear. The base defense personnel had calculated the origin of the incoming rounds and were returning fire. I hoped they got the bastards, but I realized they were probably long gone by the time our rounds landed.

As I sat in the dusty bunker, I looked around and noticed some old newspapers and a recent copy of a popular bodybuilding magazine. It was a little beat up but still readable. On the cover was a freakishly huge professional bodybuilder curling a massive dumbbell with a headline that read something like "Amazing New Secrets for Huge Arms!" I chuckled a bit and paged through the articles and advertisements inside to help pass the time. I knew it would be at least thirty minutes before the post-attack reconnaissance teams would give the all clear. Inside, I read ads for the latest protein supplements, herbal muscle builders, and pro-hormone supplements, all of which promised steroid-like gains in muscle mass almost overnight. I recognized most of the bodybuilders featured in the ads. They all either directly or indirectly credited that particular supplement for helping them build the massive muscles that won them the title of Mr. Olympia, Universe, or whatever. It didn't escape my attention that many of them had telltale signs of steroid use in the form of gynecomastia (enlarged male breast tissue).

I had given up on reading muscle magazines as a source for useful bodybuilding information years earlier, but I would occasionally get the urge to see what the latest supplements hitting the market were or who the reigning Mr. or Ms. Olympia was. I had learned long ago that these magazines had an agenda and it was not to provide me with unbiased, useful information on how to build muscle, lose body fat, and stay healthy. Most, if not all, were owned by companies that were in the business of selling nutritional supplements. Still, I couldn't help but be impressed with how slick their presentations were. The pages were made of high-quality, glossy paper; the photos of massive bodybuilders and beautiful half-naked women were everywhere. Ad slogans with key words like "Massive," "Ripped" and of course "SEX" in bold letters would draw your eyes to one advertisement or the next. All insinuated if you just took supplement X or followed Mr. Olympia's workout, you could not only get a body like his, but get the girl as well. I had to give it to the magazine editors; their product was cleverly designed to be absolutely irresistible to the under-thirty male mind. I thought about all the young soldiers I had seen in the gym two days ago. Most were twenty-one years old or younger. Against this sort of marketing, they didn't stand a chance. I couldn't be too hard on them though. Years before, when I decided I wanted to improve my body and get into shape, the same magazines lured me in as well. I read them religiously. As a result, I spent many years and lots of money spinning my wheels and not getting the results I had been working so hard to achieve. I also noticed that in the years since then, the magazines hadn't really changed. The same supplements, repackaged and remodeled, were still there. The same claims and the same hype remained. The bodybuilders were bigger, but I suspected that had nothing to do with improvements in the quality of the whey protein they were taking. The same package sold to me in my early twenties had simply been polished up and sold again to the next generation.

Fortunately, through the years, I had had the opportunity to read and educate myself, not only about nutrition and supplementation, but also about exercise science. These were subjects that I have great personal interest in but are, unfortunately, some of the most misunderstood by both the general public and physicians. As I progressed through my schooling, graduated medical school, and completed my residencies, I never lost that initial desire I developed as a teen to build my body and feel good. I took what I learned from my studies and real-world experience and fine-tuned my exercise and diet program to the point where I knew I finally had something that worked and worked extremely well.

Over the years, I had shared my insights into bodybuilding with those who asked me. Every now and then, I would strike up a conversation with a young airman in the gym who would see me working out. They almost universally wanted to know what supplements I used, what kind of workout I followed, and how I got so strong. I have never been one to proselytize, but I would always share the basics of the approach I used. Invariably, I would get a look of disbelief when I told them I rarely used any supplements at all and only lifted weights an average of two to three times a week. Most thought I was pulling their leg. Eventually, I would see them back in the gym going through the motions of the same workout they had always done. I would never push the issue but always made it clear that I was happy to help if they needed any assistance with their workouts or diets. Those who had taken me up on the offer and stuck to the system I designed for them had made outstanding progress, and through word of mouth, I became known for providing advice on bodybuilding that actually worked.

Under most circumstances, I would have flipped through that particular muscle magazine, shaken my head in dismay, and gone about my business. However, for some reason, I became more and more irritated as I read. The people publishing and advertising in this magazine were *lying*. Not only were they lying; they were also deliberately disseminating false information in order to make money. They were ripping off the same young soldiers I had seen the day before, taking their hard-earned money, and giving them pure *crap* in return. How many of them were spending two hundred dollars or more a month on supplements that these companies knew didn't work? How many of them were like I was, following the workout routines of chemically enhanced goons and spending hours a week in the gym with little to show for it? Most would give up, incorrectly assuming that they just didn't have the genetics to have the body they always dreamed of. Eventually, the next generation would come along, the same slick bullshit package would be sold to them, and the cycle would continue.

When I finished reading that magazine, I put it aside for the next person seeking shelter to read. I opened up the laptop computer that I had carefully packed away from the dust and sand and started typing. I decided it was time to precisely articulate all I had learned from my bodybuilding endeavors. I have no delusions about competing with multimillion-dollar supplement companies and their magazines. I want to give those who feel as passionately about improving their bodies as I do an unbiased source of *real* information—information that they can actually use, that will yield real results, and that is based on cutting-edge scientific research. This project isn't about money. As a physician, I make more than enough to live comfortably and support my family. It's about helping those who are willing to put forth the effort to make sense of the overwhelming amount of conflicting and contradictory information on building a stronger, healthier body. It's also about helping people see through the fog of half-truths and outright lies disseminated by slick businessmen looking to make a quick buck at the expense of the general public.

As the all-clear signal echoed overhead, I headed to my cot with a rough outline of what you are about to read safely saved on my hard drive. In the months that followed, that outline was fleshed out, written, rewritten, and edited more times than I can count. What is left is a simple, straightforward plan to help you reach your fitness goals.

Thank you for taking the time to read this book. I hope you enjoy the process of transforming your body as much as I have. Good luck!

Andrew Winge MD

When planning for a year, plant corn. When planning for a decade, plant trees. When planning for life, train and educate people.

—Chinese Proverb

WHAT IS PERSONAL EVOLUTION?

When the term *evolution* is heard, we often think of it in a scientific context as it relates to changes in a species over millions of years. Charles Darwin first popularized the notion that, over time, a species will adapt to its environment through the process of natural selection. Those members of a species best adapted to the environment in which they lived would leave more offspring than those who were not. As a result, over thousands and millions of years, a species would become fitter, better adapted, and better able to survive the rigors of daily life through the accumulation of beneficial traits passed down through the generations.

The idea of evolution, therefore, is typically thought of as something that occurs on a species level and not on an individual level. Yet, evolution, in a sense, can also occur on a personal level. Just as a species develops specific traits over time leaving it fitter, healthier, and more adapted, an individual can volitionally develop traits and behaviors that accomplish similar results. For example, by changing your diet and starting a weight-training program, you can radically change your body's ratio of fat to muscle mass. As a result, you will have more energy and be able to fight off illness better, run faster, jump higher, and perform better at a myriad of other daily activities. This process will also help you evolve intellectually and emotionally. By learning how your body works and how it responds to changes in your diet and exercise habits, you can not only develop a closer connection to your body but learn to make healthier choices that will continue your upward path toward a healthier, more vital life.

The Personal Evolution Program, or as I like to call it "The Program," in simple terms, is the fastest, most efficient, and most effective way to finally get the body you have been looking for. It is specifically designed for those of you looking to reduce your body fat and build strong, lean, healthy muscle mass in the most time-efficient manner possible. There are very few people who have the luxury of spending two hours a day in the gym six days a week, let alone taking the time to navigate the maze of conflicting information regarding nutrition. The Program is for busy people—for people with lives, families, jobs, and personal interests, who literally can't afford to spend that sort of time on their body. Fortunately, with The

Program, you won't have to. If you follow The Program to the letter, you will not only achieve the body you have always wanted; you will do so in record time. It doesn't matter if you have ten, twenty, or even one hundred pounds to lose. Personal Evolution will help get you there.

I have used the information in this program to help untold numbers of people achieve their fitness goals and improve their health and quality of life. Many of them were skeptical since some of the recommendations in The Program directly contradict what mainstream fitness experts have been preaching for years. Without exception, however, every one of these skeptics has been stunned by the virtual overnight transformation their body has gone through.

The Program is built on science. Unfortunately, much of the most useful and most important breakthroughs in the fields of nutritional and exercise science are published in obscure and highly technical journals that are not written for the average person. As a result, a breakthrough or important advancement in this area may raise a few eyebrows among scientists and academics, but rarely will it filter out into the mainstream population and make an impact on the way we are told to eat or exercise. As both a medical doctor and fitness enthusiast, I have access to and the ability to interpret some of the more obscure scientific literature and help translate that information not only into an easily understandable format but also into a practical system that yields outstanding real-world results. I originally formulated The Program for my own personal use but quickly began to share it with friends and with patients. Over the years, I have fine-tuned it based on feedback from those using it to the point where The Program has developed into a uniquely effective total-body transformation system. It is the fastest and most efficient way to achieve the goals you have for your body. It has exceeded not only my expectations, but those of everyone who has tried it.

Chalkboard Notes

In order to enhance the reader experience, most sections of the book have chalkboard notes and summaries. I recommend looking through these chalkboards to capture the essence of the chapter, and then read through the content to develop a deeper understanding of the concepts.

We can evade reality, but we cannot evade the consequences of evading reality.

—Ayn Rand

OBESITY

Obesity has become America's number-one health problem. We are by far the fattest, most out of shape nation the world has ever known. By some estimates, over 127 million Americans can be classified as obese (body mass index greater than or equal to 30).[1] The number of adults who are overweight or obese has continued to increase. Currently, 64.5 percent of US adults, age twenty years and older, are overweight and almost 40 percent are obese.[2] Severe obesity prevalence is now 4.7 percent, up from the 2.9 percent reported in the 1988 to 1994 National Health and Nutrition Examination Survey (NHANES) by the Centers for Disease Control and Prevention (CDC).

Ethnic minorities in the United States are particularly affected by this trend. Black Americans have an average obesity rate of 49.5 percent and Americans of Mexican decent have a prevalence rate of 39.1% as of 2010. This is relative to an overall 34.3 percent obesity rate among non-Hispanic whites.[3] As America's demographics change, the obesity rates among all ethnic groups are predicted to continue climbing. A study published in 2008 made the dire prediction that by 2030 up to 86 percent of all Americans will be either overweight or obese. Obesity rates among black women and Mexican-American men were predicted to exceed 91 percent.[4]

---

1   http://www.obesity.org/subs/fastfacts/obesity_US.shtml.
2   CDC/NCHS, National Health and Nutrition Examination Survey, 2009–2010
3   Flegal et. al. Prevalence of Obesity and Trends in the Distribution of Body Mass Index
Among US Adults, 1999-2010, JAMA. 2012;307(5):491-497
4   Wang, Y., Beydoun, M. A., Liang, L., Caballero, B. and Kumanyika, S. K. (2008), Will All Americans Become Overweight or Obese? Estimating the Progression and Cost of the US Obesity Epidemic. Obesity, 16: 2323–2330. doi: 10.1038/oby.2008.351

Increase in Prevalence (%) of Overweight (BMI > 25)

	1976 to 1980	1988 to 1994	1999 to 2000	2009-2010
BMI > 25	46	56	64.5	68.8
BMI > 30	14	23	30.5	35.7
BMI > 40	no data	4	4.7	6.3

Source:. Flegal et. al. Prevalence of Obesity and Trends in the Distribution of Body Mass Index Among US Adults, 1999-2010, JAMA. *2012;307(5):491-497.*

NIH, National Heart, Lung, and Blood Institute, Clinical Guidelines on the Identification, Evaluation and Treatment of Overweight and Obesity in Adults, 1998.

There are many reasons for this epidemic and therefore no simple solutions. Our technology-driven society has virtually eliminated the need to travel anywhere under our own power. High-calorie/low-nutrition foods are easily available and aggressively marketed to children and adults. Schools are cutting back on physical education requirements, and junk-food vending machines are found everywhere, including schools. Parents often lack the knowledge or the drive to provide good food choices for their kids and often set a poor example with their own dietary habits. The popularity of game consoles makes kids much more likely to spend their days in front of the TV than out playing. As a result, there is a whole new generation of Americans who have been obese their entire lives. They will develop diabetes at much younger ages and therefore suffer all the complications (heart attack, stroke, blindness, amputation) of diabetes at younger ages. There literally are not enough kidney dialysis centers available to meet the demand the booming diabetic population will create.

Let's take a look back at our population one hundred years ago. Obesity in the early 1900s was relatively rare. I have family portraits in my home of my great-grandparents and their extended families. Like many people of their day, they lived on and worked their own farms or in other professions requiring a great deal of manual labor. As I looked at these photos, I was hard pressed to find a single obese individual or even one that could be classified as overweight. Some may say that simply means we were blessed with a gene pool that lacked "fat genes." Over the years, however, our family photos have changed. Now throughout the extended family are numerous obese individuals—including children. Could our family's genes have changed so dramatically in just three or four generations? I think that is highly unlikely. Rather, as in most American families, something else has changed.

A century ago, people ate diets that were relatively high in fat, and many consumed the fruits, vegetables, and grains that they grew on their own farms. Processed flour and sugars were hard to come by and usually reserved for the rich or for special occasions. Most people who were not wealthy worked hard to make a living. They ploughed fields, they laid bricks, and if they wanted to go somewhere, they usually had to walk or ride a bike. Diseases associated with obesity, such as diabetes, were relatively rare. Then things began to change. With cheap mass production of the automobile, virtually everyone could afford to forgo walking or biking to his or her desired destination. In many areas, populations moved into the city to take advantage of jobs in industry, further limiting their opportunities to exercise. This trend has continued into the twenty-first century. Many jobs outside of construction and landscaping require nothing more strenuous than typing, using a telephone, or staring at a computer screen all day.

Perhaps the most significant event this century in terms of the obesity epidemic has been the boom in fast food. I am not just referring to fast-food restaurants but also to the proliferation of high-calorie, high-fat, high-sugar, low-nutrient prepared foods like TV dinners, snacks, and, perhaps worst of all, children's pre-made ready-to-eat school lunches. The regular consumption of these high-calories, low-nutrient items combined with a dramatic decrease in exercise levels has made the United States the fattest nation on earth. If you travel to Europe, the Middle East, or Asia, you won't see obesity on anywhere near the scale we have in the United States. Unfortunately, as fast-food companies look to expand their businesses abroad, the dietary habits that have kept the rest of the world healthy are being replaced by a more "Western" diet. The end result can only be rising obesity levels that may eventually be on par with what we see here in the United States.

There is a reason people get overweight. It rarely has anything to do with a hormonal problem or poor genetics. The bottom line is if you exercise very little and eat a typical American diet, you are almost certain to be fatter than you should be for optimal health.

The result of this booming obesity epidemic is a tremendous increase in obesity-related medical problems. These include high blood pressure, heart disease, stroke, diabetes, high cholesterol, arthritis, and kidney failure. This is in addition to the psychosocial problems often faced by overweight individuals. Failure to live up to the ridiculous standards put forth in Hollywood movies and magazines often leads overweight people to suffer from poor self-esteem and depression. Perhaps most tragically, obesity is increasing to record levels in children. The CDC estimates that from 1976 to 1980, 7 percent of children age six to eleven were classified as obese using the body mass index scale. From 1999 to 2000, that percentage increased to 15.3 percent. It used to be rare to see children suffering from obesity-related type-2 diabetes. Now it is common.

The average body fat percentage of Americans is approximately 23 percent for men and 33 percent for women.[5] Certainly, these numbers are increasing every year. While these values are considered "average," they are far from being optimal. Carrying around almost one-quarter to one-third of your body weight as fat is not healthy. That extra body fat contributes to insulin resistance (which we will discuss later), which can lead to a variety of other metabolic problems. Don't be fooled into thinking that just because you are "average" in terms of your body fat percentage that you are as healthy as you could be. Lowering your body fat percentage is one of the primary objectives you will achieve when following The Program. By doing this, you will find that many of your other goals fall into line much more easily.

There is a tremendous amount of genetic variation that influences how low and how easily you are able to reduce body fat. There is variation from individual to individual in terms of the number of fat cells you are born with. There is also variation in the size of those cells and the ease with which they store fat. As we will discuss later, fat cells do not typically divide except during certain specific stages of development during infancy and childhood. Upon reaching physical maturity, you are stuck with a certain number of fat cells and

---

5   Bailey, Covert. The Ultimate Fit or Fat. New York: Houghton Mifflin Company ©1999.

nothing short of liposuction will reduce their numbers. This is why avoiding obesity during early childhood is crucial. Overeating and lack of exercise during these critical periods can lead to an increase in both the size and the number of fat cells a person carries. For adults, the only non-surgical option for reducing one's body fat percentage is to decrease the size of one's fat cells. If you are very obese when starting The Program, you may have not only very large fat cells but also an abundant number of them. In order to achieve a very low body fat percentage, you will have to shrink those cells considerably. Don't let that discourage you. The Program will show you a number of metabolic "tricks" that can help you achieve your body fat goal more quickly than you thought possible.

There is very little consensus in the scientific literature as to what an optimal body fat percentage is. There are some better-established lower limits, especially for women, but the ideal range is still a little fuzzy. There are some guidelines out there, however, that can serve to help us. Elite athletes, such as marathon runners, sprinters, bodybuilders, and triathletes, rarely have body fat percentages over 10 percent in men and 16 to 18 percent in women. These individuals have fit, trim physiques with excellent muscle tone. If we use these individuals as examples of what is ideal, then it would seem reasonable to lower what we consider an "average" or "normal" body fat percentage to a range of 15 to 18 percent for men and 22 to 25 percent for women. One of the goals of The Program is to help you get, at the very least, down into this normal range. However, by following the guidelines set forth in the following pages, achieving the "ideal" body fat percentage of an elite athlete will be within your reach if you choose to do so. I encourage you not to settle for being "average." Set lofty goals for yourself, discipline yourself, and you will achieve them.

The following chart displays what I consider healthier reference ranges for body fat percentage:

Body Fat Content Chart for Men and Women

Body Type:	Male	Female
Athlete:	10	17
Lean:	10-15%	17-22%
Normal:	15-18%	22-25%
Above Average:	18-20%	25-29%
Overfat:	20-25%	29-35%
Obese:	25+%	35+%

As you can see, the average American is in the "overfat" category. Unfortunately, if current trends continue, virtually all Americans will soon fall within the ranges considered "obese." The Program is designed to help you fight this trend. Even in today's fast-food-friendly, sedentary society, it is possible to have the body you have always wanted. It is possible to cure yourself of conditions related to obesity and inactivity, such as diabetes, hypertension, and high cholesterol. You can achieve all this without feeling deprived and "starving" yourself. And it can be done in far less time than you think. The dietary guidelines in The Program emphasize healthy, natural foods, while discouraging high-sugar, low-nutrient items. You will learn the importance of balancing your intake of carbohydrates, fats, and proteins to "optimize" your metabolism for fat-burning and muscle building.

All life demands struggle. Those who have everything given to them become lazy,
selfish, and insensitive to the real values of life. The very striving and hard work that
we so constantly try to avoid is the major building block in the person we are today.

—Pope Paul VI

EVOLUTION OF THE PROGRAM

Mirroring this rise in obesity is an increasing confusion among both athletes and the general public regarding the best way to loose body fat and build muscle mass. The number of books, DVDs, and television shows dedicated to the subject of fitness and weight loss has grown exponentially in the past twenty-five years. If you spend more than a few minutes in a bookstore, grocery store, or library, you will notice the overwhelming number of books and magazines devoted to fitness and weight loss. There are literally hundreds of different texts advocating various methods of weight loss from crash liquid diets to yoga. More are printed every day. Yet obesity and sedentary lifestyles remain the number-one health danger in our nation. With all this information available, why is it still so difficult for people to lose body fat and stay physically fit? The truth is that there is a tremendous amount of misinformation about exercise, diet, and the way the human body responds to it. There are literally hundreds of self-proclaimed experts out there hawking diet pills, crash diets, and exercise routines. As a result, the general public has become confused and bewildered. One "expert" states all you need to do is take his/her "Magic Fat-Blocker" pill and you will transform your body. Another says you should purchase their $1,000 home gym. Some swear by juicing, some by vegetarianism, and others by high-protein, low-carb diets. In the end, for most people, these methods fail to provide lasting results. Inevitably, people become frustrated and angry and eventually lose of any hope of improving the health and appearance of their body.

The misinformation about weight loss and the difficulty in shedding unwanted pounds has led some to advocate obesity as a perfectly healthy state for the human body.[6] NAAFA (The National Association to Advance Fat Acceptance) officials state that for overweight individuals "...permanent weight loss is impossible to achieve, that dieting makes them fatter, that many of them are healthy..." As a physician, I applaud NAAFA's efforts to eliminate discrimination and boost the self esteem of overweight Americans. There is no place for the ridicule and stigmatization of overweight people. However, to promote the notion

---

6   http://www.naafa.org/documents/brochures/naafa-info.html#unhealthy

that weight loss is impossible and that obesity can be compatible with optimal health is not only false, but irresponsible.

The truth is that the scientific evidence regarding obesity and a sedentary lifestyle is very clear. Obesity is strongly associated with a shortened lifespan and an increased incidence of multiple medical problems. I see it in my medical practice every single day. The rates of high blood pressure, diabetes, high cholesterol, and heart disease are dramatically higher in my patients who are overweight. I also see many patients who are able to cure themselves of these conditions by beginning an exercise program, changing their diet, and losing weight. Many are able to come off of most, if not all, their medications by losing weight and exercising. If you have a few pounds to lose and are not exercising on a regular basis, don't fool yourself into thinking everything is okay. Being out of shape doesn't mean you're a bad person, but it does mean that you are not as healthy as you should be.

Most people would like to look better. Some may only want to improve a "problem area" on their physique; others would like to completely transform their entire appearance. Facial features aside, this almost always means increasing the size of certain muscle groups and/or reducing one's body fat. This is exactly what The Program is all about. The goal of The Program is to provide you with the most time-efficient, effective way to increase the size of your muscles while simultaneously lowering your body fat. Many exercise and diet plans promise similar results. So what makes The Program different? To answer that question, one should look at all the other weight-loss and fitness programs available in a given book-store or those advertised on TV. They each promise weight loss, increased energy, and improved health and strength. Yet they also espouse radically different ways to reach that goal. In terms of diet, some say a high-carbohydrate/low-fat diet is best for losing body fat and increasing muscle mass. Others insist a veg-etarian diet is supreme or a high-fat/low-carbohydrate plan is ideal. As much confusion as there is about diet, it gets even worse when we look at training. Some say Pilates or yoga is best. Or is it high repetition, light weightlifting at home? Cross-Fit perhaps? Maybe training every day or every other day is the best way to build and strengthen a muscle?

The bottom line is that it is impossible for all these different approaches to lowering body fat and increasing muscle size to be equally effective and provide results at the same rate. Will each of them produce some results? Certainly they will. But such radically different philosophies and approaches to exercise cannot all be the *best* way. Fortunately, there is information available that can help you sort through this confusing quagmire of conflicting theories and claims. Unfortunately, much of that infor-mation is published in obscure scientific journals aimed primarily at researchers and physicians and not the general public. Occasionally, you will see supplement companies quoting scientific studies that appear to show benefit from consuming their products. Unfortunately, they typically exaggerate and distort the results of those studies to show their product in the best possible light. For the most part, *real* information is difficult to access and often presented in such a way that makes applying it in the real world difficult. What I have done for you in this book is attempt to sort through the scientific and medi-cal data regarding fat loss and muscle building. I have spent countless hours scouring research journals to extract practical information and distill it down into a form you can actually use. The information I will be presenting comes directly from these sources as well as my own personal experience applying it in a practical fashion.

One of the fundamental principles of medical science is that human beings are virtually identical physiologically. Certainly, there are variations in metabolism, muscle mass, exercise capacity, blood pressure, and a myriad of other bodily functions. But these are nothing more than variations within narrow parameters that all human beings possess. The truth is that every human being has cells, tissues, and organs that operate in fundamentally the same way. It is this fact that allows me to prescribe medication and be able to accurately predict the results that medication will have on its recipient. If everyone's cells and organs functioned uniquely, medical science and the study of anatomy and physiology, pharmacology, and a myriad of other sciences simply could not exist. It is the knowledge that the human body—any human body—will respond in a predictable way to a given stimulus that has allowed medical and sports science to progress. The fact that every human being is essentially identical from a physiologic standpoint suggests that there must be an ideal way to stimulate muscle mass and an ideal way to lower body fat that will work for everyone. Notice that I say "ideal." Many approaches will yield results to some degree, but they cannot all simultaneously be the most effective and most efficient way. There has to be one method that is superior to the rest. The Program was created based on this principle. It is the result of years of painstaking research and experimentation in many fields including medicine, exercise physiology, nutrition, sports medicine, and pharmacology. The Program integrates important theories from all these fields and applies them to a single goal: lowering body fat and increasing muscle strength and size in the most time-efficient manner possible.

Like many people, I developed an interest in fitness and bodybuilding as a teenager. I knew that I wanted to develop a more muscular physique but didn't have the slightest clue how to achieve my goal. I knew enough to know I would have to lift weights and eat more food. Beyond that, training was a mystery. I started with a home dumbbell set and Weider bench press at age fourteen. I followed the simple training program and faithfully trained each body part twice a week with five to ten sets each. Over the following year, I did gain some muscle mass and quickly found that my home gym was inadequate for my needs. I became serious about weight training when, for Christmas, I received Arnold Schwarzenegger's *Encyclopedia of Modern Bodybuilding*. Finally, I would have all the information I needed to build my body in Arnold's image—or so I thought.

I began on the recommended introductory program, training six days a week with five to ten sets per body part. Sundays were deemed as rest days. Why Sunday? That was never mentioned. My workouts averaged about two hours. I continued to grow bigger and stronger in the months after starting this regimen, but eventually my strength and size gains slowed and eventually stopped. I took this as a sign that I needed to increase my workload and progress to the intermediate program. Surely after a full two years of training, I would be ready for the increase in sets this program provided. I began faithfully performing twelve to twenty sets per body part six days a week with as much intensity as I could muster. What I discovered was that I could barely make it through the marathon workouts provided in the book. Instead of growing bigger and stronger, I became fatigued, weak, and irritable. I was already spending over twelve hours a week lifting weights, and now it had increased to fourteen to fifteen hours. All this time, I was attempting to do well in school and play rugby and football. Despite my lack of formal training, I intuitively sensed that something was wrong with this type of training. I knew on some level that I was over-training and that continuing to train in this manner would only lead to failure. What I failed to realize at the time was that the Arnold program was not based on science at all. There was no evidence or proof provided in the book that this type of training was superior to any other. I believed in Arnold's regimen only because it was Arnold's, and, obviously, he used it successfully so why couldn't I do the same? What I didn't know at the time was that Arnold and the other bodybuilders who successfully used this type of training were not only genetically gifted but also using large amounts of steroids. This allowed them to push their bodies past normal limits and enhanced their recovery ability so that they did not overtrain. Non-steroid-using individuals would be hard pressed to make any long-term increases in muscle size on such a program, and they would be spending hours and hours in the gym each week for the gains they did achieve.

Not until I entered college, was I able to incorporate and articulate what my intuition revealed to me as a teenager. As a premed student majoring in exercise science, I was introduced to various exercise theories. Through courses in biochemistry, exercise physiology, and anatomy, I learned about the body's adaptive response to exercise and, most important, what happens when the level of exercise out-paces the body's ability to recover from it. I gradually realized that I had been performing workouts that were far too long and far too frequent. I vowed that if I was going to spend all this time and effort on my body, I would find the most effective and efficient way to exercise. Fortunately, I stumbled across a book by former Mr. Universe Mike Mentzer. In his book, Mr. Mentzer clearly stated what I was beginning to understand: that weight training is an intense stimulus that must be delivered in precise amounts in order to efficiently build muscle. If any more or any less exercise than is required is performed, the results will be less than optimal. I devoured all of Mr. Mentzer's books and began applying the principles he discussed to my own training. Now, instead of training six days a week for two hours a session, I was only in the gym two to three days a week for thirty minutes or less per session. This decrease in training came at a perfect time, as I was just about to start medical school and did not have much time to train. As I used this new approach, my size and strength increased dramatically. I bulked up to over 250 pounds and routinely performed reps of squats and deadlifts with over 600 pounds. I managed this despite working 80 to 120 hours a week as a medical student and resident.

However, the more I read of Mentzer's work, the more I realized he had missed a critical part of the puzzle. His training system was excellent. He properly identified the biological fact that optimal muscle growth requires high-intensity stimulation. He was absolutely correct that most bodybuilders grossly overtrain. However, his dietary recommendations were overly simplistic and would not lead to the optimal gains in muscle mass that his training system could provide. Mentzer was a believer in the "a calorie is a calorie" fallacy, meaning that he thought that the human body responded similarly to a single unit of food energy, a calorie, in essentially the same way, no matter if that calorie came from protein, carbohydrate, or fat. This was why his advice for losing weight never went much beyond "eat less than you burn" and why he reportedly included things like ice cream in his pre-contest diet. Mentzer didn't understand that food is **more than just a source of energy and raw materials; it is a potent manipulator of the entire metabolism. In a very real sense, food is a drug, and as such, it can be manipulated to bring about a desired effect.** In his defense, Mentzer, despite his considerable intellect, was not a scientist. He wasn't trained in the detailed biochemistry of the human body; nor did he have the ability to evaluate research articles critically and apply them to real-world bodybuilding problems. He developed his ideas in the trenches, by experimenting with his own training and that of his clients to come up with something that worked extremely well compared to the other available training approaches of the time. This was where I knew I could fill in the gaps and create a complete system. The Program is the result of years of effort in integrating the fundamentals of high-intensity weight-training exercise with the latest scientific advancements in the field of diet and metabolism.

The purpose of The Program is not to provide yet another weight-loss gimmick. It is designed to provide you with a comprehensive set of tools you can use to transform your body. Whether your goals are to simply drop a few pounds and tone up before a reunion or if you want nothing less than the Mr. Olympia title, The Program will help you achieve your goals. Its purpose goes beyond transforming your body, however. I hope to provide you with the knowledge to see through all the false advertising, bogus testimonials, and outright fraud that prevail in the diet and exercise industry. The Program starts with explanations of some of the fundamental processes that govern how your body gains and loses both fat and muscle mass and what it does with the calories you consume. You will also read about the role of exercise and, most important, how to exercise to build muscle mass and burn fat in the shortest possible time. Much of what I will share with you will seem controversial and some of it in direct opposition to what you have been told your whole life. Don't worry. I don't expect you to accept what I say blindly without evidence to back it up. All of the theories I will present have solid backing in the medical and sports literature and have been used with great success by others and myself over the years. I will attempt to explain these concepts in a clear and straightforward manner, but I won't spoon-feed you. Learning new ideas always takes effort. If you are tired of hype and have the drive and motivation to reach your goals, The Program can start you down the road to improving your health and appearance.

Fraud and falsehood only dread examination. Truth invites it.

—Samuel Johnson

THE DIET INDUSTRY

Losing weight in the United States is big business. Americans spend millions every year on various weight-loss supplements, programs, and equipment. With all this expenditure, you would think that America's waistlines would be shrinking. Unfortunately, as we have seen, precisely the opposite is occurring. Obesity is on the rise. This problem has created a fertile field for businesses to exploit in their pursuit of profit. Quick-fix weight-loss products have literally flooded the market. Some promise that you can burn fat without any exercise or lose weight while you sleep. Despite their outrageous claims, the general public, for the most part, believes in them and continues to spend their hard-earned money on these pie-in-the-sky products. The same can be said for home exercise equipment. Late-night television is literally swamped with infomercials for products like the Ab-lounge, Thigh-Master, Gazelle, Bow-Flex, and many more. They all show trim and muscular models effortlessly working out and having a great time as they build their bodies. Some of these machines have some merit and, when used properly, can be a good way to exercise in your home. Most are woefully inadequate for those who need to lose a significant amount of weight or wish to build a significant amount of lean muscle. They are often expensive and, unfortunately, once the initial enthusiasm of owning one wears off, they often end up collecting dust or functioning as an expensive place to hang your dirty clothes.

Most companies that sell weight-loss aids know that their products don't work. Their primary focus is not so much on effectiveness, but in profit. And profits in this industry are usually very good. Most people who purchase these products use them once or twice, realize they don't work, and move on to something else. Therefore, companies have a constant turnover of potential customers. They are continually looking for the new generation to come along and make a one-time purchase. You would think that no company could survive for long with this type of situation, but they do. Unfortunately, the population of obese Americans is growing every day, but the dissemination of accurate and trustworthy information on weight loss and health isn't keeping pace. Therefore, there will always be a large pool of potential customers for diet supplement companies to target.

I have been focusing mostly on weight-loss products, but the same can be said for bodybuilding supplements. Bodybuilding magazines are full of advertisements for the latest protein powders, weight gainers, fat burners, and other supplements. They target a slightly different population—young males who are desperate to build their bodies as quickly as possible. These companies have, in many ways, an even better racket than the mainstream diet industry. Many bodybuilding supplement companies are also in the business of publishing bodybuilding magazines. Weider publishes *Flex* and *Muscle and Fitness*, and there are many others. These magazines are loaded with articles written by bodybuilders (in reality, most are written by shadow writers and the bodybuilder has no input) or other "experts" who espouse the benefits of a particular supplement the company produces. Some even claim to provide "scientific proof" in the form of carefully contrived clinical studies (sponsored by the company, of course—if they took place at all). Many males in their teens and twenties devour the information in these magazines and take it as gospel. The supplement companies strictly control what information is put in their magazines and deliberately omit any data that would suggest their products are in fact no better than placebo for building muscle, burning fat, etcetera. I'm not saying that these magazines are useless. They occasionally contain some useful dietary tips and are a good source of inspirational photos, but they should be looked at for what they are: an advertising medium for the supplement company that publishes them. In no way should they be considered a reliable, unbiased source of information on nutritional supplements or training.

The weight-loss industry knows Americans are looking for quick-fix solutions to their weight problems. We have been conditioned to expect rapid solutions to our problems. Hungry? You can go through a fast-food drive-through and get a burger, fries, and soda in less than five minutes. Need information? Get on the Internet, and any search engine will give you what you need in seconds. Not happy with your love handles? Any plastic surgeon will be happy to liposuction them away. Morbidly obese? Just go get a gastric bypass. Need to drop a few pounds before your reunion? Go to any nutritional outlet, turn on the TV, or pick up a magazine, and you'll find dozens of pills and potions that promise to help. It is this impatience and desire to look for an easy way to fix your problems that has allowed much of the diet industry to prosper.

There is a little secret the hawkers of fad diets and weight-loss supplements don't want you to know is that they *don't* want you to lose weight! Well, not for good anyway. Sure, they'll help you take off a few pounds here and there, but they know their products and systems are flawed and can never lead to permanent weight loss. They want you to gain the weight back because that is what keeps them in business. It's the constant turnover of new customers and the continuous return of old ones who have regained the weight they lost that makes them billions of dollars annually. As long as you stay fat, your weight yo-yos up and down, and you keep giving these snake-oil salesmen your money, they are happy. If they actually showed you how to lose weight and keep it off, they would put themselves out of business.

As a result, sources that offer realistic, rational, and healthy ways to lose weight and stay fit are few and far between. They also lack the big budgets for advertising that other companies have. Their message is drowned out by all the background noise that permeates the diet industry. What most Americans fail to realize is that they didn't get out of shape overnight. In the vast majority of cases, obesity is a result of years of poor diet and a sedentary lifestyle. Therefore, it is unrealistic to expect that in a matter of days or weeks, some pill or crash diet is going to burn off the fat you put on your body through years of neglect.

Nature is relentless and unchangeable, and it is indifferent as to whether its hidden reasons and actions are understandable to man or not.

—Galileo

WHY CONVENTIONAL DIETS FAIL

Most overweight individuals have attempted to lose weight through dieting at least once. Many have tried dozens of times with brief periods of success followed by failure as the lost weight returns and more is added. The same can be said for those attempting to gain weight. They have tried various crash weight-gain plans often with more fat gained than muscle. There are various reasons why these plans fail. Most often, it is because they are not sustainable and lead to unfavorable metabolic changes that encourage, instead of discourage, the deposition of body fat. Most people have heard of individuals losing significant amounts of weight on very low-calorie liquid diets. These diets often restrict calorie intake to less than a thousand calories per day, primarily in the form of liquid protein and vitamin shakes. The body is quickly placed into a state of controlled starvation and turns to its stored body fat and muscle mass to make up the missing calories needed to sustain bodily functions. It certainly is possible to lose a tremendous amount of weight on these plans, but it becomes nearly impossible to keep the weight off after discontinuing them.

The reason for this is that your body is operating under the control of genes that evolved to keep you alive forty thousand years ago. In those days, humans hunted and foraged for food and often had prolonged periods of starvation to deal with. In that environment, it was to your advantage to store as many excess calories away as fat as possible for use later when food became scarce. Fat was a lifesaver, so much so that during periods of calorie restriction, the human body evolved to preferentially metabolize muscle tissue for energy over fat. To complicate matters further, humans have also evolved an innate preference for calorie-dense foods like fats, heavy starches, and sweets. These sorts of foods were highly sought after by our ancient ancestors because they were dense in calories and were easily and efficiently stored as body fat. Of course, back then, you usually had to work for your food. Our ancestors walked and ran many miles per day; they jumped, sprinted, stretched, and climbed to secure their next meal. As a result, our Paleolithic brethren were lean and muscular and virtually devoid of many of the chronic medical problems that plague our society today. In fact, there is good anthropologic evidence that as humans settled into larger communities and began making grains a larger part of their diet, they developed weaker bones, shorter stature, and developed increased rates of dental disease, smaller brains, hypertension, atherosclerosis, and heart disease. In modern society, where high-sugar, high-fat foods are available everywhere and where the need for physical exercise is greatly diminished, our genes are backfiring on us.

On a conventional calorie-restricted diet, your body doesn't know that you are trying to lose body fat. It responds as if it doesn't know when your next meal will come along and activates a series of mechanisms to ensure your survival. To ensure adequate blood-sugar levels, amino acids from proteins are metabolized and used as energy. The primary source of these proteins is muscle tissue. Various hormones and enzymes are activated to burn body fat as well, but at least at first, muscle tissue is consumed preferentially. If this calorie-deficient state persists, the body's overall metabolic rate decreases. Eventually, weight loss will slow and then cease as you reach a new steady state. Further weight loss will require another decrease in calories. Eventually, metabolism will slow further and another steady state will be reached. At the conclusion of a typical calorie-restricted diet, most dieters have lost a significant amount of weight. However, much of that weight has been in the form of precious muscle tissue. In fact, in terms of overall body fat percentage, they may actually be fatter than when they started. To compound this problem, they are now left with a greatly slowed metabolic rate. When they return to a more normal diet, even if it is lower in calories than their pre-diet intake, the body senses this abundance of calories and rapidly stores those calories away as body fat in anticipation of the next period of starvation. This is the primary reason why severely calorie-restricted diets fail in the long run. They are a short-term solution to weight loss. The number of dieters who can maintain their weight loss six months or a year after they cease their diet is very low.

The Program will provide you with the tools to avoid many of the problems with conventional diets. You will be focusing less on body weight and much more on body composition. For those of you looking to cut fat, The Program will boost your metabolic rate to allow continuous, around-the-clock fat metabolism. Those of you who are already gifted with a lean physique and who want to add additional muscle will learn how to accelerate your muscle growth while minimizing the addition of body fat. You will be provided with a highly efficient weight-training program that will not just preserve your all-important muscle mass but actually help you build new muscle tissue while you burn body fat. As your muscle mass increases, so will your metabolic rate. As a result, you will burn more body fat and not need to continually decrease your calorie levels to continue losing weight. With proper control of the amounts and types of nutrients you ingest, you will learn to manipulate your primitive caveman genes into working with you instead of against you in your quest for a leaner, more muscular physique.

You cannot be disciplined in great things and undisciplined in small things. Brave undisciplined men have no chance against the discipline and valor of other men.

—General George S. Patton Jr.

DISCIPLINE

The first step on the road to getting in shape is to take responsibility for the current state of your body. One of my favorite infomercials is for one of the so-called cortisol blockers. In it, the salesman claims "It's not your fault you're overweight. It's a nasty little stress hormone called cortisol." As you will learn later, this statement is completely false. The truth (barring some unavoidable illness or injury) is if you are out of shape, there is only a single root cause for your condition: *You.* Your body is the end result of all the things you have been doing wrong. Don't blame genetics; your undiagnosed, under-active thyroid; your stressful job; or a "slow metabolism," even if these things really are contributing to the problem. Take responsibility, make a decision to change, get the knowledge you need, and move forward.

Following The Program is not easy. If you are looking for an easy way to build a lean, muscular body, prepare to be disappointed. You will need a lot of discipline and dedication to reach your goals. There are no cutting corners or shortcuts if you want to transform your body permanently. If you are at a point in your life where you don't think you can summon the dedication to stick to a nutrition and exercise program, then I would recommend that you stop reading right now. The Program is not for you. Put the book away until you are really ready to make a change.

There will be days when you want to cheat on your diet, skip workouts, or slack off. That is completely normal. The good news is that you will generally feel so good on The Program, that your cravings for sweets and other prohibited items will be low. Regardless, you must be able to generate a minimum amount of self-control in order to successfully follow The Program. If you can't do that, then no system will work for you, no matter how well designed it is. If you "fall off the wagon" here or there, it's not the end of the world. It happens to everyone, but you must be able to pick yourself up and get back on track quickly. More importantly, look at what factors led you to cheat on your diet or exercise program in the first place. Did you skip a meal and out of shear hunger reach for an easily available candy bar? If so, try to plan your meals a little better so that you don't face that situation again. Did you bow to peer pressure from friends who are shoving fast food in your face? Maybe you need to explain to your "friends" that you need their support and they can show that by not sabotaging your diet. If you get the occasional powerful craving for a doughnut, learn to quickly redirect yourself to something else—get up and go for a walk, take a drive, watch a movie, or go to the gym, whatever you need to do to take your mind off the junk food you are craving.

The ideal candidates for The Program have several characteristics in common. They are unhappy with their bodies and have been for some time. Many have tried other methods of diet and exercise and have experienced frustration at not meeting their goals. Most important, they have made, often in a split second, the decision that they have to change and are willing to do whatever they must to do so. Despite their previous failures, they are open to new ideas and demonstrate a willingness to change their lifestyles. The fact that you are reading this at all indicates that you have the desire to change your body for the better. Unfortunately, it takes more than desire to accomplish your goals. Simply wanting something badly enough won't help you get it. You must acquire the specific knowledge needed to reach your goals.

It is common to see young trainees in the gym devoutly following a workout they gleaned from a muscle magazine and following it to the letter for months and years. Their desire to grow bigger muscles is so strong that they have no doubt they will succeed if they just train hard enough and never waver. The same is true for dieters following some of these ultra-restrictive low-calorie diets. Unfortunately, they couldn't be more wrong. Eventually, their wild enthusiasm will falter as they see they are not reaching their goal, and they will ultimately slip into despair and cease their efforts. They fail not because of a lack of will but rather a deficiency in their knowledge. It is admirable to shoot for the moon, but if you don't know the first thing about physics and engineering, you won't be able to build the rocket that will get you there—no matter how badly you want to make the trip. Take the time before you begin The Program to read it in its entirety. Try your best to understand the reasons why you will be doing the things that are asked of you. Feel free to reference other sources like medical websites and textbooks if you want to obtain an even deeper level of understanding. The more you understand how your body works, the more successful you will be at directing it to give you what you want.

A lie gets halfway around the world before the truth has a chance to get its pants on.

—Winston Churchill

DIET AND EXERCISE MYTHS

Before beginning any exercise program, it's important to review some of the popular myths that surround both dieting and exercise. Unfortunately, these myths continue to be propagated among athletes, physicians, and the general public. This is by no means a comprehensive list but does include some of the most common myths you will encounter as well as the scientific research that refutes them.

"A calorie is a calorie."

A calorie is a unit of heat energy. It is defined as the amount of energy needed to raise the temperature of a gram of water by one degree Celsius at standard atmospheric pressure. Fats, carbohydrates, and protein are assigned standard caloric values per gram. In 1900, Wilbur Olin Atwater at the Connecticut Agriculture Experiment Station assigned the following caloric values to fat, protein, and carbohydrates, respectively:

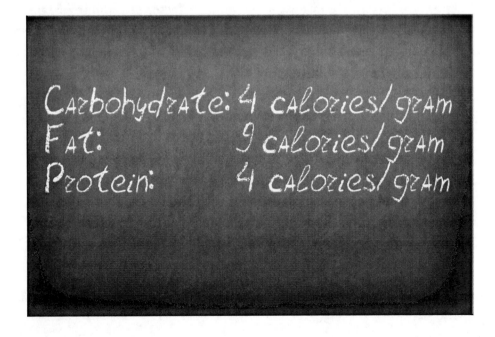

Carbohydrate: 4 calories/gram
Fat: 9 calories/gram
Protein: 4 calories/gram

These values are still used today. According to this definition, all three basic food types are capable of producing heat energy, with fat being the most calorically dense. This has led to the assumption that all calories are created equal—i.e., it does not matter where your calories are coming from per se, as long as you are meeting your body's energy/caloric requirements. Following this logic, one can therefore assume that restricting calories, regardless of their type, to below maintenance levels will result in weight loss. And this is true. Unfortunately, this has led some to assume that the composition of a diet is less important than the total number of calories it contains. This is partially true. If you cut your calories below maintenance levels, you will lose weight regardless of the percentages of fat, carbohydrate, and protein that the diet contains. And if you are taking enough anabolic steroids, you will hold onto most of your muscle mass and lose fat almost exclusively, even if your diet consists of cookies, cake, and ice cream.

This idea, however, fails to take into account the metabolic effects of protein, carbohydrates, and fats. Five hundred calories from carbohydrates do not have the same metabolic effects as five hundred calories from fat or protein. Ingesting a meal of, say five hundred calories, exclusively from carbohydrates, as we will learn in greater detail later, triggers a hormonal cascade that places the body into "storage mode." Carbohydrates can only be utilized in the presence of insulin, which further encourages the storage of not only carbohydrates, but fat as well. Ingestion of similar caloric levels of protein and fat do not trigger the same insulin response. Protein and fat do not require significant amounts of insulin to be metabolized and, in fact, create a metabolic environment that is conducive to fat burning. Several studies have demonstrated that diets containing equal numbers of calories, but varying amounts of carbohydrates, fats, and proteins do not lead to equal amounts of weight loss. If caloric restriction was of primary importance in weight loss, then it shouldn't matter the composition of the diet. The trend in these studies is that, in general, the greater the degree to which carbohydrate intake is limited, the greater the amount of weight loss seen. For example, in a study published in *The American Journal of Clinical Nutrition*, demographically similar obese male subjects were placed on one of three diets. All contained 1,800 calories but one contained 30 grams total of carbohydrate, another 60 grams, and the last 104 grams per day. Over nine weeks, the subjects on the 30 grams of carbohydrate diet lost an average of 3.6 pounds of fat per week, the 60 gram group lost 2.5 pounds of fat per week, and the 104 gram group an average of 2 pounds per week.[7] One would think that if caloric intake were the primary factor determining degree of weight loss, then all groups should have lost equal amounts of weight. Clearly, all calories are not created equal when it comes to dieting for fat loss. To the contrary, the percentages of fat, protein, and carbohydrate are critically important in maximizing fat loss while dieting.

"The Spot Reduction Myth"

Spot reduction is the notion that localized deposits of fat on the body can be selectively reduced by intensely working the surrounding muscles. For example, if you carry a little extra fat on your belly, then doing extra sets of sit-ups, according to spot reduction theory, should result in increased fat loss from the abdominal area. This notion has been thoroughly discredited. Fat lost from exercise and dieting generally comes from all areas, with some minor exceptions, equally. It is true that some folks have "stubborn

---

7   Young, C.M., Scanlan, S.S., Im, H.S., et al., "Effect on Body Composition and Other Parameters in Obese Young Men of Carbohydrate Level of Reduction Diet," The American Journal of Clinical Nutrition, 24, 1971, pages 290–296.

areas" of localized fat deposits that tend to resist shrinking. Men for example tend to lose the fat around their belly and "love handles" last, while women will hold onto the fat around their hips and buttocks more stubbornly. These are genetically mediated traits, often with a hormonal component, and no amount of additional sit-ups, lunges, or squats will accelerate the fat loss in those areas at the expense of others.

"Low-fat foods help you lose weight."

As mentioned above, the composition of one's diet is of primary importance when it comes to fat loss. Despite this fact, the diet industry and most food manufacturers have cashed in on the myth that reducing fat intake will lead to weight loss. As we will discuss later, Americans are indeed eating less fat in their diets but are still fatter than ever. Close inspection of the nutritional content of the many low-fat food items hawked in grocery stores will show that most of them have as many or more calories as their traditional counterparts and, in many cases, have more sugar added. Often, these low-fat foods are actually worse for you than the regular versions. There are some low-fat foods that obviously will be useful additions to your diet, but don't be fooled into thinking that an item marketed as "low fat" is automatically better for you than one that isn't. Read labels carefully and only include those items that meet your dietary requirements.

"Eating all that cholesterol is bad for you."

There is often concern raised in the media regarding the high intake of cholesterol in our diets. The preponderance of data—though there is still some controversy in this area—suggests that high levels of low-density lipoprotein (LDL) are associated with increased risk for heart disease and stroke. Most studies show that as the intake of cholesterol in the diet increases, there is a correlation with rising cholesterol levels in the blood.[8]

The problem is that most of these studies have also had subjects on diets high in saturated fat. It is well documented that diets high in saturated fats, especially in the setting of high concomitant intake of carbohydrate, are associated with elevated serum cholesterol levels. This occurs even when the intake of cholesterol is not particularly high. Therefore, it's not entirely clear whether it is the actual cholesterol in the food that is causing the elevated blood cholesterol levels or rather the effects of excess saturated fat and carbohydrate in the diet. Regardless, total calories and saturated fat, as well as carbohydrate, seem to play a more important role in determining your serum cholesterol than does your total cholesterol intake. Most foods that are high in cholesterol are also high in saturated fats, with the exception of organ meats and shrimp. These are high in cholesterol but very low in saturated fat. It is estimated that dietary cholesterol can contribute anywhere from 20 to 40 percent of the serum cholesterol level.[9] There is a limit

---

8   Rianne M. Weggemans, Peter L. Zock, and Martijn B. Katan. Dietary Cholesterol from Eggs Increases the Ratio of Total Cholesterol to High-Density Lipoprotein Cholesterol in Humans: A Meta-Analysis, American Journal of Clinical Nutrition 73(5): 885–891 (May 2001).
9   Colon, W. E., R. E. Hodges, R. A. Bleiler. The serum lipids in men receiving high cholesterol and cholesterol-free diets. J.C/in. Invest. 40: 894, 1961.

to the intestine's ability to absorb cholesterol, however, and it appears that ingesting more than about six hundred milligrams per day does not cause further significant elevations in serum cholesterol.[10]

It is very likely that you will be consuming higher than normal levels of cholesterol in your diet on the Endomorphic Diet. This is unavoidable but largely something that shouldn't worry you. While on the diet, you will be keeping your saturated fat intake to a modest level and losing weight, which will actually improve your cholesterol levels.

As discussed later, many indigenous peoples consume high-fat, high-cholesterol ketogenic diets and have favorable lipid profiles and very low rates of heart disease. The bottom line is that the jury is still out on how much dietary cholesterol should be ingested and how much it actually contributes to your serum cholesterol when you are consuming a carbohydrate-restricted diet. Before starting The Program, you should have your cholesterol checked by your physician and have it checked again at some point during your diet so you can accurately track your progress and make any adjustments if necessary.

"Vegetarians can't build muscle."

I have heard this many times: "You have to eat meat to gain muscle!" Now, let me state up front that I am not a vegetarian. I love a good steak as much as anyone, and meat does make up a significant portion of my diet. However, there is much to be said about consuming a vegetarian diet in terms of promoting health, but I will not go into great detail on that now. The most common problem I see, not only with vegetarian bodybuilders, but with many vegetarian athletes, is inadequate variety in terms of their protein sources. Meat eaters have it easy. All meats contain high levels of all the essential and nonessential amino acids. It is almost impossible to develop a deficiency in this area if you consume meat. Vegetarians have to be a little cleverer. Ensuring adequate intake of all essential amino acids and high-quality protein in general, often requires combining vegetable protein sources together to create a complete protein. The upside to this is that you can greatly expand the number of tasty items in your diet and combine them in new ways for added flavor. It just takes a bit more work on your part. A complete guide to vegetarian dieting for bodybuilding is beyond the scope of this book, but there are multiple resources available for those who wish to pursue this course. Former Mr. Olympia Bill Pearl is a well-known vegetarian bodybuilder. He is living proof that one can build and maintain a fantastic physique well into one's seventies while consuming a vegetarian diet. Check out his books for a detailed approach to vegetarian bodybuilding. The Endomorphic Diet is the only diet in this book that can present a challenge to the pure vegetarian. The very low carbohydrate requirements can still be achieved with a little planning and research, however. If you wish to pursue a vegetarian lifestyle, I certainly have no objections. I think you will find that with a little extra preparation and creativity, you can build just as much muscle and burn as much fat as your carnivorous counterparts.

---

10 Wilson, J. D., Lindsey, C.A, JR. Studies on the influence of dietary cholesterol on cholesterol metabolism in the isotopic steady state in man. I. C/in. invest. 44: 1805, 1965.

"Fast food is always unhealthy and should be avoided."

There is a lot of truth to this statement. Most items on the menu at fast-food restaurants are loaded with the deadly combination of saturated trans fats and highly refined sugar. They should be avoided at all costs even if you have no interest in losing weight or building muscle. Fortunately, there are a few options that you can choose from that are reasonably healthy and can be included in The Program, regardless of which diet variant you decide to undertake. Most fast-food restaurants have websites where you can look up the nutritional information for their menu items. You may be surprised to find that most of the major fast-food chains in the United States have at least a few items that can be consumed while on any of the diets in The Program.

"Eating meat is bad for you."

Meat has gotten a bad rap in the past few decades. There have been a number of studies published in various scientific journals that showed consumption of meat products was directly linked to elevated risk of cardiovascular disease and several cancers. As a result, various government agencies began recommending that Americans decrease their intake of meat, particularly red meat, as a way to reduce the risk of having a heart attack or a stroke or developing colon cancer. The general public has listened and consumption of meat has declined over the past two decades. The funny thing is, the rates of heart disease and cancer did not decline. Is meat really so bad after all?

It turns out that the issue is more complicated. If high animal meat intake were associated with elevated prevalence of cardiovascular disease, then the populations with the highest intake would logically have the greatest prevalence of these diseases. Close examination of the dietary habits of thirteen indigenous populations shows that meat makes up an average of 65 percent of their dietary energy intake, while plant-based sources made up only 32 percent.[11] Ironically, these same populations have very low rates of cardiovascular disease and cancer; this is true even among native Alaskans and Greenlanders whose diets are well over 90 percent animal-fat and protein derived. These people were also fit, lean, and virtually free of many of the chronic ailments that plague our modern society. Ironically, as these populations adapt to more Western diets with fewer animal products and higher percentages of refined carbohydrates, their disease rates are matching if not exceeding those of Western Europeans.

There are a number of explanations for these findings. The meat of wild game consumed by our hunter-gatherer brethren is nutritionally quite different than what you purchase in the grocery store. Wild game typically has much less fat by weight than domesticated meats (4 percent versus up to 25 percent). Domesticated animals are usually fed high-calorie grain-based diets that not only increase the amount of fat they contain, but lower the amount of healthy omega-3 fatty acids as well. Western cooking practices, such as cooking red meats at temperatures high enough to cause charring, as well as smoking and preserving meats, release a variety of carcinogenic chemicals that have been implicated in stomach, colon, prostate, and breast cancers.

---

11   Cordain, L, Eaton SB, Miller JB, Mann N, Hill K. The paradoxical nature of hunter-gatherer diets: meat-based, yet non-atherogenic. Eur J Clin Nutr, 2002;56(suppl 1): S42–S52.

What can be gleaned from the research to date is that it is not the consumption of meat per se that raises the risk of heart disease and cancer, but rather its composition that makes the difference. In the West, meat consumption is closely tied to high saturated-fat intake, and it is this saturated fat (in combination with excess carbohydrate intake) that contributes to the high rates of cardiovascular disease and cancer that we see in our population. There are multiple studies that support this idea. In an Australian study, when subjects were taken off their typical Western diets and placed on a traditional aboriginal diet that was high in kangaroo meat (a very low-fat meat), they had marked improvements in their cholesterol and triglyceride levels.[12] In another interesting five-week study, subjects were fed a diet rich in vegetables and grains and five hundred grams per day of lean beef in which all visible fat was trimmed. Within one week, they experienced an average 24 percent reduction in their LDL cholesterol levels. Each week thereafter, an additional 10 percent of calories from saturated fat (in the form of beef drippings) were added. Total calories were kept constant by reducing the percentage of calories from carbohydrate. With each passing week, the subject's LDL cholesterol levels steadily rose without significant changes in their HDL cholesterol levels. This study shows clearly that it is not the addition of beef itself (indeed, the addition of lean beef *improved* LDL cholesterol levels) but rather the addition of saturated animal fat to a diet already relatively high in carbohydrates (approximately 60 percent of calories in this study were from carbohydrates) that led to elevations in LDL cholesterol.[13]

So don't shy away from including meat in your diet. Just remember, if possible, always to choose the leanest cuts available. If you have access to meat from wild game, then all the better. Wild game meat is leaner, higher in omega-3 fatty acids, and free of hormones and other chemicals found in domesticated meats.

"Ketosis is unhealthy and unnatural."

In the world of medicine, *ketosis* is bad word. Physicians are trained from very early in their careers to recognize and treat one of the deadly complications of diabetes—diabetic ketoacidosis (DKA)—as well as another dangerous, but less deadly, form of ketosis known as alcoholic ketoacidosis (AKA). In DKA, the body is profoundly insulin deficient. This primarily occurs in type 1 diabetics, who, for a variety of reasons, do not have enough insulin in their system to meet their body's demands. Many times, patients with type 1 diabetes will present with this condition as the first manifestation of their disease. Sometimes, a minor infection, trauma, or noncompliance with their daily insulin regimen will tip them over the edge into DKA. In DKA, patients develop very high blood glucose levels, but because they lack insulin, they are unable to dispose of it in their cells. The osmotic effect of such high glucose levels in the kidneys and urine pulls water with it and leads to profound dehydration. As the body's cells acutely starve for glucose, they begin to undergo anaerobic metabolism and fat stores are broken down to form ketones in an inadequate attempt to provide fuel to the brain and other organs. As a result, the blood becomes increasingly acidic and overwhelms the body's normal pH buffering system. The downward spiral of worsening

---

12 O'Dea K. Marked improvement in carbohydrate and lipid metabolism in diabetic Australian aborigines after temporary reversion to traditional lifestyle. Diabetes 1984; 33:596–603.

13 O'Dea K. Traianedes K, Chishoim K, Leyden H, Sinclair A. Cholesterol-lowering effect of a low-fat diet containing lean beef is reversed by the addition of beef fat. AmiClinNutr 1990;52:491–4.

dehydration and acidosis leads to severe electrolyte disturbances, and, if appropriate intervention is not initiated, to death.

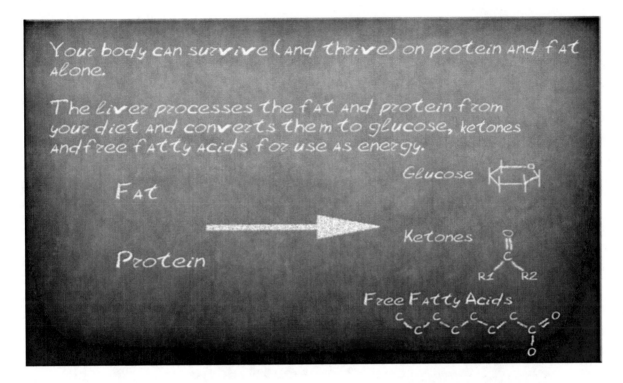

AKA is a different animal. The typical AKA patient is a chronic alcoholic who has relatively poor baseline nutrition. These people will go on a drinking binge where most of the calories consumed come from alcohol and very little from regular food. They may then develop nausea, vomiting, diarrhea, or abdominal pain that further limits their calorie intake. Their body, deprived of calories and typically quite dehydrated, enters a starvation state. Large amounts of ketones are produced, and because of a lack of the chemical NAD+, lactic acid builds up, further lowering the pH of the blood beyond the ability of the blood's buffering system to correct. The liver's production of glucose is impaired due to both calorie deprivation and problems converting pyruvate into glucose. As a result, serum glucose levels may be low, which contrasts with DKA, in which glucose levels are almost always elevated. Fortunately, AKA is usually not fatal, though there can be some serious complications like kidney failure and pancreatitis that can lead to death. Treatment is aimed at restoring adequate hydration and providing glucose and other nutrients to reverse starvation.

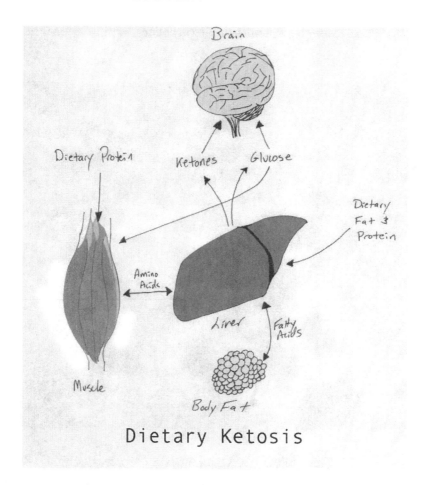

Dietary Ketosis

Unlike DKA and AKA, dietary ketosis is a normal physiological adaption to dietary carbohydrate restriction. When liver glycogen stores are depleted and the majority of ingested calories come from fats and proteins, the body switches to its alternative fuel source: ketones. Additionally, glucose is produced at modest levels from various amino acids from either dietary sources or from existing muscle tissue. Through this mechanism, the body's energy needs are met and blood glucose levels remain stable. There is a slight increase in overall acid production, but the blood's innate buffer system is easily able to neutralize this acid and maintain serum pH within normal limits. Both dietary and stored fats are continuously broken down to provide energy, and as long as the body's nutrient requirements are met, no harm will result. Unlike DKA and AKA, dietary ketosis can be continued safely for prolonged periods of time and could theoretically continue indefinitely as long as caloric and micronutrient requirements are met.

Therefore, don't be fooled when people claim that all forms of ketosis are dangerous. Even medical experts often confuse DKA/AKA with dietary ketosis and assume that the latter is harmful. Their prior experience with patients suffering from DKA/AKA causes them to raise a red flag when the word *ketosis* is mentioned. Dietary ketosis is not a harmful or dangerous condition. Understanding the differences between these very different conditions can help you discuss the matter more intelligently with your doctor as well as help lay to rest any concerns that your friends or family may have about your dietary habits.

"High-protein diets cause kidney stones."

This topic remains controversial. In general, physicians have recommended that patients with recurrent kidney stones avoid high-protein ketogenic diets. A number of studies, many using animal models, have shown that a high-protein diet does lead to a decrease in urinary pH and transient increase in urinary calcium levels. The controversy is whether these changes actually lead to increased kidney stone formation or not. People with recurrent kidney stones often have one or more genetic defects that lead to higher rates of stone formation. These include renal tubular acidosis; various defects in the production and excretion of calcium, uric acid, oxalate, and citrate; and many other problems. This is why kidney stones often run in families.

There are very few studies examining whether normal, healthy individuals, without any known genetic predisposition toward kidney stone formation, who consume a high-protein, ketogenic diet have higher rates of kidney stone formation than those who follow a typical Western diet. There is some limited data in epileptic children whose seizures are controlled with long-term ketogenic diets that shows that they do seem to have higher rates of kidney stone formation. This conclusion is also somewhat controversial, as several medications used in children to control seizures are also known to raise the risk of kidney stone formation. The available data in this area shows that children on a long-term ketogenic diet consisting of a 3:1 or 4:1 ratio of fats to protein and carbohydrate for control of epilepsy have an approximately 5 to 6 percent risk of developing kidney stones over a six-year period.[14] Translating these results into practical advice for healthy adults is problematic. Epidemiological data looking at indigenous populations who consume high animal-protein diets seem to suggest that rates of kidney stone formation are actually lower than Western averages. Native Greenland Eskimo populations who followed their traditional diet and some Japanese populations who also consume a large amount of protein from fish sources have very low incidence of kidney stone formation. In these cases, it may be the high levels of essential oils in fish and wild game that help to prevent kidney stone formation.[15]

Probably the most important factor in kidney stone formation, regardless of underlying etiology, is fluid intake. Maintaining adequate hydration is a key in avoiding recurrent kidney stones as well as maintaining optimum athletic performance. It is well documented that the risk of stone formation is increased with urine volumes of less than one liter per day, and it is probably ideal to maintain your urine output to at least two liters per day.[16] Does this mean you have to carry around a measuring cup and measure your daily urine output? Of course not. Just strive to consume one to two glasses of fluid (preferably water) with each meal and keep your urine relatively clear throughout the day. Avoid excess soda consumption, as this is thought to increase the risk of stone formation in some cases.

The bottom line regarding high protein/ketogenic diets and kidney stone risk in healthy adults is that we just don't know with certainty if they increase the risk. It is quite possible that they do, but hard data is

---

14 A Sampath, EH Kossoff, SL Furth, PL Pyzik, EG Vining. Kidney Stones and the Ketogenic Diet: Risk Factors and Prevention. J Child Neurol 2007; 22; 375.

15 Buck AC, Jenkins A, Lingam K, et al. The treatment of idiopathic recurrent urolithiasis with fish oil (EPA) and evening primrose oil (GLA)—a double blind study. J Urol. 1993;149:253A.

16 Robertson WG, Peacock M, Heyburn PJ et al: Epidemiological risk factors in calcium stone disease. Scand J Urol Nephrol 1980; 53 (suppl): 15–28.

lacking in this area. At this time, if you are an otherwise healthy adult with no family or personal history of kidney stones, then I would not shy away from any of the diets presented in The Program. If you have a history of recurrent stones or are otherwise considered high risk for stone formation, then consult with your doctor and discuss the issue with him or her.

"The weight loss is all water."

This claim just doesn't make sense. It is true that the first few pounds lost while on a low-carbohydrate diet (or any diet for that matter) may come largely from water. This is a short-lived phenomenon that occurs early in dieting and reflects the natural shifts in body water that occur with depletion of glycogen stores in muscle and liver. Glycogen is a very polar molecule, meaning that it attracts and holds on to water wherever it is found. However, attributing the long-term weight loss (often in excess of thirty pounds) experienced by many low-carbohydrate dieters to water loss is simply preposterous. If water loss accounted for the bulk of the weight loss, then we would not expect to see the phenomenal improvements in blood sugar and cholesterol levels that accompany adherence to a low-carbohydrate diet, not to mention the measurable decrease in body fat percentage. Additionally, if this myth were true, it would be possible to regain all the weight one has lost simply by increasing one's water intake. Clearly, water weight loss plays a negligible role in the overall weight loss experienced by low-carbohydrate dieters. The vast majority of weight loss can clearly be attributed to reduction in body fat.

"Eating fat will make me gain weight."

This is a clearly false but, unfortunately, all too common misconception. No particular macronutrient, be it fat, carbohydrate, or protein will make you gain weight in and of itself. Eating any one of those in excess, however, will cause weight gain. It all comes down to the balance between energy consumption and energy expenditure. If you consume calories in excess of what your body can burn, then you will gain weight. The nature of the calories you consume and the type of exercise you perform can greatly influence what type of weight you gain, be it muscle or fat tissue.

You shouldn't have any fear about consuming protein, fats, or carbohydrates in your diet. Once you understand how your body uses these nutrients, you will know how to include them in your diet in precise quantities to achieve your goals, whether that is fat loss, muscle gain, or both.

"My cholesterol will get worse on a low-carbohydrate diet."

There has been a great deal of research on low-carbohydrate diets and their effects on serum cholesterol and triglyceride levels. Even critics of low-carb diets have been forced to admit that they are highly effective in improving cholesterol profiles. One of the cardinal features of the obesity-associated metabolic syndrome is an unfavorable shift in lipid levels. High insulin levels associated with high carbohydrate intake have been consistently linked to elevated triglyceride levels; low HDL cholesterol; and changes in

LDL cholesterol to small, dense, more atherogenic (artery-clogging) forms.[17] Several studies have demonstrated that when individuals switch to the conventional high-carbohydrate, low-fat diet recommended by most dieticians, they begin to suffer from carbohydrate-induced hypertriglyceridemia. This phenomenon appears to occur when even as little as 10 percent of dietary fat is replaced with carbohydrate.[18] A number of factors seem to influence the degree to which carbohydrate intake increases triglyceride levels. These include obesity, insulin resistance, post-menopausal state, and genetic predisposition. Therefore, if you are already overweight (and therefore have a certain degree of insulin resistance), you are at particularly high risk for elevating your triglyceride levels with high carbohydrate intake.

Multiple studies have demonstrated that low-carbohydrate diets can significantly lower triglyceride levels as well as increase HDL levels even when carbohydrate levels are only moderately restricted. Any diet that leads to weight loss, especially when combined with exercise, generally will improve triglyceride, HDL, and LDL levels. However, a low-carbohydrate diet appears to have an additive effect beyond just weight loss. Even when subjects lost similar amounts of weight, those on low-carbohydrate diets showed superior improvements in lipid profiles when compared to those on conventional high-carbohydrate, low-calorie diet plans.[19]

LDL levels tend to decrease on both low-carbohydrate and conventional diets, as long as there is weight loss. Low carbohydrate diets appear to have one important advantage, however. LDL particles vary in size and density. Small, dense LDL particles appear to be more likely to lead to atherogenic plaques in the arterial walls of the heart and other organs. Low-carbohydrate diets have been shown not only to decrease LDL levels but also to increase LDL size, making it less likely to adhere to arterial walls and lead to atherosclerosis.[20]

Before starting any of the diets in The Program, I encourage you to have your cholesterol profile measured. This will give you some insight into your current metabolic state and your risk for heart disease. Repeat the measurement eight to twelve weeks after starting the diet and exercise program. You will be pleasantly surprised at the improvements you have made.

"Low-carb/high-protein diets cause osteoporosis."

This myth has been perpetuated for a number of years. It originated with a few studies showing that the urinary calcium levels increased during the first few days in test subjects who consumed a high-protein diet. Urinary calcium levels then returned to normal. This observation was taken out of context and extrapolated into the unfounded conclusion that this would lead to osteoporosis or premature bone thinning.

17 A Garg, SM Grundy, RH Unger: Comparison of effects of high and low carbohydrate diets on plasma lipoproteins and insulin sensitivity in patients with mild NIDDM. Diabetes 1992, 41:1278–85.

18 EJ Parks: Effect of dietary carbohydrate on triglyceride metabolism in humans. J Nutr 2001, 131:2772S–2774S.

19 L Stern, N Iqbal, P Seshadri, KL Chicano, DA Daily, J McGrory, M Williams, EJ Gracely, FF Samaha: The effects of low-carbohydrate versus conventional weight loss diets in severely obese adults: one-year follow-up of a randomized trial. Ann Intern Med 2004, 140:778–85.

20 P Seshadri, N Iqbal, L Stern, M Williams, KL Chicano, DA Daily, J McGrory, EJ Gracely, DJ Rader, FF Samaha: A randomized study comparing the effects of a low-carbohydrate diet and a conventional diet on lipoprotein subfractions and C-reactive protein levels in patients with severe obesity. Am J Med 2004, 117:398–405.

Fortunately, there is a good deal of research that clearly refutes this conclusion. The general consensus among various studies looking at bone mineral density and protein intake has shown that there is no effect on bone density in relation to protein intake in subjects who had adequate calcium intake.[21] There is even evidence that consuming a higher protein diet may actually be protective against hip fractures in elderly women.[22]

Examination of modern-day hunter-gatherer societies, as well as studies of our Paleolithic ancestors, both of whom generally consume or consumed a significant amount of meat and high-fiber, low-carbohydrate vegetables, consistently show bone mineral densities on par or superior to humans consuming a typical modern diet. The most important factor in avoiding osteoporosis for women is adequate calcium intake. Unfortunately, young girls and teens rarely consume the required 1,500 milligram minimum of calcium. It is during the teen years that the bulk of your bone density is deposited.

An inadequate supply of bone's building blocks will result in thinner bones and the eventual development of osteoporosis in later life. Therefore, it is recommended that all women and young girls consume a calcium supplement of some sort to help protect bone mineral density as much as possible. If you are post-menopausal, you should consult with your physician regarding the need for a bone mineral density test to determine your risk.

"Low-carb diets aren't as good as low-fat/high-carb diets for fat loss."

Until relatively recently, there was little data comparing the various popular weight-loss plans on the market today. In 2007, however, a study performed at Stanford University's Prevention Research Center actually compared four popular commercial diet plans head-to-head over one year.[23] Their purpose was to answer, once and for all, which diet led to the greatest amount of weight loss. The researchers recruited 311 overweight premenopausal women and divided them into four groups. Each group was randomly assigned to one of four different diets: the Atkins diet, Zone diet, LEARN diet, or the Ornish diet. For those of you not familiar with these diets, you can read more about them on their respective web pages. Briefly, the Atkins diet is a low-carbohydrate diet with a period of ketosis at the initiation of the diet followed by gradually increasing carbohydrate intake. Only the first two weeks of the diet are ketotic for most individuals. The Zone diet emphasizes complex lower glycemic carbohydrates and low-fat protein sources but does not result in dietary ketosis. The LEARN diet (Lifestyle, Exercise, Attitudes, Relationships, and Nutrition) as well as the Ornish diet are high-carbohydrate and very low fat (10 percent total calories) diets.

Study participants were followed weekly for the initial two months of their diets and then followed up at six and twelve months to assess their progress. Mean weight loss for the Atkins group was greatest at twelve months with 10.3 pounds lost. Zone dieters lost 3.52 pounds, LEARN dieters lost 5.7 pounds, and

21   Massey LK. Does Excess Dietary Protein Adversely Affect Bone? Symposium Overview. Journal of Nutrition, June 1998; 128 (6): 1048–1050.

22   Munger R.G., et al. Prospective Study of dietary protein intake and risk of hip fracture in postmenopausal women. American Journal of Clinical Nutrition, 2000; 72: 466–471.

23   Gardner C, et al. The A to Z Weight Loss Study: A Randomized Clinical Trial. JAMA. 2007;297:969–977.

those on the Ornish diet lost 4.8 pounds.[24] Analysis of the subjects' diets showed that they all consumed approximately the same number of calories per day and their daily energy expenditures were similar as well. The researchers also looked at other markers of cardiovascular health like cholesterol, insulin, and glucose levels as well as blood pressure. The Atkins group also showed the most improvement in these parameters as well. An interesting point regarding this study was that by the twelve-month point, most of the dieters were not 100 percent compliant with their diets. In fact, all groups lost the maximal amount of weight by six months and in the final six months of the study actually started gaining some of their weight back. This simply demonstrates that it is very difficult to stay on any diet for a prolonged period of time. The take-home lesson here is that lower-carbohydrate diets not only appear to lead to more weight loss than higher-carbohydrate, low-fat diets but show no evidence of any deleterious health effects during long-term use. These findings are supported by a number of other similar studies comparing low-carbohydrate diets with high-carbohydrate, low-fat diets. Lower carbohydrate intake consistently leads to greater weight loss and improvement in other health markers when compared to calorically similar low fat, high-carbohydrate diets. For this reason, those of you wishing to lose the greatest amount of body fat possible should consider the Endomorphic Diet. This diet takes what I believe to be the best features of the currently available low-carbohydrate, ketogenic diets on the market today and gives you a framework from which you can reach your fat-loss goals.

"The ADA (American Diabetes Association) doesn't recommend a low-carb diet so it must not be good."

Be cautious about what the government and large, organized dietetic groups say regarding dietary recommendations. They are notoriously slow to recognize new scientific data that refutes their long-established guidelines. They are also under constant pressure from high-paid lobbyists from the food and drug industry. These lobbyists are there to ensure the financial well-being of their companies, not your personal health.

"My doctor doesn't follow a low-carb diet so why should I?"

Don't be so sure about that. As more and more research is done on the metabolic effects of limiting carbohydrate intake and replacing carbohydrates with lean protein sources and healthy fats, more and more physicians are recommending these diets to their patients and using them themselves. Dr. Atkins was probably the first MD to popularize low-carbohydrate eating as not only a method of weight loss but for treatment of a variety of medical conditions like high cholesterol, heart disease, and diabetes. However, several other physicians discovered the benefits of low-carbohydrate eating many years before him. In 1967, Dr. Irwin Stillman published *The Doctor's Quick Weight Loss Diet* and Austrian physician, Dr. Wolfgang Lutz, published his book *Leben Ohne Brot* (Life without Bread). I have been treating diabetics and patients at risk for diabetes with low-carbohydrate eating plans for many years and have had excellent results in those willing to stick to the plan. Anecdotally, many of my colleagues now recommend the same sort of dietary approach for their overweight patients and report similar results. Most of the "test

---

24   Gardner CD, et al. Comparison of the Atkins, Zone, Ornish, and LEARN diets for change in weight and related risk factors among overweight premenopausal women: the A to Z Weight Loss Study: a randomized trial. JAMA Mar 7: 297 (9):969–77.

subjects" I used while developing The Program were, in fact, medical doctors and colleagues. Most got involved in this project in the same way. In between patients, or while kicking back and relaxing after a busy shift, they would ask me, "What sort of workout program are you on?" or "How do you stay in such great shape with our awful work schedule?" After discussing my ideas and the project I was working on, they would invariably ask if I could help them with a diet and exercise program. After explaining the details most would look a little bewildered. You could sense the hesitation they were experiencing about embarking on such a radical change in their eating patterns. After all, these ideas flew in the face of conventional wisdom and the official recommendations of the American Diabetes Association, the FDA, and a variety of other nutrition "authorities." Most had tried the typical low-calorie, low-fat approach in the past with varying degrees of success, and some were a little nervous about embarking on what seemed to be the antithesis of that approach. However, now that a few interested researchers are taking a second look at low-carbohydrate diets and publishing their results in reputable medical journals like *JAMA*, the *New England Journal of Medicine*, and *American Family Physician*, I was able to provide them with objective scientific literature on the subject. I'm pleased to say that, without exception, everyone who helped me develop The Program by following the system I developed for them experienced results far in excess of their expectations.

An important point to remember when discussing weight-loss diets with your physician is that most physicians are *not* dietary or exercise experts. Most of the physicians I know, across a wide range of specialties, are out of shape, don't exercise, and consume a terrible diet. They don't get enough sleep, live off sugar and coffee, and some even smoke! In medical school, I sat through endless hours of lectures on heart disease, diabetes, cancer, and surgery but not a single lecture on arguably the most important factor impacting a patient's health: *nutrition*! I suspect my experience is not unique. What little doctors do know about nutrition often comes from governmental bodies that notoriously lag decades behind the medical literature and practically require acts of Congress in order to change their dogmatic positions. So don't feel discouraged if your pudgy MD tries to talk you out of following a low or moderate carbohydrate diet for fat loss. The best thing you can do is educate yourself by reading the latest research on the subject. I've provided a number of references that are easily found online that you can bring to your physician as well. Who knows? Maybe you can teach him/her a thing or two about nutrition.

"Low-carb diets are not safe long term."

As more research is published regarding the effectiveness of low-glycemic/low-carbohydrate diets, the debate regarding their effectiveness is beginning to quiet. What continues to be a hot issue is the long-term safety of these diets. Opponents of low-carbohydrate diets raise concerns about the potential for increased rates of coronary artery disease and various cancers linked to high saturated-fat intake. These concerns are difficult to address since there is a near complete lack of unbiased studies looking at the long-term effects of these diets. We do know, from the available research, that low-carbohydrate diets are safe and effective for up to one year.[25] Subjects on a low-carbohydrate diet for up to twelve months showed substantial fat loss as well as improvements in their lipid panels. This would seem to indicate

---

25   Stern L, Iqbal N, Seshadri P, Chicano KL, Daily DA, McGrory J, et al. The effects of low-carbohydrate versus conventional weight loss diets in severely obese adults: one-year follow-up of a randomized trial. Ann Intern Med 2004;140: 778–85.

that even longer durations of low-carbohydrate dieting would also be safe. There is no data showing that long-term low-carbohydrate dieting is harmful. The concerns raised by critics of these diets are, at this time, speculative. They raise concerns about the long-term risks of increased rates of cancer, heart disease, hypertension, kidney failure, and so on but are unable to produce a single study to support their assertions. They can't because these studies don't exist. Similarly, I cannot tell you with certainty that these diets are safe for long-term use either. Unfortunately, for a variety of reasons, there is currently no good data looking at sustained low-carbohydrate dieting for over one year, and it's doubtful there ever will be. It is nearly impossible to recruit a group of people who will agree to undergo over a year's worth of dieting of any kind, especially under the strict supervision of dietary researchers, as would be required for any sort of legitimate, controlled study. Most people who stick to a low-carbohydrate diet reach their weight-loss goals in under a year anyway and then either return to their previous dietary regimen or on to a more calorically balanced diet. Additionally, staying on any diet, especially a low-carbohydrate diet, for over a year is mentally tough. It requires an extraordinary degree of self-discipline; therefore, any study looking at truly long-term effects of these diets would be riddled with non-compliant subjects and a very high dropout rate.

As we discussed earlier, a number of native populations (namely Alaskan/Canadian Inuit populations) consume low-carbohydrate diets for most of their lives. Until relatively recent times, there simply wasn't any significant source of carbohydrate available to these people, and therefore, they relied primarily on animal sources high in protein and fat for their survival. These populations are known to have low rates of both heart disease and cancer. Therefore, it would make sense to conclude that long-term adherence to this type of diet is not atherogenic or carcinogenic.

At this time, I cannot back up the statement that long-term adherence to a low-carbohydrate diet is safe with definitive, randomized, controlled scientific studies. Indeed, I doubt if such studies will ever be performed for the reasons already mentioned. With this in mind, I will reiterate that if you plan on starting a very low carbohydrate diet like the Endomorphic Diet and staying on it for more than about two months, then you should undergo a complete physical beforehand and have regular visits with your physician to follow your progress.

"High-protein diets will damage your kidneys."

This myth originated from studies showing that patients with preexisting kidney failure seemed to benefit from a diet lower in protein. One of the products of protein metabolism is urea. Urea is filtered by the kidneys but can build up to toxic levels in patients with dysfunctional kidneys. Unfortunately, some authors have taken this phenomenon out of context and suggested that increased protein intake would damage normal kidneys. All studies looking into the effects of a high-protein diet on subjects with healthy kidneys have failed to show any sign of harm.

In March of 2000, a study published in the *International Journal of Sports Nutrition and Exercise Metabolism* compared renal function among bodybuilders and other athletes. Some subjects consumed greater than two hundred grams of protein per day and had been doing so for years. In all subjects, measures of kidney function were well within normal parameters.[26] Multiple other studies have confirmed this finding. If you have normal kidney function, there is no evidence that consuming a high-protein diet will have any deleterious effects at all. If you do have a history of kidney dysfunction, then I advise you to discuss your condition with your physician before starting any diet and exercise plan.

"Low-carb diets cause heart disease."

There simply is no evidence that low-carbohydrate diets cause heart disease. In fact, the vast majority of studies looking at dietary effects on traditional risk factors for heart disease like hypertension, cholesterol, glucose intolerance, C-reactive protein, and others have shown that all these parameters improve on low-carbohydrate diets. In some cases, they actually improve even when subjects did not lose significant amounts of weight.

"You can eat all you want on a low-carb diet and still lose weight."

Yeah, don't I wish that were true? Low-carbohydrate diets are the optimal diets for losing body fat, but they still can't violate the laws of nature. If you eat more calories than you burn, on *any* diet, you are going to gain weight to some degree. On a low-carbohydrate diet, you will be less hungry than you would be on a traditional calorie-restricted diet. You will also feel full sooner and for a longer period of time. This will make cutting calories much easier, but that doesn't mean you can tie on the feedbag, down five cheeseburgers and a steak with every meal, and expect to lose weight. It's not going to happen.

"Low-carb diets don't have enough fiber."

A common misconception about low-carbohydrate diets is that they, by their nature, are also low-fiber diets. Some people have the erroneous impression that following a low-carbohydrate diet involves eating nothing but meat and eggs. Nothing could be further from the truth. Dietary fiber, because of its negligible effects on blood sugar, is a crucial part of any healthy low-carbohydrate diet. High dietary fiber intake not only keeps the colon healthy, but as an added bonus, most high-fiber foods are also rich in antioxidants and other nutrients. While on any of the diets detailed in The Program, you should be consuming a minimum of thirty to forty grams of fiber, preferably from natural sources like raw vegetables. These foods provide large amounts of bulky insoluble fiber with relatively little absorbable carbohydrate. This will allow you to eat large amounts of vegetables while still keeping your carbohydrate intake under control. For those of you who wish to consume added fiber or for some reason just can't get enough from your diet, there are a number of commercial soluble fiber drinks available on the market. These shouldn't be used to replace the dietary fiber you get from natural sources but rather should only be used as a supplement.

---

26 Poortmans JR, Dellalieux O. Do regular high protein diets have potential health risks on kidney function in athletes? International Journal of Sports Nutrition and Exercise Metabolism, Mar. 2000;10(1):28–38.

"If you want to look like a pro bodybuilder, you have to train like a pro bodybuilder."

Muscle magazines are full of workout articles written by professional bodybuilders detailing how they work out various body parts. The vast majority of professional bodybuilders look the way they do for three very important reasons. First, without a doubt, they put in a tremendous amount of hard work, discipline, and dedication to their sport. For a professional bodybuilder, achieving "the look" is an all-encompassing passion. Secondly, these individuals are genetically gifted. By this, I mean they are born with a bone structure and muscle shape that provides a framework for an aesthetic, muscular appearance. They are also blessed with a far better-than-average ability to build muscle mass. Your average Joe with the same amount of dedication, even with steroids, could not achieve a Mr. Olympia-caliber physique. This brings me to the third reason today's professional bodybuilders look the way they do. Steroids, lots of steroids. This is perhaps the single biggest factor that has turned today's pro bodybuilders into the muscle monsters that we see on stage. Compare today's bodybuilders with those in the 1970s. Steroids were around back then too, but their use, along with a myriad of other hormones, diuretics, and other agents, has pushed the envelope well beyond anything achieved by Arnold and the bodybuilders of his era. Even in the best shape of his life, Arnold would be hard pressed to win a top amateur event these days.

Given these facts, why in the hell would you take a pro bodybuilder's advice about how to work out? Their workouts are multi-hour marathons fuelled by steroid-assisted recovery and growth. If non-steroid-using athletes attempted these workouts for any length of time, they would find themselves grossly over trained, very likely injured, and making no progress. If you are using massive amounts of steroids and have great genetics to boot, you could probably use just about any workout regimen you like and still build tons of muscle and look great. For the rest of us, however, a more rational approach needs to be taken.

Unfortunately, the same bad advice that was being put into muscle magazines when I was first training is still showing up in print and now on the Internet. The following is a sample workout I lifted from a website called freedomfly.net. (http://www.freedomfly.net/workouts/workout2.htm) written by a fellow called Marc David.[27] This is a sample "advanced" workout for an experienced bodybuilder. There are many different workouts espoused in the muscle mags and online that supposedly are for "advanced" bodybuilders. This is just one example, but it is largely typical of the high-volume marathon workouts that are pushed in the magazines and elsewhere. Let's take a closer look at it.

Monday
(45–60 minutes of some type of cardio before workout)
Body Part Exercise Sets Reps
Abdominals Crunches 4 sets 25–30 reps
Hanging Leg Raises 4 sets 25–30 reps
Standing Bent-Over Twists 2 sets 50 reps
Chest Bench Press (*warm up*) 1 set 15 reps
Bench Press (*superset w/flys*) 4 sets 10, 8, 8, 6 reps
Dumbbell Fly 4 sets 10, 8, 8, 6 reps

---

27   http://www.freedomfly.net/workouts/workout2.htm

Incline Press 4 sets 10, 8, 8, 6 reps
Dumbbell Incline Fly 4 sets 10, 8, 8, 6 reps
Decline Bench Press 4 sets 10, 8, 8, 6 reps
Dumbbell Decline Fly 4 sets 10, 8, 8, 6 reps
Machine Flys 2 sets 15–20 reps
Triceps Dips behind Back 5 sets 10 reps
Triceps Pushdowns 4 sets 8–10 reps
Rope Extensions 4 sets 8–10 reps
Skull Crushers 3 sets 10–12 reps

So let's review…after walking on a treadmill, stair-climber, or some other cardio machine for up to an hour, you are going to perform ten sets of abdominal exercises, twenty-five sets of chest work, and sixteen sets of triceps work. That should take you all of at least three hours…

Tuesday

(45–60 minutes of some type of cardio before workout)
Body Part Exercise Sets Reps
Abdominals Crunches 4 sets 25–30 reps
Hanging Leg Raises 4 sets 25–30 reps
Standing Bent-Over Twists 2 sets 50 reps
Back Deadlift *(warm up)* 1 set 15 reps
Deadlift *(superset w/cable rows)* 4 sets 10, 8, 8, 6 reps
Cable Rows 4 sets 10, 8, 8, 6 reps
Lat Pull Downs (to front) 4 sets 10, 8, 8, 6 reps
T-Bar Rows 4 sets 10, 8, 8, 6 reps
T-Bar Rows *(negatives)* 4 sets 10 reps
Biceps Preacher Barbell Curls *(wide grip)* 3 sets 10, 8, 8 reps
Preacher Barbell Curls *(close grip)* 3 sets 10, 8, 8 reps
Incline Dumbbell Curls 3 sets 10, 8, 8 reps
Concentrated Curls 2 sets 10–12 reps

With no rest day, you are back in the gym again for back and biceps. On this day, you will perform another ten sets of abdominal exercises, twenty-one sets of back exercises, and only eleven sets of biceps work…

Wednesday Day Off

Unfortunately, you will be too sore and overtrained to do much with your day off.

Thursday

(45–60 minutes of some type of cardio before workout)
Abdominals Crunches 4 sets 25–30 reps

Hanging Leg Raises 4 sets 25–30 reps
Standing Bent-Over Twists 2 sets 50 reps
Quads/Hams Squats (warm-up) 1 set 15 reps
Squats 5 sets 10, 8, 8, 6, 6 reps
Leg Press 4 sets 10, 8, 8, 6 reps
Leg Extension 5 sets 10, 8, 8, 6, 6 reps
Leg Curls 5 sets 8, 8, 6, 6, 4 reps
Barbell Lunges 4 sets 8, 8, 6, 6 reps

After a whole day off to recover from approximately six hours of exercise over the past two days, you will perform the obligatory cardio followed by ten sets of abdominal work and twenty-four sets of leg exercises! Assuming you can still walk you, you get to go home and rest for a few hours.

Friday

(45–60 minutes of some type of cardio before workout)
Abdominal Crunches 4 sets 25–30 reps
Hanging Leg Raises 4 sets 25–30 reps
Standing Bent-Over Twists 2 sets 50 reps
Shoulders Military Shoulder Press (to front) 1 set 15 reps
Military Press (to front) 4 sets 10, 8, 8, 6 reps
Barbell Upright Rows 4 sets 10, 8, 8, 6 reps
Side Dumbbell Lateral Raises 4 sets 10, 8, 8, 6 reps
Seated Bent-Over Dumbbell Laterals 3 sets 10, 8, 8 reps
Calves Standing Calf Raises (warm-up) 1 set 15 reps
Standing Calf Raises (Toes In) 3 sets 10 reps
Standing Calf Raises (Toes Out) 3 sets 10 reps
Seated Calf Raises 3 sets 10, 8, 8 reps

Ah, Friday…the weekend is here. If you have managed to survive and not put yourself into kidney failure with the past three workouts, then perhaps you can cut loose and have some fun.

But not before you perform yet another cardio session, ten sets of abs (abs four times per week?), and sixteen sets of shoulder work followed by ten sets of calf exercise (make sure you point your toes the right way…that makes all the difference!).

Saturday Day Off

Sunday Day Off

Unfortunately for you, you were so overtrained and exhausted that you spent your two days off lying on the couch, popping Motrin and wondering how long you will have to perform this sadistic workout before you start looking like Mr. Universe.

I think this workout plan would yield outstanding results for steroid-using athletes. With the assistance of these drugs, they should be able to recover adequately between workouts with the assumption that they are getting enough sleep and proper nutrition. If you are not a steroid-using bodybuilder, then this program and others like it will run you into the ground. If you don't believe me, try it for two weeks and see how you feel and also record how long it takes you to finish. I trained this way for years as a teenager and wondered why I barely made any progress. Fortunately, there is a better way. The Program will give you, the non-steroid-using athlete, results you are looking for in a fraction of the time.

"You have to do three to five sets per exercise to build strength in the gym."

This has been bodybuilding dogma for years. Where did it come from? Probably from the Joe Weider camp or perhaps even earlier when home dumbbell sets were sold with small instructional booklets that gave sample exercise routines. Over the years, the multitude of fitness experts have recited the "three to five sets per exercise" mantra so often that pretty much everyone believes it. I personally don't think you should do something just because everyone else is doing it. You should have good reasons for doing the things you do—preferably reasons you can back up with scientific evidence. This is why after a few years of blindly accepting the idea that three to five sets were optimal, I actually took a look at what the scientific literature had to say about it. It turns out that what these so-called experts were espousing for years was actually wrong! They just made it up, and everyone else followed along. I go into the specific studies in a more detailed manner in the training chapters of The Program, but suffice it to say that it turns out three to five sets per body part is *not* the most efficient way to build strength and muscle mass. Equal or better results can be achieved with far less exercise and in a much shorter period of time than previously thought. While on The Program, you will be performing only *one* and in some cases two sets per body part and getting fantastic results.

"There is no such thing as over-training, just under-eating."

This myth was bantered around in some of the muscle magazines a few years ago and occasionally pops up again on Internet forums and other places. The idea is that you can compensate for higher and higher volumes of exercise by consuming higher and higher volumes of food. It suggests that the primary thing limiting your ability to recover from prolonged exercise is the number of calories you can take in. On first pass, this might make sense to a few folks. Your body needs protein, fat, and carbohydrate to recover from exercise and build up additional muscle mass, right? It should follow that the more you eat, the faster you can recover and thereby extend the amount of time you train. If you follow this argument to its extreme, you can see how ridiculous it is.

Very ill patients in the hospital are often unable to eat for prolonged periods of time. Obviously, prolonged starvation needs to be avoided in order for them to recover. To get around this problem, at least until they are able to use their gut again, they are often given TPN (total parenteral nutrition). TPN is an intravenous formulation of proteins, fats, carbohydrates, vitamins, and minerals, sometimes mixed with insulin, which provides nutrition to patients who cannot eat for prolonged periods of time. If there really was no such thing as overtraining, just under eating, then it would be possible, according to this theory, to hook up athletes to several huge bags of TPN and infuse it at a high rate and this would allow them to exercise virtually non-stop. They could literally perform squats, for example, with maximum weight continuously without rest! If they began to fatigue, you could simply dial up the rate of TPN infused and keep on going! If caloric intake were the only thing limiting your ability to train, then simply pumping in more calories would allow you to exercise indefinitely. Obviously, this is ludicrous.

Recovery from intense exercise takes time. As you train, not only are microscopic muscle fibers torn and collagen disrupted, but the very substrate that your muscle uses for fuel, ATP, is depleted. Muscles grow after the damage training creates has been repaired, and this takes time. The process requires synthesis of new proteins, a complex task requiring transcription of RNA and assembly of proteins on the ribosomes within your cells. The synthesis of new proteins is not a rapid step, it takes from hours to days to complete. Simply forcing more substrate in the form of calories into your body will not accelerate this process. The best way to avoid overtraining…is *not to overtrain*! Perform the precise amount of exercise that you need to stimulate the growth you want and then get out of the gym and rest. Feed your body what it needs to repair the damage you cause and enough to build the muscle you want, and that's it. Overstuffing yourself with tons of extra calories in the misguided attempt to speed up your recovery will only leave you fat, tired, and no closer to your goals.

"If you stop working out, all your muscle will turn to fat!"

I won't spend too much time on this one even though it's probably the single most common myth I've heard thrown around by people who don't know the first thing about exercise. Usually, it was directed at me by some overweight fifty-something-year-old couch potato who would say something like, "Once you get older and stop working out, all that muscle is just going to turn to fat, you know!" My usual response was to simply smile. It wasn't worth the time to explain the facts about actual muscle cell physiological processes to justify the effort. It is literally impossible for a muscle cell to turn into a fat cell.

What the myth refers to is the case of athletes who in their youth had very well-muscled physiques with little body fat but after retirement or an injury, lost much of their muscle mass and gained lots of additional fat. What happens in these cases is what happens to anyone who stops exercising. In response to exercise, your muscles will adapt and hypertrophy. When you stop exercising, they will atrophy. If you continue to take in more calories than you burn, once you stop exercising, then naturally, you will gain weight in the form of fat. This doesn't mean that your muscle tissue "turned into" fat! Your muscle cells and fat cells differentiated from each other very early in your embryological development. Once that change happened, the genes that told a muscle cell to be a muscle cell turned on and the ones that told it to be a fat cell were turned off. Barring some breakthrough in genetic manipulation, this change is permanent. It therefore is impossible for a muscle cell to spontaneously turn into a fat cell, a nerve cell, a skin cell, or any other kind of cell. A muscle will atrophy with disuse, but it will never become a fat cell. So my answer now to the above comment is "Well, I won't have to worry about that because I'm never going to stop working out!"

"I'm not fat; I'm just 'big-boned.'"

Most people have heard this somewhat tongue-in-cheek comment on a number of occasions. It goes without saying that "big bones" have nothing to do with the amount of body fat you are carrying around.

Sure, some obese individuals have thicker, stronger bones, but that is an adaption to the increased weight they are forced to carry day in and day out. The "big-boned" excuse really is a humorous example of a more common problem that many people who are overweight tend to have and that is to rationalize or explain away their excess weight. By doing so, they avoid taking responsibility and attribute their weight issue to something outside of their control. It's a common coping mechanism. Unfortunately, it's a strategy that keeps us from examining our behavior and our motivations, and that can consistently keep us from reaching our goals. You need to stop trying to fool yourself and not make excuses. In order to reach your goals, you have to make the difficult step of looking at yourself and your body objectively — something that isn't easy to do. Once you have the courage to take this step, however, you will be on your way to making the changes you need. Be willing to take the risk and give yourself permission to succeed.

"Lifting weights makes you less flexible."

This myth used to be common among athletic coaches in the 1970s and earlier. Football and track and field coaches would routinely warn their athletes that lifting weights would make them "muscle bound" and hamper performance. Fortunately, this fallacy has been thoroughly discredited and it's rare for a coach in any sport today not to encourage his or her athletes to weight train.

Rather than make you less flexible, lifting weights through a full range of motion will actually make you more flexible. This has been demonstrated in multiple studies. For example, in 2001, the *International Journal of Sports Medicine* published a paper on the changes in hamstring, low back, hip, shoulder, elbow, and knee flexibility in older adults who were placed on a resistance training program. Those assigned to the weight-training group performed eight exercises (chest presses, leg extensions, shoulder presses, leg curls, lat pull-downs, leg presses, arm curls, and tricep extensions) on a Universal machine. Over the course of sixteen weeks, the number of sets and intensity (as a function of their one-rep maximum) was increased. All subjects gained a significant amount of strength and lean body mass as compared to controls who did not exercise. Not surprisingly, their flexibility in all joints measured also improved significantly.[28]

This study confirms the findings of several others that showed that the flexibility of a given joint can be enhanced by moving it through its full range of motion against resistance. As part of your warm-up and cool-down, you will be performing a variety of stretches in addition to your weight training. The combination of the two will help keep you flexible and limber.

What has not been studied adequately, in my opinion, is the effect of partial-range-of-motion weight training on flexibility. There are several authors who recommend performing "heavy partials," where very heavy weights, often in excess of an athlete's one-rep max, are moved through an incomplete range of motion. For example, when performing a bench press, a power lifter may set the bars on a power rack high enough that he can only lower the weight to about six inches off his chest. In this manner, he is focusing on the second half of the movement or "lockout." It is my suspicion that performing only this type of

---

28 Fatouros, I.G., Taxildaris, K., Tokmakidis, S.P., Kalapotharakos, V., Aggelousis, N.,Athanasopoulos, S., Zeeris, I., Katrabasas, I. (2001). The effects of strength training, cardiovascular training and their combination on flexibility of inactive older adults. International Journal of Sports Medicine. 23, 112–119.

training could potentially limit one's flexibility. I don't have scientific proof of this, but it seems logical. I don't want to discourage you from using heavy partials. They are an excellent high-intensity technique, but I would be cautious about making them the cornerstone of your training if you are concerned about maintaining optimal flexibility.

For men are not equal: thus speaks justice.

—Friedrich Nietzsche

GENETICS AND BODY TYPES

Thus far, I have been trying to convince you that as human beings, we are all virtually identical. As you look around, however, you can see that the similarities we all share only go so far. In truth, the statement "All men are created equal" is biologically false. There are obvious differences among all of us. Even identical twins have subtle differences that set them apart from each other. Some people are tall; some are short. Some are thin and others fat. Some have large muscles, while others have long, thin muscles. Some are able to build muscle mass very quickly while others do so slowly. There are also obvious metabolic differences. We all know people who can eat huge amounts of food, even if it is pure junk, and not gain any significant amount of fat. Yet there are those who eat a relatively "normal" diet and still gain unwanted body fat.

In the 1940s, the American psychologist William Sheldon attempted to classify human bodies into three general body types or *somatotypes*: endomorphs, mesomorphs, and ectomorphs. Through a series of observations, he noted that most individuals favored one of these three basic body types. He also attempted to associate specific body types with behavioral attributes. While his observation of different body types does provide a useful context in which to classify human physiques, his claims that specific psychological characteristics could be assigned to them has been proven false. Individuals who conform exactly to one particular somatotype are not common. Most people favor one particular type while possessing various qualities inherent in the others. In reality, somatotyping is somewhat of an artificial distinction, and you can be fooled. Someone may have the outward appearance of an endomorph due to years of poor diet and exercise habits, but when exposed to a proper exercise and diet, he or she begins to show that his or her real genetic tendency is toward a mesomorphic physique.

Despite its inherent limitations, somatotyping can serve as a useful starting point when deciding how to start off The Program. Understanding which somatotype you favor can help you decide not only which diet to choose but also what types of gains in muscle mass you can expect.

Endomorphs

The classic endomorph has a tendency to hold a greater than average amount of body fat while at the same time having large muscles capable of great strength. A typical NFL lineman or competitive heavyweight power lifter is usually an endomorph. Body fat is carried primarily in the abdomen for men and hips and buttocks for women. Endomorphs also may store a greater amount of fat around their internal organs. Metabolically, endomorphs have a greater capacity to store calories as fat. They tend to have a greater degree of insulin resistance and tend to develop diabetes and heart disease at greater rates than other body types. The good news about being a classic endomorph is that most can build a significant amount of muscle mass. The downside is that body fat is easily accumulated and somewhat more difficult to burn. The Endomorphic Diet was designed specifically to tackle this problem.

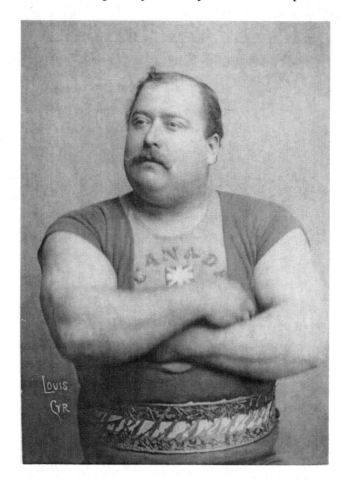

Canadian strongman Louis Cyr. A classic endomorph.

Mesomorphs

Mesomorphs have physiques that most people strive to achieve. They tend to carry a well-proportioned amount of muscle mass with a low amount of body fat. Many are quite athletic and have powerful, lean physiques. They tend to build muscle easily and have to overeat significantly in order to put on body fat. The goal of The Program is to help you achieve a mesomorphic appearance. You may be starting off as an endomorph or ectomorph, but with proper training and diet, you will ultimately take on the appearance of a mesomorph. Mesomorphs tend to have low levels of insulin resistance due to their increased muscle mass.

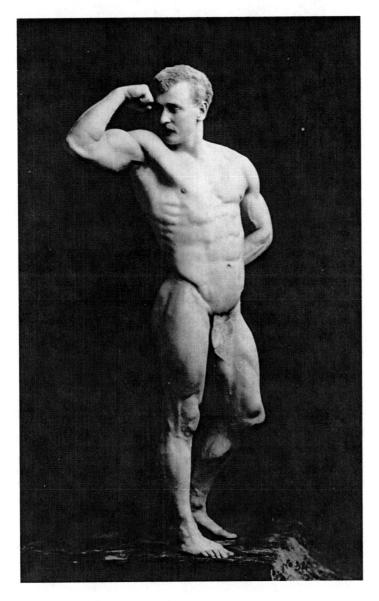

Eugene Sandow: pure mesomorph

Ectomorphs

Ectomorphs have long, thin muscles and very low body fat percentages. Many are also tall with long limb lengths. In general, they tend to have higher percentages of slow-twitch muscle fibers (see training chapter for a full description of muscle-fiber types). Ectomorphs tend to have difficulty building significant amounts of muscle mass but generally have no problem staying lean. They have metabolisms that resist the deposition of body fat. Typical ectomorphs include marathon runners or other long-distance running athletes. Ectomorphs do respond to high-intensity weight training but typically at a slower pace. They also tend to require longer recovery periods between workouts.

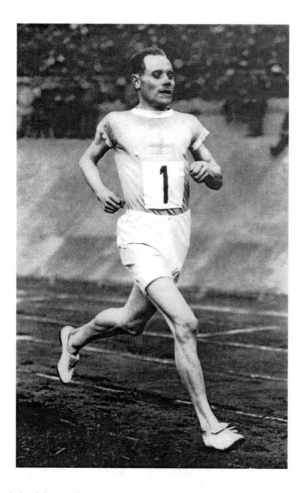

**Finnish Olympic distance runner Paavo Nurmi. Like
all great distance runners, Nurmi was a true ectomorph.**

Genetic Differences in Metabolism

Delving into the complex genetic differences among people regarding metabolism is far beyond the scope of this book. However, I think it is important to cover a few basic principles since the study of human genetics is rapidly accelerating our understanding of the variations in human physiology.

As stated earlier, on a genetic level, all human beings are virtually identical. But you can look around the room and tell right away that we are not all the same. We all have twenty-three chromosomes; each with multiple genes, but it is the different versions of those genes that you inherit from your parents that set you apart from your fellow man. When it comes to genes influencing body size and shape, there are literally thousands of known variations in the gene pool. It is estimated that about 45 to 75 percent of the variation we see among individuals in terms of body fat percentage can be attributed to inheritance and not to environmental factors.[29]

---

29 Maes HH, Neale MC, Eaves LJ. Genetic and environmental factors in relative body weight and human adiposity. Behav Genet 1997; 27: 325–351.

What we know so far regarding genes and obesity is that your body type is greatly influenced by heredity. Twins reared apart usually end up with very similar body types, and adopted children's body types are highly correlated with that of their biological parents and not with their adopted parents.[30] We all come into the world with a genetic blueprint inherited from our parents and our ancestors going back millions of years. Under normal circumstances, your body will follow that blueprint more or less exactly. This does not mean that just because both your parents were obese you can't have a set of six-pack abdominals. You may have inherited genes from your parents that make you more efficient at disposing of calories as body fat, but your body will still respond to a low-glycemic, quality-protein diet and high-intensity weight training. You may have to be a bit stricter in terms of your caloric intake, but you can still look just as good as people whose metabolism allows them to eat whatever they want.

There is intense ongoing research trying to find "fat genes" that make some people obese while others remain thin or of normal body weight. There have been a number of promising discoveries in this area that are particularly interesting. One of the recurring themes in these discoveries is that many of these "fat genes," particularly those found in the "super-obese" (those with BMI's of 50), have little whatsoever to do with how people metabolize foods. Rather they are genes influencing neurobehavioral portions of the brain. Specifically, these genes control things like satiety, hunger, and food cravings. Fortunately, these genes are relatively rare, even among the super-obese and cannot be blamed for the current obesity epidemic. There are a number of genes that also control nutrient partitioning. This refers to the way in which the body disposes of its calories. When a given number of calories are consumed, a certain percentage of those calories are stored as either fat or glycogen, while others are used as fuel or to assist in the building and repair of various bodily tissues. The degree to which the body shunts calories to these various functions is influenced by both environmental and genetic factors. Genes that code for more efficient shunting of calories into fat tissue, especially when combined with poor diet and lack of exercise, likely have a greater degree of influence in the general population than the "fat genes" researchers have recently discovered. (If you are really interested in this field and want to learn more about genetic causes of obesity, check out the Obesity Gene Map Database at http://obesitygene.pbrc.edu/.)

Having said all that, I don't think it's productive to spend too much time focusing on the genetics of obesity or muscle mass for that matter. You can't change your genetics, and too often, I see "poor genetics" blamed for poor conditioning and poor effort. What you do have control over is what you do with your body and what you put into it. That should be your focus. For the average man or woman without a strong family history of obesity, it is lifestyle that is largely to blame for the sorry state of his or her physique.[31] Am I contradicting what I just said above? Not really. Remember, I said under "normal" circumstances, your body will follow the blueprint inherited by your parents. If you think you inherited a crappy blueprint, then there isn't much you can do about that. But you *can* change the circumstances under which that blueprint is translated. It's up to you set up some "abnormal" circumstances in the form of a metabolically favorable diet and an intense exercise program to make the most of your blueprint. (I hesitate to call our culture's current sedentary, junk-food lifestyle "normal" when in fact it the most "abnormal" lifestyle our species has ever undertaken.) The only thing you can do is exert your free will and change your environment. It is genetics that loads the gun, but it's you who pulls the trigger.

---

30   Stunkard, A.J., J.R. Harris, N.L. Pederson, and G.E. McClearn. The body-mass index of twins who have been reared apart. N. Engl. J. Med. 322:1483–1487, 1990.

31   M van Rossum[1], B Hoebee[2], et al. Genetic factors as predictors of weight gain in young adult Dutch men and women. Int Journal of Obesity. April 2002, Volume 26, Number 4, Pages 517–528C.

No price is too high to pay for the privilege of owning yourself.

—Friedrich Nietzsche

CHOOSING THE RIGHT EATING PLAN FOR YOU

There are three diet plans presented in The Program. Each has its own metabolic effects and is designed with certain goals in mind.

The Endomorphic Diet

This diet is designed for maximum fat loss. It significantly lowers insulin levels and turns your body into a round-the-clock fat-burning machine. Those of you with a significant amount of body fat to lose or those looking to achieve the lowest possible body fat levels should try this diet. Through having you control the amount of carbohydrate you eat and consume mostly high-quality protein and the right kinds of fats, this diet will get you ripped faster than any other while at the same time preserving and building your muscle mass. The Endomorphic Diet is designed for those who:

- Have a significant amount of body fat to lose
- Have or possess a tendency toward significant insulin resistance or type 2 diabetes.
- Are already fairly lean but want to obtain an extremely low body fat percentage either for bodybuilding competition or personal reasons.

The Mesomorphic Diet

This diet is a natural transition from the Endomorphic Diet. It is designed not only to maintain low body fat levels but also to create an environment conducive to building muscle mass. The Mesomorphic Diet is also designed to be a diet you can follow for life. It contains the right amount of calories and the correct balance between proteins, fats, and carbohydrates. The Mesomorphic Diet is designed for those who:

- Are already lean and muscular and want to continue building muscle mass while maintaining a low body fat percentage

- Have made significant progress on either the Endomorphic or Ectomorphic Diet and want to transition to a long-term diet to maintain and continue to build upon their gains.
- Want to or need to take a temporary break from the demands of the Endomorphic Diet without regaining the fat that has already been lost.

The Ectomorphic Diet

This diet is designed for those looking to gain as much muscle mass as they possibly can. If you are thin and looking to pack on quality mass or are already muscular and want to build even more, this is the diet for you. You will learn to consume the right kinds of foods and supplements to create the optimal anabolic environment. The Ectomorphic Diet is designed for those who:

- Are thin and have difficulty gaining weight
- Want to gain as much muscle mass as possible and are not concerned about gaining some body fat along the way.

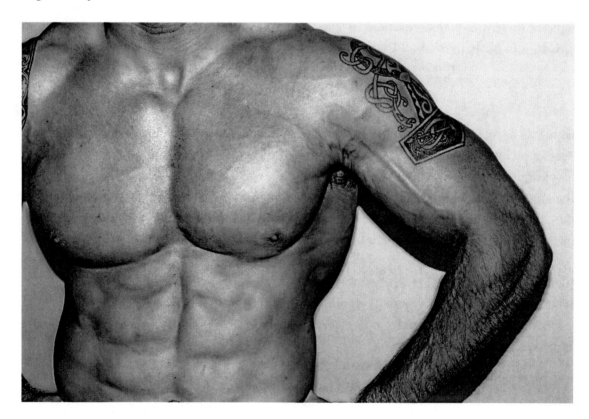

WHAT YOU CAN EXPECT

The Program is designed to be the most efficient means of achieving the goals you set for your body. It is designed with the simple idea that to meet those goals, you have to use what works and discard the rest. As with any discipline, when the proper knowledge is applied to a project, the results achieved should be predictably successful in all cases. As a result, when properly applied, The Program can provide dramatic and consistent changes in body composition and muscular strength, far beyond those resulting from other diet and exercise programs.

It is not uncommon for overweight individuals on the Endomorphic Diet to lose well over five pounds in their first week of dieting, and in many cases, they lose over ten pounds in the first week with no loss in muscle mass or strength. This rapid weight loss in the one to two weeks eventually begins to level off, of course, as the burning of that much body fat without the sacrifice of muscle tissue is difficult if not impossible for the non-steroid-using athlete. However, it is not uncommon to average a loss of over two pounds of fat per week. Overweight dieters on the Endomorphic Diet can expect to lose eight to ten pounds of fat per month if they follow The Program precisely. One physician colleague of mine, who was very obese, lost over eighty pounds in less than five months while on the Endomorphic Diet. Your overall body weight may not reflect this loss, as you will be gaining new muscle tissue, but the fat loss will be very noticeable, not only in the mirror, but also in the way your clothes fit. As one's body fat levels enter the low teens and single digits, then, obviously, such dramatic fat loss will not be possible. The body will attempt to hold onto its stored fat deposits both subcutaneously and internally. At this stage in your dieting, average fat loss rarely exceeds one pound per week but in some cases may be much less. Fat loss greater than this rarely occurs without sacrificing some muscle tissue.

Results on the Mesomorphic Diet are variable depending on the goals of the dieter. Mesomorphic eating is ideal for lifelong maintenance of low body fat levels and heavy muscularity but can be adapted for either fat loss or for additional muscle gains. The Mesomorphic Diet generally will not result in quite the same dramatic fat loss seen with the Endomorphic Diet but can still lead to steady one- to two-pound-per-week fat loss in overweight individuals if the necessary caloric deficit is achieved. Similarly, surplus calories can be included for individuals who wish to gain muscle mass without the risk of putting on additional body fat.

The Ectomorphic Diet is designed to provide an optimal nutritional environment for maximal muscle growth. The amount of muscle mass an individual may gain and the speed with which he or she may gain it, however, is genetically predetermined. The goal of the Ectomorphic Diet, combined with the training regime provided later, is to provide the proper stimulus and all the necessary building blocks so an individual may gain muscle mass at as close to the upper limit of his or her genetic potential as possible. Since athletes vary in their ability to build new muscle tissue, it stands to reason that giving precise predictions for muscle mass gains that apply to all athletes is difficult. However, even the most stubborn ectomorph can and will make substantial gains in muscle mass and strength while on the Ectomorphic Diet. It is not unreasonable to expect a young, novice athlete to gain a pound of solid muscle per week. Some will gain more, and gains of up to twenty to thirty pounds in two months are not unheard of. If you are age thirty or greater then these sorts of gains are probably not realistic. Your ability to build muscle tissue dramatically declines after age thirty. For older athletes a gain of ten to twenty pounds of muscle over the course of a year would be a reasonable expectation for the novice trainer. If you are in your forties and beyond your gains will be much less but can still be quite substantial.

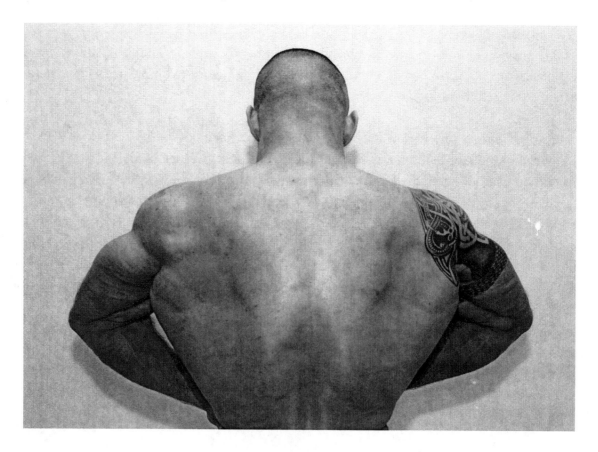

Let food be thy medicine and medicine be thy food.

—Hippocrates

WHAT YOUR BODY DOES WITH ITS FOOD

Most people don't give a second thought to the events that occur immediately before and after they eat. They consume their meal or snack and move on with the rest of their day. The process of consuming and digesting food, however, is incredibly complex. From the first bite to the eventual return to the outside world, there are literally millions of complex chemical processes taking place that allow your body to extract the necessary nutrients from your food. A detailed description of these processes is far beyond the scope of this book. Nevertheless, a fundamental understanding of what happens to your food (and what your food does to you) will provide you with a deeper level of understanding and make it clear why The Program is designed the way it is.

The body prepares for the digestion of food before it even enters your mouth. A region in the brain known as the lateral hypothalamic area produces the sensation of hunger and stimulates an intense desire to seek out and consume food. This area is activated by various stimuli, such as falling glucose levels, contraction of the stomach, neuropeptides like leptin, gastrointestinal hormones, stress, temperature, and a host of other factors that are only now being partially understood by scientists. Psychological factors also play an important role in our desire to consume food. We all have experienced times when we craved certain foods even though we were not hungry or turned to food for comfort during stressful or emotional periods.

Once you have acquired the food of your choice, the digestion process begins with chewing. This breaks the food into smaller, more digestible pieces. Enzymes in the mouth begin to break down carbohydrates in the food into simpler sugars even before we swallow. After we swallow, food transits through the esophagus to the stomach where powerful acids are secreted to further break it down. This mass of partially liquefied food then passes into the small intestine where digestive juices from the pancreas and gallbladder are introduced to further the digestion process. In the small intestine, fats, carbohydrates, and proteins are broken down into simple, easily absorbable components. Most of the body's vitamin and mineral absorption occurs here too. The remaining food mass then passes into the large intestine (or colon) whose primary job is to reabsorb water and create a solid waste that is able to pass into the rectum and eventually out of the body.

The process above is a brief description of the overall digestive process. A basic understanding of what happens at the microscopic and molecular level, however, is helpful in understanding how the various eating plans presented in The Program work and how they use your body's internal mechanisms to help you burn fat and build muscle.

METABOLISM OF CARBOHYDRATES

The process of digesting and metabolizing carbohydrates begins in the mouth. The enzyme amylase is secreted in your saliva and begins to break down starchy foods into a simpler, sweeter sugar known as maltose. You can experience this process firsthand by keeping a small amount of starchy food like a cracker or biscuit in your mouth for a few minutes without swallowing it. After a minute or so, you will notice the food tastes a little bit sweeter than it did when you first put it in your mouth. Since most people don't keep food in their mouths for this long, very little of this sugar is produced or absorbed into the bloodstream.

In the stomach, carbohydrates are further liquefied as they mix with stomach acids, but there are no enzymes in the stomach to actually digest carbohydrate. Eventually, the liquefied carbohydrate mixture exits the stomach and enters the small intestine. If your carbohydrate source was high in fiber, then the process of exiting the stomach will proceed more slowly and the sensation of fullness you experience after eating will last longer.

In the small intestine, enzymes secreted by the pancreas break down dietary carbohydrates (usually in the form of long chains of glucose molecules called polysaccharides) into shorter glucose chains. Before they are absorbed into the bloodstream, nearly all carbohydrates have been broken down into single sugar molecules (glucose, galactose, or fructose). As these sugar molecules enter the bloodstream, they raise blood glucose levels. This is detected by the pancreas, which begins to secrete insulin. Insulin's primary role is to allow the body's cells to take in glucose and utilize it for various purposes. This eventually reduces the blood glucose level back down to normal. Both the rate of insulin production and the total amount of insulin produced are influenced by how quickly the blood sugar rises and by how much total carbohydrate is consumed. Simple sugars require very little breakdown and quickly enter the bloodstream leading to a rapid and high insulin level very quickly after consumption. This occurs, for example, after eating a candy bar or white bread or drinking fruit juice or regular soda. The rise in insulin levels is much slower and occurs to a lesser degree when you consume complex carbohydrates. These carbohydrate sources have long, complex glucose chains and often contain a significant amount of fiber, which cannot be absorbed. As a result, it takes longer for the carbohydrate to be broken down, and it trickles into the bloodstream at a much slower rate. The slow secretion of insulin follows this pattern and leads to a much more gradual rise and subsequent fall in blood glucose levels.

In the presence of insulin, the body's cells take in precisely what they need to meet their energy demands. Any additional carbohydrate ingested beyond this basic level is processed in one of several ways. The liver absorbs some glucose and converts it into a storage form known as glycogen where it is available for use later. The liver can store enough glucose in the form of glycogen to supply the body's needs for about twelve hours. This is the primary source of glucose when you are sleeping. The brain absorbs and utilizes about 15 to 20 percent of the carbohydrate you ingest. All this carbohydrate is burned, as the brain does not have the ability to store glucose in the form of glycogen. Muscle cells also take in glucose and store it as glycogen for their own use. Up to 50 percent of the glucose that reaches the bloodstream under normal conditions is taken up by muscle cells. The primary difference between the liver and muscle in this regard is that once a muscle cell takes in a glucose molecule, it is never released back into circulation. It remains there to provide energy for that particular muscle cell. Additional carbohydrate intake, above and beyond that needed by the liver and muscle, has a far less desirable destination—fat. The liver, under the influence of insulin, is very efficient at transforming glucose into fatty acids through a series of complex chemical processes. These fatty acids are eventually shuttled into the body's fat cells with the encouragement of insulin for long-term storage. Clearly, this final step is something that should be minimized for those of you trying to lose body fat.

> After you digest carbohydrates from your diet they are converted to glucose and enter the bloodstream.
>
> From there, with the help of insulin, glucose is either stored in the liver or muscle, converted to fatty acids and stored as fat, or burned by the brain as fuel.

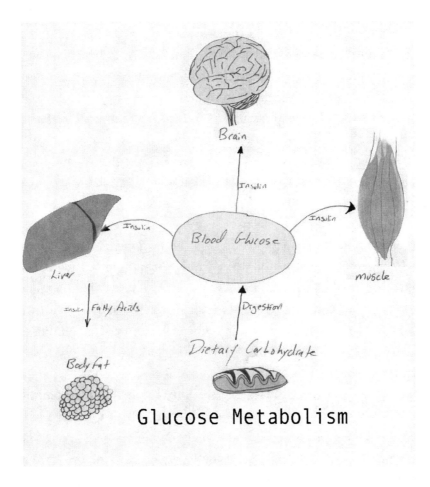

Glucose Metabolism

Maintaining Blood Glucose Levels: Insulin and Glucagon

Your body is genetically programmed to maintain your blood glucose levels within fairly narrow parameters. This provides a constant, steady supply of glucose to the working cells of the body. When glucose levels get too high, insulin is secreted to bring them back down. Conversely, if glucose levels get too low, the hormone glucagon is secreted by the pancreas to correct the problem. It is this constant balance between glucagon and insulin that is primarily responsible for the maintenance of blood glucose levels even in the face of very little or no carbohydrate intake.

Insulin

Insulin is an anabolic hormone released into the bloodstream by the beta cells of the pancreas. It has important effects on carbohydrate, protein, and fat metabolism. Like many hormones, it is a polypeptide (a series of amino acids put together in a precise arrangement). The primary factor regulating insulin secretion is blood glucose. The primary function of insulin is to help maintain normal blood glucose levels. Insulin performs this task by suppressing the production of glucose in the liver but also by increasing the uptake of glucose into muscle, fat, brain, and other tissues. Insulin exerts a number of other important effects beyond glucose disposal, however. Insulin is highly anabolic, meaning that it promotes the growth and buildup of bodily tissues. In terms of preventing protein breakdown and promoting the uptake of amino acids and subsequent synthesis of new proteins in muscle tissue, it is arguably the body's most anabolic hormone. Insulin's ability to inhibit the breakdown of muscle tissue is well known in medicine. Severely burned patients experience rapid and profound catabolic states and can lose a tremendous amount of lean mass after their injury. The term "catabolic" refers to the breakdown of bodily tissues into various smaller subunits. Intravenous insulin infusions are commonly used in these patients, not only to control high blood sugar levels, but also to promote protein synthesis and retention of lean mass. In some cases, insulin infusions have resulted in a doubling of protein synthesis in burn patients and halted the expected increase in protein breakdown.[32] Insulin exerts its anabolic properties on protein synthesis through a variety of mechanisms including increased transcription of messenger RNA (mRNA) and increased activity of cellular ribosomes (cellular protein factories) as well as through the stimulation of new ribosome formation to further increase cellular protein output.

Insulin secretion by the pancreas occurs twenty-four hours a day and not just in response to changes in blood glucose. Insulin secretion occurs at a "basal" rate, meaning at a low, constant level in between meals and even at night or during fasting conditions. It is estimated that about 50 percent of the total insulin secreted in a twenty-four-hour period is secreted in this manner.[33] Insulin levels rise quickly after a carbohydrate meal and peak within about sixty minutes. This peak can vary depending on the glycemic index of the foods consumed, as can the total amount of insulin secreted. Insulin, however, is not just secreted as a large bolus after each meal. Rather, it is released in pulses. There are short, rapid pulses occurring every eight to fifteen minutes as well as slower pulses every eighty to one hundred and fifty minutes.[34] After a meal, there may be between two and three pulses of insulin rather than one large pulse released at the beginning of the meal. Insulin pulses also occur at night when food is not being consumed. Normal nocturnal insulin pulsations (an average of almost four) occur between 11:00 p.m. and 6:00 a.m. as well as in the three hours before breakfast. These pulses are likely related to increased secretion of growth hormone and cortisol during nighttime hours. Both these hormones lead to increases in blood glucose levels.

The early morning insulin pulse after breakfast appears to be the largest of the day. It is during this time that pancreatic beta cells seem to be the most sensitive to blood glucose levels. Identical lunch or dinner meals result in less insulin secretion than one eaten at breakfast time. The practical implication for the Endomorphic dieter is that the breakfast meal should be the lowest carbohydrate meal of the day. Other low-carbohydrate diets have often recommended that the morning meal contain the bulk of the day's carbohydrates. With what we know about morning insulin secretion, this doesn't make much sense. If the goal is to keep insulin levels low and thereby promote fat loss, it would make sense to eat your higher-carbohydrate meals later in the day (like just before your workout) to limit the amount of post-meal insulin secretion. On the other hand, on the Ectomorphic Diet, consuming a generous amount of carbohydrate in the morning can let you take advantage of this phenomenon; you can boost insulin levels and thereby increase protein synthesis and muscle glycogen storage.

The overall pattern of insulin secretion is unaltered in obese subjects compared with normal subjects with two important exceptions. Firstly, the amplitude of these pulses after meals is much higher. Obese

---

32 Ferrando AA, Chinkes DL, Wolf SE, et al: A submaximal dose of insulin promotes net skeletal muscle protein synthesis in patients with severe burns. Ann Surg 229. 11–18. 1999.

33 Kruszynska Y, Home PD, Hanning I, Alberti KG: Basal and 24-h C-peptide and insulin secretion rate in normal man. *Diabetologia* 1987;30:16–21.

34 Polonsky KS: Lilly Lecture 1994. The beta-cell in diabetes: from molecular genetics to clinical research. *Diabetes* 1995; 44:705–717.

individuals tend to secrete more insulin for a given amount of carbohydrate than non-obese individuals. This occurs as a mechanism to overcome obesity-related insulin resistance. For a given amount of carbohydrate ingested, more insulin is required in the obese individual to drive blood glucose levels back to normal when compared to non-obese individuals. Obese individuals also tend to have an oversensitivity of their pancreatic beta cells to blood glucose. This means that independent of the degree of insulin resistance, obesity leads to internal changes within the beta cells of the pancreas that cause them to release more insulin than normal. Essentially, the internal cellular machinery in the beta cells is ramped up and adapted to maximize insulin production. Basal rates of insulin secretion are also higher in non-diabetic, obese individuals. In fact, there is a strong correlation between rising body mass index and level of basal insulin secretion, with obese individuals secreting three to four times the amount of insulin as the non-obese.[35]

A few other factors also influence insulin secretion. Certain amino acids are known to stimulate insulin secretion even in the absence of glucose. The primary insulin stimulating amino acids are the essential amino acids leucine, arginine, and lysine, with leucine being the least potent.[36] In practical terms, the amount of insulin secreted by ingesting these amino acids is not important in your overall fat loss or muscle-gaining program. Do not limit your intake of these important nutrients over fear of excess insulin secretion. You will need a healthy intake of essential amino acids to build and maintain your muscle mass on all three Program diets.

The brain also appears to influence insulin secretion. Merely tasting something sweet, even if it is a zero-calorie sweetener like saccharine, can trigger a small release of insulin. This process is called cephalic phase insulin release (CPIR). This burst of insulin secretion occurs very quickly, before blood glucose levels even have a chance to raise and acts to prepare the system for an impending meal. Simply put, the brain has a sweet recognition based trigger affecting insulin levels before blood sugar spikes. So, CPIR is a preparation for an increase in blood sugar.

Fats have a much less pronounced effect on insulin secretion. Studies looking specifically at ketone bodies have shown conflicting results but most seem to indicate that they can stimulate small amounts of insulin secretion from the pancreas. Long-term ketosis can actually suppress insulin secretion triggered by spikes in blood glucose, at least in animal models. The bottom line is that both fats and ketones play a minimal role in stimulating insulin secretion and your main focus should be on your carbohydrate intake in this regard.

To review, insulin is one of the key hormones responsible for metabolizing and maintaining normal blood sugar levels and is absolutely necessary for life. Type 1 diabetes is a condition in which the body's own immune system attacks and destroys the beta cells in the pancreas. These beta cells are responsible for creating and releasing insulin. Without multiple doses of synthetic insulin daily, patients with type 1 diabetes would quickly enter a state of severe metabolic derangement known as diabetic ketoacidosis and eventually die.

35　Byrne MM, Sturis J, Sobel RJ, Polonsky KS. Elevated plasma glucose 2 h post-challenge predicts defects in beta-cell function. Am J Physiol 1996;270:E572–E579.

36　Fajans S, Floyd J: *Stimulation of islet cell secretion by nutrients and by gastrointestinal hormones released during digestion.* In: Steiner D, Freinkel N, ed. *Handbook of Physiology. Section 7. Endocrinology*, Washington, DC: American Physiological Society; 1972:473–493.

> # insulin
>
> Insulin is the body's primary "storage hormone." It is essential for life and is secreted by the pancreas in response to rising blood glucose levels. Important metabolic functions of insulin include:
>
> 1. Stimulates the production of glycogen from blood sugar in the liver and muscles.
>
> 2. Stimulates cholesterol-producing enzymes.
>
> 3. Slows the breakdown of fat and promotes the storage of fat.
>
> 4. Increases the uptake of proteins into the muscles and encourages muscle growth while preventing muscle breakdown.
>
> 5. Allows glucose to enter body cells

For those of you trying to lose body fat, however, insulin has a darker side. Insulin's primary action as a "storage hormone" can work against you in your quest to lose body fat. That is, it promotes the storage of calories from all sources as fat. It blocks the burning of fat for energy and increases the body's production of cholesterol. As you may have guessed, high insulin levels make losing body fat much more difficult. Obese individuals consuming a "normal" diet, even those who do not clinically have diabetes, have chronically elevated insulin levels. In response to the rise in blood sugar after eating, they secrete larger than normal amounts of insulin with every carbohydrate-containing meal. The higher and faster the rise in blood sugar, the higher the rise in insulin. This insulin spike drives blood sugar into the cells of the body. In fat cells, it triggers a series of enzymes that put those cells into "storage mode," meaning they take in blood glucose, amino acids, and fats and turn them into fatty acids for long-term storage. For the obese individual who is consuming large amounts of carbohydrate with every meal, insulin levels remain chronically elevated. They maintain a level of insulin so high that their fat cells are in permanent fat storage mode. Their insulin levels never drop low enough to trigger those fat cells to release their fat stores for use as energy, even when they are exercising regularly.

Underlying insulin resistance not only makes weight loss more difficult but also can predispose one to a number of serious health problems including cardiovascular disease. Elevated insulin levels have been strongly associated with elevated levels of LDL (bad cholesterol), which contributes to cholesterol plaque buildup in the arteries of the heart. Elevated insulin levels also appear to affect the "fight or flight" (sympathetic) nervous system, resulting in increased secretion of adrenaline from the adrenal glands. As a result, elevated insulin levels can result in an exaggerated blood pressure response to stress. Adrenaline causes intense constriction of blood vessels and may limit blood flow to various parts of the body. This phenomenon partially explains why so many obese individuals develop high blood pressure.[37]

After a carbohydrate meal is consumed, the sugars it contains are broken down in the gut and enter the bloodstream as glucose. The rate at which blood glucose levels rise depends on several factors, the primary one being the carbohydrate's glycemic index (more on that later). This rise in blood sugar is detected by the beta cells in the pancreas. Insulin is secreted in order to allow the body's cells to take in that glucose thereby lowering blood glucose levels back down to normal. In an insulin-resistant state, a variety of factors make the body's tissues less responsive to insulin. As a result, blood glucose levels remain elevated for longer periods of time and greater amounts of insulin are required to eventually bring glucose levels back down to normal. Over the years, chronically elevated insulin levels contribute to excess body fat production, which in turn worsens insulin resistance. This downward spiral eventually reaches a point where the pancreas can no longer keep up with the persistently elevated blood glucose levels and even fasting glucose levels remain elevated. This leads directly to type-II diabetes. Without dramatic lifestyle changes, most people who reach this point will eventually burn out most of their beta cells from years of overuse. They will require insulin injections to control their blood sugar. As you may have guessed, the time to correct this problem is not after you have reached frank diabetes, but years before, when those first few excess pounds start showing up.

The goals of the Endomorphic and Mesomorphic Diets are to control insulin levels and ultimately keep them relatively low most of the time. This will create a favorable environment for fat loss. The Ectomorphic Diet, however, is designed to take advantage of some of insulin's beneficial effects, namely its ability to greatly increase protein synthesis and thereby increase muscle mass. Within minutes of its secretion, insulin accelerates the transport of amino acids into muscle cells and activates various preexisting enzymes that are necessary for the synthesis of new protein. It also stimulates the transcription of messenger RNA, which directly accelerates protein synthesis. Ideally, one would want to take advantage of insulin's anabolic effects in regards to stimulation of muscle protein synthesis and minimize its effects on accelerating fat storage. With a little clever manipulation of your diet and the timing of your meals, you can use your body's own insulin to maximize gains in lean muscle mass while minimizing its fat-storing properties.

The body's sensitivity to insulin is not constant throughout the day. It varies based not only on time of day but also on your activity. The body's sensitivity to insulin is greatest in the early morning. During this time, the liver, which has been maintaining your blood glucose in a stable range while you slept, is relatively depleted of its stored glycogen. Insulin receptors in the muscle cells are up-regulated and ready to bind any available insulin and speed the transport of amino acids and glucose into waiting muscle cells. As mentioned above, the beta cells of the pancreas are also more sensitive to changes in blood glucose levels during this time. For a given amount of carbohydrate ingested, they will secrete more insulin than at any other time of the day. Therefore, a morning meal rich in high-quality protein *and* carbohydrate will maximize insulin secretion and amino acid transport while one is on the Ectomorphic Diet.

---

37   Sung, BH; Moderately Obese, Insulin-Resistant Women Exhibit Abnormal Vascular Reactivity to Stress. *Hypertension.* 1997;30:848–853.

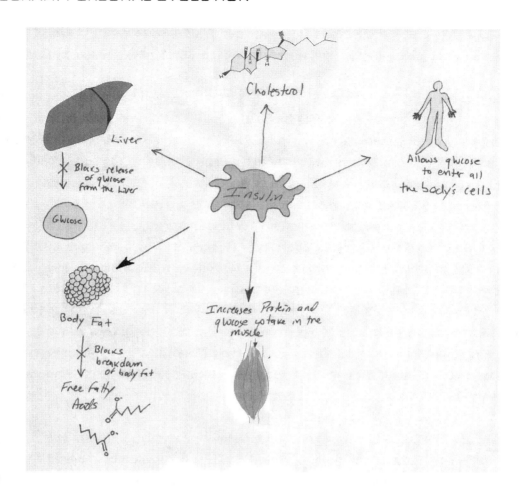

A brief word of caution about a disturbing trend I have seen in some aspiring bodybuilders: in an attempt to speed gains in muscle mass, some athletes have resorted to using injectable insulin as part of their training and diet regimen. With the ever-growing number of diabetics in this country, insulin in both short- and long-acting versions is readily available. This practice is incredibly dangerous. With all the hype surrounding the dangers of anabolic steroids and other performance-enhancing drugs, illicit insulin use hasn't received much exposure. This is unfortunate, because its misuse can kill. As any diabetic can tell you, sudden drops in blood sugar wreak havoc on the body and brain. Every now and then, you will hear stories on the news of a bodybuilder who passed out in a restaurant, had a seizure, or ended up in a coma as a result of a sudden drop in blood sugar linked to insulin use. This is no joke. Sudden hypoglycemia can literally destroy brain cells. As I learned in medical school, "hypoglycemia doesn't just stop the machine; it wrecks it." Most bodybuilders using insulin have no idea what they are doing. They have little understanding of the differences between Lantus, Novolog, Lispro, Regular, NPH, or 70/30 insulin, let alone how much additional carbohydrate they must ingest to avoid becoming hypoglycemic. Insulin is a potent anabolic hormone, but your body makes all you will ever need. Injecting additional insulin is like playing Russian roulette. Eventually, you are going to lose.

Improving Insulin Sensitivity

There are a few simple things you can do to maximize your muscles' sensitivity to insulin using diet and exercise. It is important on The Program's three diets to keep muscle sensitivity to insulin high. This will shunt any ingested carbohydrate and protein preferentially into muscle cells and minimize the amount converted to fatty acids and stored in fat cells.

Exercise is one of the most potent ways of increasing muscle sensitivity to insulin. Even a single exercise session can acutely increase the transport of glucose and amino acids into muscle cells.[38] This effect occurs through both insulin-dependent and insulin-independent mechanisms. Up to two hours after a single bout of exercise, glucose transporters (known as GLUT4 transporters) move to the surface and provide channels for glucose to enter.[39] This process is stimulated both by repeated muscle contraction and low muscle oxygen levels that occur during exercise. This means that relatively high repetition sets taken to full muscular failure are perfect for enhancing glucose transport into muscle cells after exercise. The Program's workout is designed precisely to take advantage of this effect.

Improved insulin sensitivity actually lasts for up to sixteen hours after exercise in both healthy individuals and those with insulin resistance. In addition to the translocation of GLUT4 channels during and immediately after exercise that occurs whether insulin is present or not, the depletion of muscle glycogen levels as a result of exercise and low carbohydrate intake triggers muscle cells to create additional GLUT4 channels, thereby further improving insulin sensitivity. Over time, repeated bouts of intense exercise will stimulate the growth of additional capillaries, improving blood flow to working muscles, and increase the density of muscle mitochondria. These changes all serve to improve energy efficiency and the uptake of both glucose and amino acids.

The Right Carbs at the Right Time

The building of new muscle tissue is complex and requires the complex interaction of multiple hormones, external stimuli, and availability of the appropriate raw materials. Some of these factors are genetic in nature, meaning you have little control over them. For example, for all practical purposes, you can't change the overall number of muscle fibers you were born with, nor can you change the relative proportion of muscle fiber types. No matter how hard he or she tries, someone with 80 percent slow-twitch muscle fibers will not be able to change those fibers to fast-twitch fibers. The good news is that there are a number of factors that *can* be changed to tip the scales in your favor in terms of building muscle mass. As discussed in the training chapter, you can increase your testosterone and growth-hormone levels by following a high-intensity weight-training regimen like the one in The Program. You can also influence the amount of another very potent anabolic hormone that often gets overlooked. Testosterone and, to a slightly lesser extent, growth hormone (GH) get most of the press when it comes to anabolic hormones, but insulin is actually just as potent, if not more so, when it comes to its ability to build new muscle tissue.

To review, insulin is the primary hormone responsible for the driving of blood sugar, in the form of glucose, into the body's tissues. It stimulates the formation of glycogen in muscle tissue and the liver while simultaneously inhibiting its breakdown as well. Of equal importance, however, are the effects it

---

38   Holloszy JO, Schultz J, Kusnierkiewicz J, Hagberg JM, Ehsani AA. Effects of exercise on glucose tolerance and insulin resistance. Brief review and some preliminary results. Acta Med Scand Suppl 1986; 711:55–65.

39   Goodyear LJ, Hirshman MF, King PA, et al: Skeletal muscle plasma membrane glucose transport and glucose transporters after exercise. *J Appl Physiol* 1990; 68:193–198.

has on muscle tissue. Elevated insulin levels drive amino acids into muscle cells and significantly elevate protein synthesis while simultaneously inhibiting the breakdown of muscle tissue.[40] This dual function as an anabolic and anti-catabolic hormone can be taken advantage of at certain times of the day to help increase overall protein synthesis and the building of new muscle tissue. As discussed previously, there is a continuous basal level of insulin that is secreted from the pancreas twenty-four hours a day, which fluctuates in a predictable manner.

Independent of diet, the pancreas in healthy individuals typically releases a larger than normal pulse of insulin after 11:00 p.m. as well as approximately three hours before the morning meal. This is a natural response to naturally rising early morning cortisol levels. Insulin secretion in response to a given amount of carbohydrate is also highest in the early morning. This means that a slice of bread, for example, eaten in the morning, will cause a larger amount of insulin to be secreted than the same slice of bread in the late afternoon. Similarly, insulin sensitivity, the ability for peripheral tissues like muscle and liver to take up blood sugar and amino acids in response to insulin, is higher in the early morning as well. This presents us with two windows of opportunity (there are others too) to spike insulin levels with a high-glycemic carbohydrate and quality protein and thereby significantly raise levels of protein synthesis.

> ## Manipulating Insulin
>
> 1. Your body releases more insulin in the morning for a given amount of carbohydrate than it does in the afternoon. Keep those morning carbs low on the Endomorphic Diet and high on the Ectomorphic Diet!
>
> 2. Insulin also spikes about three hours before you wake up in the morning.
>
> 3. Spiking insulin levels with a simple carbohydrate and a quality protein immediately after a workout will boost your muscles' protein synthesis by 400%!

---

40   Biolo G, Declan Fleming RY, Wolfe RR. Physiologic hyperinsulinemia stimulates protein synthesis and enhances transport of selected amino acids in human skeletal muscle. J. Clin Invest. 1995 Feb; 95(2):811–9.

The third time when you can manipulate insulin levels to accelerate your muscle growth is in the immediate post-workout period. Consuming a quality protein with all the essential amino acids immediately after an intense workout can boost protein synthesis by up to 200 percent. Consuming that same protein with as little as thirty-six grams of simple sugars can boost protein synthesis by up to 400 percent. [41] Interestingly enough, consuming carbohydrate alone after intense exercise does little to boost protein synthesis, so a good supply of essential amino acids is crucial.[42] The Ectomorphic Diet is built around taking advantage of insulin's potent anabolic and anti-catabolic properties through consumption of specific types of carbohydrates at key times as well as providing an ample and steady supply of essential amino acids for maximum protein synthesis around the clock.

Glucagon

The effects of glucagon are opposite to those of insulin in nearly every instance. While insulin lowers blood sugar, glucagon's primary role is to trigger the elevation of blood glucose levels through a variety of mechanisms. It is glucagon that is responsible primarily for the prevention of low blood sugar during fasting or other carbohydrate-deprived states. Glucagon stimulates the breakdown of glycogen stored in the liver. When blood glucose levels are high, the liver takes up large amounts of glucose. Under the influence of insulin, much of this glucose is stored in the form of glycogen. Later, when blood glucose levels begin to fall, glucagon is secreted and acts on hepatocytes to activate the enzymes that break down glycogen and release glucose.

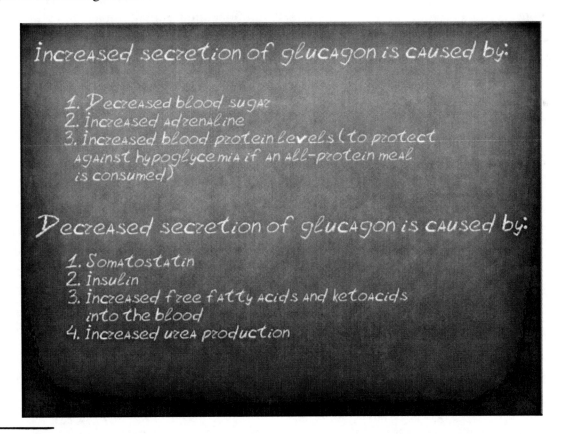

Increased secretion of glucagon is caused by:

1. Decreased blood sugar
2. Increased Adrenaline
3. Increased blood protein levels (to protect against hypoglycemia if an all-protein meal is consumed)

Decreased secretion of glucagon is caused by:

1. Somatostatin
2. Insulin
3. Increased free fatty acids and ketoacids into the blood
4. Increased urea production

41   Rasmussen B, Tipton K, et al. An oral essential amino acid-carbohydrate supplement enhances muscle protein anabolism after resistance exercise. J. Appl. Physiol. 88:386–392, 2000.

42   Roy, B.D., Tarnopolsky, J.D., et al. The effect of glucose supplement timing on protein metabolism following resistance training. J. Appl. Physiol. 82:1882–1888, 1997.

Glucagon activates the liver production of glucose (gluconeogenesis). Gluconeogenesis is the pathway by which non-sugars such as amino acids, are converted to glucose. As such, it provides another source of glucose for blood. This is especially important in animals like cats and sheep that don't absorb much if any glucose from the intestine—in these species, activation of gluconeogenic enzymes is the chief mechanism by which glucagon does its job.

Knowing that glucagon's major effect is to increase blood glucose levels, it makes sense that glucagon is secreted in response to hypoglycemia or low blood concentrations of glucose.

Two other conditions are known to trigger glucagon secretion:

1. Elevated blood levels of amino acids, as would be seen after consumption of a protein-rich meal: In this situation, glucagon would foster conversion of excess amino acids to glucose by enhancing gluconeogenesis. Since high blood levels of amino acids also stimulate insulin release, this would be a situation in which both insulin and glucagon are active.
2. Exercise: In this case, it is not clear whether the actual stimulus is exercise per se or the accompanying exercise-induced depletion of glucose.

In terms of negative control, high levels of blood glucose inhibit glucagon secretion. It is not clear whether this reflects a direct effect of glucose on the alpha cell or perhaps an effect of insulin, which is known to dampen glucagon release. Another hormone well known to inhibit glucagon secretion, amongst other functions, is somatostatin. Also known as growth hormone inhibiting hormone, this primarily functions to balance the secretion of pancreatic and pituitary hormones, and gastric enzymes. Unless, there are very specific diseases or disorders such as acromalegy to address, there isn't any need for intentional attempts to manipulate levels of somatostatin.

The Glycemic Index and Glycemic Load

The Glycemic Index (GI) is a research tool invented by Dr. David Jenkins in 1981. Its purpose is to provide a standardized tool with which to measure and predict the effects of certain foods on blood sugar. In particular, the GI assigns a numerical value that shows how rapidly fifty grams of a particular food item are converted to blood sugar as compared to an established standard. The established standard is typically glucose or white bread and is assigned a value of 1.0 (or sometimes 100). The GI is written as a percentage of that value. The more rapidly a food is broken down and enters the bloodstream as glucose, the higher its' GI. Conversely, the longer it takes to break down a given food and the slower blood glucose rises, the lower its' glycemic index. This is important because insulin is the body's primary fat-storage hormone. By controlling not only the number of carbohydrates you consume but their quality based on glycemic index/glycemic load, you will be able to influence your body's insulin levels and use that to help reach your goals. Foods with a high glycemic index/glycemic load tend to cause large and rapid spikes in insulin levels, while those with lower values tend to cause smaller and more gradual rises in insulin levels.

Multiple factors influence the GI. The manner in which foods are processed and the amount of fat and fiber all have significant effects on a food's GI. In general, foods with a high GI should be ingested in limited quantities. Having said that, choosing foods based solely on GI is not the wisest way to construct your diet. There are certain foods that despite being high on the GI can easily be included in all three diets outlined in The Program. One of the primary flaws in the GI is that it fails to take into account the amount of carbohydrate in a standard serving size of a given food. For example, carrots have a glycemic index of approximately 0.9 to 1.30 (90 to 130) depending on the reference source. Based on this value, carrots are almost as bad as white bread, or pure glucose, when it comes to rapidly elevating blood sugar. Remember though that that GI value is based on consuming fifty grams of carbohydrate from carrots—which translates into almost a pound of carrots! Nobody eats that many carrots in a sitting. Therefore, not only the GI but also the amount of carbohydrate in a given serving of food must be examined. Fortunately, the concept of glycemic load (GL) takes into account both these factors and gives a more accurate measurement of a given food's impact on blood sugar. The GL can help you make better decisions about whether to include that food in your diet. While on the Mesomorphic Diet, the bulk of your carbohydrate intake will come from foods with a relatively low glycemic load.

The GL is the product of the amount of total available carbohydrate in a given food (minus fiber, of course) multiplied by its glycemic index. Therefore, the higher the GL a food possesses, the higher the expected elevation in blood sugar and greater the degree of insulin secretion it would cause. When using the GL to take another look at carrots, we find that the GL of carrots is actually quite low. A given serving of a half cup of cooked carrots has approximately eight grams of carbohydrate. When this is multiplied by its GI of up to 1.3, the product is the GL of 10, which is actually quite low. To compare, a half cup of white rice has a GI of 0.81 (or 81) but a GL of 28! When glycemic index is expressed based on the glucose standard of 100, instead of 1.0, the result is the same when the glycemic index is divided by 100 and then multiplied by its available carbohydrate content. You will see glycemic index values listed in both these ways. They are really the same thing, so don't let that confuse you.

GL = (grams of carbohydrate per serving x glycemic index)

Food	Glycemic Index	Glycemic Load
Glucose	100	50
Watermelon	72	8
Oranges	48	6
Instant white rice	46	19
Bean sprouts	25	1
Peanuts	14	2

Note how some common foods can vary in their respective glycemic index and glycemic load. Watermelon, for example, has a high glycemic index but low glycemic load, whereas instant white rice has a lower glycemic index but very high glycemic load.

I encourage you to purchase or download a book of glycemic values and look up the foods you plan to include in your diet. In practical terms, the GL is of primary significance only while on the Mesomorphic Diet. Though carbohydrate intake is strictly limited on the Endomorphic Diet, its total intake is so low that its source is not quite as important. When consuming thirty grams or less per day of carbohydrate, don't fret too much if some of your carbohydrate intake comes from high GI or GL sources. Ideally, you should be consuming most of your carbohydrate from low-glycemic vegetables, but if you consume the occasional hard candy or other sweet item, it won't be the end of the world. Just keep your total carbohydrate intake under thirty grams for the day. The only caveat to that would be if you are going to consume high GI/GL carbohydrates on the Endomorphic plan, try to consume them later in the day, preferably before your workout, rather than in the morning. This will help minimize the amount of insulin secreted resulting from these carbohydrates.

The Mesomorphic Diet allows more carbohydrate, but it is critical that insulin levels remain controlled. Therefore, it's worth your while to investigate your carbohydrate sources with a standardized reference and make sure that you choose low GL items.

On the Ectomorphic Diet the GI/GL is not of primary importance. You will be allowed to consume approximately 25 percent of your carbohydrates from high GI/GL sources. You should still examine your food items with a standard reference, however, to ensure you do not exceed this amount.

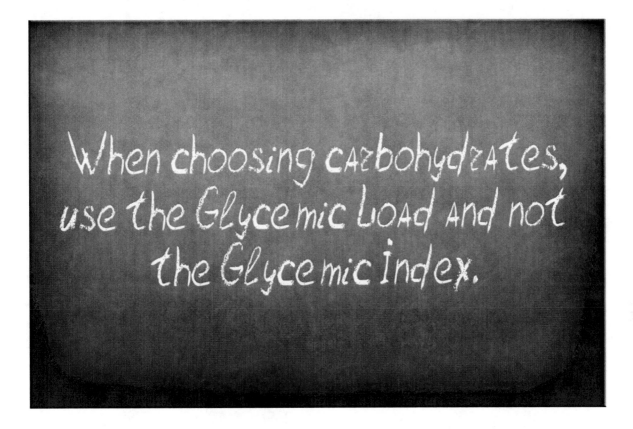

PROTEIN METABOLISM

Proteins are long strands of individual amino acids that form the basic structural units within the body. They are found in every tissue and perform a myriad of different functions. Some proteins provide tensile strength to tissues while others form enzymes that carry out complex chemical reactions. Altogether, protein constitutes about 17 to 20 percent of your total body weight.

Proteins are manufactured throughout the cells of your body on little factories known as ribosomes. These ribosomes assemble proteins by sequencing individual amino acids in precise order as dictated by the instructions they receive from your DNA. Amino acids, therefore, are the fundamental building blocks of all proteins. The human body uses twenty different amino acids to build proteins. Of these twenty, ten are considered essential amino acids, meaning that your body cannot synthesize them on its own and they must be obtained through dietary sources. The consumption of protein has been given paramount importance in bodybuilding circles for many years. Indeed, most of the major supplement companies continue to generate the bulk of their revenue from the sale of protein supplements. Despite the popularity of these supplements, or perhaps because of it, there continues to be a considerable amount of confusion regarding which type of protein is best for those wanting to build as much lean muscle mass as possible. There is debate about which type of protein is best absorbed in the gut, which is more readily incorporated into muscle tissue, which tastes better, which type of whey protein is best, and so on. Fortunately, there are answers to these questions. In this chapter, I discuss the details of protein metabolism with the goal of enlightening you on how to proceed when making choices for your diet.

> Your body needs all the amino acids to build muscle mass but the essential amino acids can only be obtained from your diet.

Digestion of Protein

Protein digestion begins in the stomach. The acidic environment of the stomach begins to break apart the peptide bonds that hold individual amino acids together. The enzyme pepsinogen begins the process of breaking down proteins into two and three amino acid chains called dipeptides and tripeptides as well as individual amino acids. Once they are in the small intestine, the pancreas secretes other proteolytic enzymes to continue this process. Enzymes on the surface of the epithelial cells lining the intestine also contribute to this process. These cells absorb both free amino acids and di- and tripeptides. Inside the cell, these peptides are broken down into individual amino acids and then diffuse out of the cell and into the bloodstream. From the bloodstream, individual amino acids travel to the body's tissues where they are either used to synthesize new protein (like muscle tissue) or are further metabolized into glucose or ketones to be used as energy. Unlike fats and carbohydrates, the body cannot store amino acids. They must either be used to synthesize new proteins or converted into a usable fuel source like glucose or ketones. Most amino acids are considered glucogenic, meaning that they are preferentially converted to glucose when present in excess of the body's requirements. In fact, it is estimated that up to 60 percent of the body's endogenous glucose production comes directly from amino acids. The exceptions to this rule are leucine and lysine. These amino acids are more suited to conversion to ketone bodies rather than glucose. Once converted into ketones, they are then utilized for energy. There are some amino acids that can be converted to either glucose or ketone bodies depending on the body's needs.

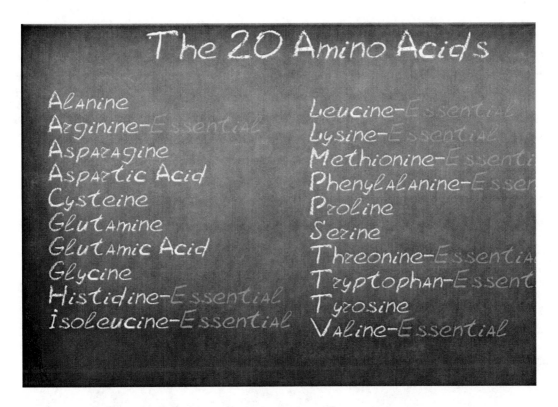

This fact has particular relevance for those on the Endomorphic Diet. During periods of carbohydrate restriction, amino acids from dietary protein will help maintain a normal blood glucose level. One pitfall that is occasionally encountered on the Endomorphic Diet is consumption of excessive amounts of protein, particularly from sources rich in glucogenic amino acids. This tends to promote the production of excess glucose. When glucose remains plentiful, the body is less willing to resort to ketones for fuel and fat loss will decrease. Some individuals, despite greatly restricting their carbohydrate intake, still have difficulty maintaining ketosis.

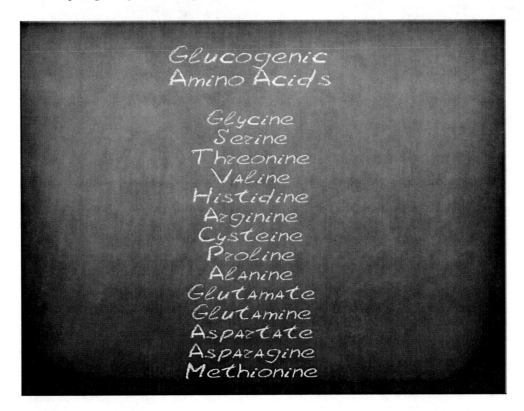

A closer look at their diets reveals, in many cases, that they were consuming too much protein, particularly from sources high in the glucogenic amino acids, in relation to their fat intake. With some minor modifications, their protein intake can be decreased and those calories replaced with healthy fats and protein sources higher in the ketogenic amino acids leucine and lysine. This quickly restores ketosis and promotes further fat loss. The following is a by no means inclusive list of some common foods that are high in lysine and leucine. If you are having difficulty maintaining ketosis despite adequate carbohydrate restriction, consider replacing some of your protein sources with some of the following food items.

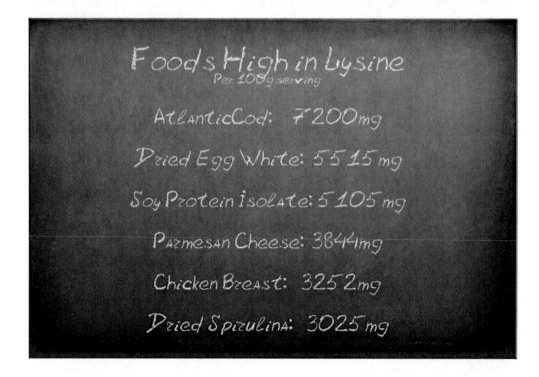

Foods High in Leucine
Per 100g serving

Soy Protein Isolate:	7200mg
Dried Egg White:	7172mg
Atlantic Cod:	5105mg
Whitefish:	4110mg
Dried Spirulina:	4947mg
Beef:	1760mg

Foods High in Lysine
Per 100g serving

Atlantic Cod:	7200mg
Dried Egg White:	5515mg
Soy Protein Isolate:	5105mg
Parmesan Cheese:	3844mg
Chicken Breast:	3252mg
Dried Spirulina:	3025mg

Fast and Slow Proteins

One would think that given their small size, free amino acids that are not linked to other amino acids by peptide bonds would be the most rapidly absorbed form of protein. It turns out that short amino acid chains, such as dipeptides and tripeptides, are absorbed much more quickly into gut epithelial cells than free amino acids. Once inside, they are then broken down into their individual amino acids and enter the bloodstream, which takes them to the liver and out into the peripheral tissues. This difference in absorption rates between free amino acids and amino acids linked in short peptide chains allows us to classify protein sources as either "fast" or "slow" proteins. Fast proteins are those that are rapidly absorbed from the gut and enter the bloodstream very quickly leading to a spike in blood amino acid concentration within three to four hours after consumption. Slow proteins lead to a more gradual rise in serum amino acid levels over many hours. Slow proteins tend to clump or congeal in the acidic environment of the stomach, thereby slowing their entry into the small intestine. Their relatively long peptide chains require more time to be broken down by the digestive enzymes released from the pancreas, further slowing down the absorption process. Fast proteins tend to be already made up of solitary amino acids and rapidly absorbable di- and tripeptides that require very little additional breakdown in the stomach or intestine.

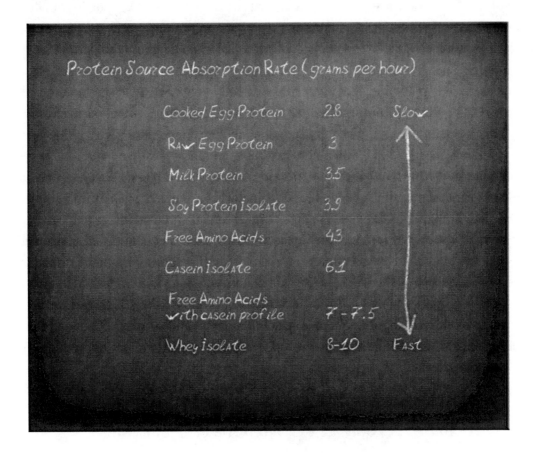

Metabolic Effects of Fast and Slow Proteins

The effects of fast and slow proteins go beyond simply their relative rates of absorption. The rate of absorption also strongly influences overall body protein synthesis and breakdown. Muscle cells are in a perpetual cycle of breaking down and building up their intrinsic proteins. Depending on the needs of the body, the relative balance between anabolism and catabolism can shift to favor one or the other. It may also remain neutral, where the rate of protein breakdown equals the rate of new protein synthesis and there is no net gain in muscle mass. During periods of heavy exercise and/or protein deficiency, muscle proteins are broken down and used as fuel. During recovery from intense exercise, muscle protein synthesis increases in the presence of an adequate supply of dietary amino acids. In an ideal situation, there would be a net increase in protein synthesis over protein breakdown leading to the growth of new muscle tissue.

Protein synthesis refers to the process of constructing new proteins. The first step in protein synthesis is the copying of instructions from DNA onto an mRNA molecule in a process known as transcription. The mRNA then attaches to tiny protein factories known as ribosomes, which link amino acids in the precise order encoded by mRNA. The end result is a complex protein that performs a specific function required by the cell. Protein synthesis occurs in all cells and not just in muscle tissue, though for our purposes, this will be the primary area we are concerned with. Fast-absorbing proteins, like whey protein, that lead to a rapid spike in serum amino acid levels actually stimulate protein synthesis by up to 68 percent while having a minimal effect on protein breakdown.[43] Slower proteins like casein, on the other hand, can inhibit protein breakdown by up to 30 percent for up to seven hours after ingestion while having a minimal effect on protein synthesis. On the surface, it would seem that the fast proteins like whey would be far superior to slow proteins like casein in terms of stimulating a net gain in protein synthesis. However, the increase in protein synthesis stimulated by fast proteins is offset to a certain degree by their tendency to accelerate amino acid oxidation. This means that more of the amino acids absorbed from, for example, whey protein are diverted for use as energy by the body rather than directly contributing to the building of new muscle protein. The net result is that fast proteins induce less overall protein gain than slow proteins when consumed alone. This property changes when fast proteins are consumed along with either fats or carbohydrates. In this situation, the spike in blood amino acid concentration is slowed and total protein synthesis appears to be higher over time than when fast proteins are consumed alone. This property has important practical implications. When a rapid spike in blood amino acids is desired, such as immediately before and after a workout, then fast proteins like whey or free-form essential amino acids should be consumed alone. During other parts of the day, if fast proteins are consumed, then they should be consumed along with carbohydrates and/or fats. Obviously, Endomorphic dieters will be consuming added fats and restricting carbohydrates, while Mesomorphic and Ectomorphic dieters will have more freedom to include additional carbohydrates. During times when you do not want to consume additional calories or carbohydrates, a slow-acting protein like casein or egg protein consumed alone would be ideal. Knowing this, you will be able to take advantage of the different properties of each type of protein and apply them for maximum stimulation of muscle growth.

Protein Timing
Taking Advantage of "Windows of Opportunity"

It is often stated that "timing is everything." This couldn't be truer when it comes to optimizing your muscle growth. The human body responds to its environment and the stresses it encounters by adapting

---

43 Boirie, Y., M. Dangin, P. Gachon, M.P. Vasson, J.L. Maubois, and B. Beaufrere. Slow and fast dietary proteins differently modulate postprandial accretion. Proc. Natl. Acad.Sci. 94: 14930–14935, 1997

its physiology to compensate and prepare for further stressors. When exposed to excess sunlight, light-skinned individuals perceive this stressor and trigger a complex cascade of chemical signals that ultimately results in increased melanin production. The end result is a suntan. Similarly, exercise, especially high-intensity weight training, is a severe stressor that triggers a myriad of hormonal and metabolic changes designed to adapt the body to further training episodes. The most important adaptation for our purposes is, of course, the growth of new muscle tissue.

Muscle growth, as well as muscle breakdown, does not occur at a fixed rate twenty-four hours a day. During intense resistance exercise, as well as endurance activities like biking or running, muscle breakdown exceeds synthesis of new muscle tissue for an overall net negative nitrogen balance. Amino acids from muscle are oxidized for use as energy and also used to form glucose via gluconeogenesis. Intense weight training, especially when involving a heavy negative component (lowering of very heavy weights against gravity), causes widespread microtrauma throughout muscle tissue, which leads to further protein catabolism. In this situation, the loss of existing muscle tissue exceeds the creation of new muscle tissue. Immediately after intense resistance exercise, there is a significant increase in protein synthesis. However, in the absence of a ready pool of available amino acids to boost this process, the overall net effect is still negative nitrogen balance and a net loss of muscle tissue. Obviously, your goal should be to maintain a positive nitrogen balance so that net protein synthesis exceeds protein breakdown for as much of the day as possible.

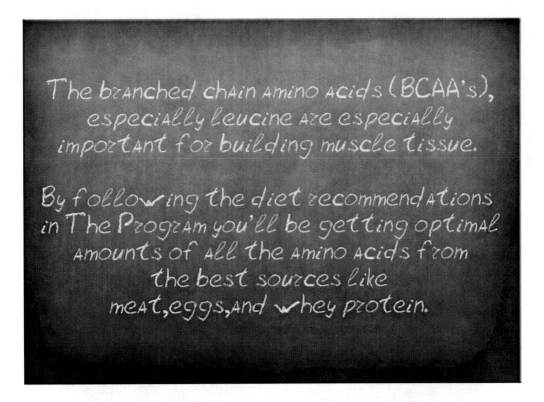

The branched chain amino acids (BCAA's), especially leucine are especially important for building muscle tissue.

By following the diet recommendations in The Program you'll be getting optimal amounts of all the amino acids from the best sources like meat, eggs, and whey protein.

It is the branched chain amino acids (BCAAs) leucine, isoleucine, and valine that appear to play the key role in stimulating protein synthesis. While certainly all the amino acids are important for optimal gains in muscle mass, it is the BCAAs that constitute about one-third of skeletal muscle protein. BCAAs are also unique in that the enzyme required for their degradation is absent in the liver. Most other amino acids are taken up by the liver and broken down into various other substances, but the BCAAs infuse directly into the blood and are absorbed by muscle tissue completely intact. Studies looking at the infusion of BCAAs in humans at rest have shown that they not only stimulate new muscle protein synthesis but also inhibit the breakdown of muscle tissue. These effects are seen not only at rest but also with exercise. Aerobic exercise and high-intensity resistance exercise, as discussed, can produce significant protein catabolism. Consumption of protein rich in BCAAs prior to exercise can significantly attenuate this effect. Of particular importance to those on the Endomorphic Diet, they also appear to delay muscle glycogen depletion during intense exercise. This may allow individuals consuming very little carbohydrate to exercise for longer periods of time and to delay the onset of muscle fatigue.

Of the three BCAAs, it appears that leucine is the most important in terms of triggering muscle protein synthesis. Leucine has the unique ability to activate a complex molecule known as mTOR (mammalian target of rapamycin). mTOR indirectly stimulates protein synthesis by increasing the concentration of various initiation factors that then "turn on" the ribosomal protein factories within your cells. In addition to stimulating muscle protein synthesis, leucine also appears to inhibit protein breakdown though not to the same degree as insulin. The exact mechanism by which this occurs is unknown.

The optimal amount of leucine intake has yet to be determined. The recommended dietary allowance (RDA) is only sixteen milligrams per kilogram per day. For a seventy-kilogram male, it would come out to around 1.1 grams. I don't need to tell you by now that there is a big difference between the RDA for a given nutrient and what is considered optimal intake for those interested in building as much muscle mass as possible. Studies looking at leucine's effects on protein synthesis have found benefits with as little as three grams per meal. Most studies have used upward of sixteen grams and have also shown benefit. Given leucine's many roles in the body and its low toxicity, even at very high doses, a reasonable goal for daily intake would be around twenty grams for athletes training at peak intensity. Divided between five to six meals, this would yield a rough goal of three to four grams per meal. This works out well because leucine's effects on protein synthesis only last about two to three hours, which is about how long you will have between meals anyway.

> Attempt to eat at least 20 grams of leucine per day. Divided over 5-6 meals this will be around 3-4 grams per meal. You can do this easily with a quality whey protein or soy protein supplement. Certain fish like Atlantic cod are also high in leucine.

Leucine, however, is rarely consumed alone. It usually comes with various quantities of the other BCAAs as well as essential and non-essential amino acids. While it has been shown that leucine when take alone can indeed increase protein synthesis, it seems to work a lot better when combined with a mixture of essential amino acids (EAAs). The optimal ratio of leucine to EAAs is around five to one.[44] That is, for every gram of leucine, five grams of a mixture of essential amino acids should also be consumed to maximize protein synthesis. This is a ballpark figure, of course. The precise ratio has yet to be determined, but based on available scientific literature, this appears to be a reasonable estimate for most hard-training athletes. In natural foods, such as meats, the ratio of leucine to the other BCAAs isoleucine and valine is about 2:1:1. That is, of the total amount of BCAAs in, for example, red meat, 50 percent of the total is made up of leucine while equal parts isoleucine and valine make up the remainder.[45] This is the ratio you should aim for if you are using a tablet or powdered BCAA supplement.

LEUCINE AND BCAA CONTENT IN VARIOUS FOODS

	% LEUCINE	% BCAA
WHEY PROTEIN ISOLATE	13	26
MILK PROTEIN	10	21
EGG PROTEIN	8.5	20
MEAT	8	18
SOY PROTEIN ISOLATE	8	18

Protein before Exercise

As we discussed previously, intense resistance exercise leads to a decrease in protein synthesis and increase in protein breakdown in the absence of an adequate pool of essential amino acids. Your goal, therefore, going into each and every workout, is to prime your system to minimize the amount of acute exercise-induced protein breakdown and to have, on demand, a pool of essential amino acids to rapidly take advantage of the increased rates of protein synthesis that will occur immediately after the workout. Most athletes are aware of the fact that the body will absorb greater amounts of protein and carbohydrate

---

44   Layman DK. The Role of Leucine in Weight Loss Diets and Glucose Homeostasis J Nutr. 2003 Jan; 133(1):261S–267S.
45   Garlick, P. J. The Role of Leucine in the Regulation of Protein Metabolism. J. Nutr. 135:1553S–1556S, 2005.

after a workout. What is not well known is that the meal *prior* to your workout is of just as much importance in terms of stimulating muscle protein synthesis. Several studies have shown that ingesting a high-quality whey protein supplement before exercise can markedly improve overall protein synthesis as well as reduce signs of protein breakdown.[46]

While on any of the three diets presented in The Program, you should endeavor to consume a minimum of six grams of BCAAs with each meal, at least three of which should be from leucine. This should occur about thirty to sixty minutes before your workout. When taken in the form of a commercial protein supplement, this will likely give you a total of somewhere between thirty and forty-five grams of protein. This pre-workout meal should consist almost entirely of "fast" proteins like whey. If you are really cutting calories, you could consider taking BCAAs in tablet form. Fortunately, if you are supplementing with a good-quality whey protein isolate powder, you don't have to think too hard about this. A typical serving will get you within this range.

We have not discussed much about carbohydrate intake in relation to protein intake either before or after exercise. Endomorphic dieters will be strictly limited in the amount of carbohydrate they can consume in a given day. For them, the following information does not apply. Just stick to the above recommendations regarding protein intake. Those of you on the Mesomorphic or Ectomorphic Diets, however, should pay attention. Proper timing of carbohydrate intake, especially when combined with high-quality protein as described above can have an additive effect on inhibiting protein breakdown and boosting protein synthesis.[47] Multiple studies have demonstrated that insulin is a potent inhibitor of protein breakdown. If our goal is to shift the balance of protein breakdown to protein synthesis to favor the later as much as possible, then it would make sense to take advantage of this phenomenon. We already know that protein, especially the BCAAs, can significantly increase protein synthesis. Addition of a modest amount of high-glycemic carbohydrate to a pre-workout drink will spike insulin levels during the workout and further shift our ratio toward a net positive gain. The optimal amount of carbohydrate to add to your pre-workout protein supplement is a bit unclear. It is likely dependent on multiple factors including the duration of exercise, body weight, and overall fitness level. Most studies have used between twenty and one hundred grams of a high-glycemic carbohydrate (usually maltodextrin) and have shown positive results with all dosages. As a general recommendation, while on the Mesomorphic Diet, your pre-workout carbohydrate and protein beverage should probably not exceed forty to fifty grams of carbohydrate. The Ectomorphic Diet is less restrictive, and up to one hundred grams may be taken in a pre-workout beverage though lower amounts would be just fine. There are a number of ready-to-drink protein/carbohydrate beverages on the market right now that easily fit within these boundaries. Find one that you like, and use it.

---

46   Willoughby DS, Stout JR, Wilborn CD: Effects of resistance training and protein plus amino acid supplementation on muscle anabolic, mass, and strength. *Amino Acids* 2007, 32:467–477

47   Tipton KD, Rasmussen BB, Miller SL, Wolf SE, Owens-Stovall SK, Petrini BE, Wolfe RR: Timing of amino acid-carbohydrate ingestion alters anabolic response of muscle to resistance exercise. Am J Physiol Endocrinol Metab 2001, 281:E197–E206.

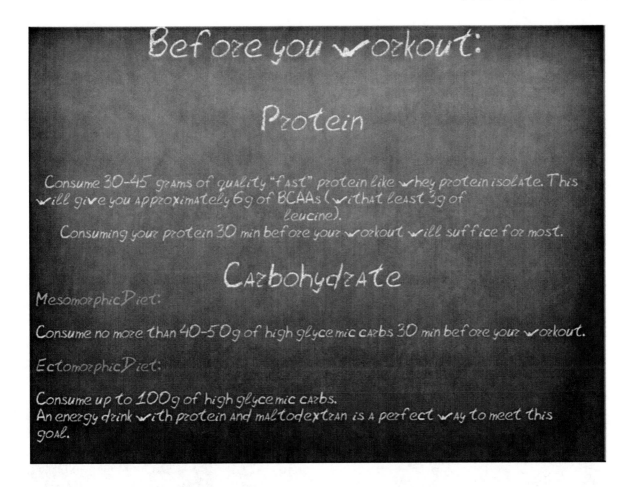

Before you workout:

Protein

Consume 30-45 grams of quality "fast" protein like whey protein isolate. This will give you approximately 6g of BCAAs (with at least 3g of leucine).
Consuming your protein 30 min before your workout will suffice for most.

Carbohydrate

Mesomorphic Diet:

Consume no more than 40-50g of high glycemic carbs 30 min before your workout.

Ectomorphic Diet:

Consume up to 100g of high glycemic carbs.
An energy drink with protein and maltodextran is a perfect way to meet this goal.

Protein during Exercise

For prolonged bouts of exercise, whether it is anaerobic high-intensity weight training or low-intensity aerobic activity like running or biking, there appear to be benefits in terms of improved protein synthesis when athletes supplement with a carbohydrate and protein beverage during exercise. There are also benefits in terms of maintaining muscle glycogen stores. As a result, most experts recommend that you sip one of these beverages during the course of your workout. While of interest to athletes who perform prolonged bouts of exercise, this information does not apply well to those of you performing brief, high-intensity training sessions like those recommended in The Program. Once you become familiar with the exercises, your weight-training workouts will usually last well under thirty minutes. If you have prepared adequately before your workout by following the advice described above, then you will have more than an ample supply of amino acids and glucose to maximally support growth and recovery during your workout. If you are going to perform an aerobic exercise session either after your weight training or on the days between your weight workouts, then I would recommend you consume your post workout meal (see below) at the conclusion of your weight workout before you begin your aerobic training. This will help offset some of the muscle breakdown that will occur with prolonged aerobic exercise while still allowing you to burn body fat.

In conclusion, while weight training, do not worry too much about consuming a protein or carbohydrate supplement. Just make sure you stay properly hydrated between your sets. If you then move on to cardiovascular exercise after your weight workout, give your body a quick boost of high-quality protein with (if you are on the Mesomorphic or Ectomorphic Diets) some simple sugars to maintain a ready pool of amino acids to promote growth and inhibit protein breakdown while you burn fat.

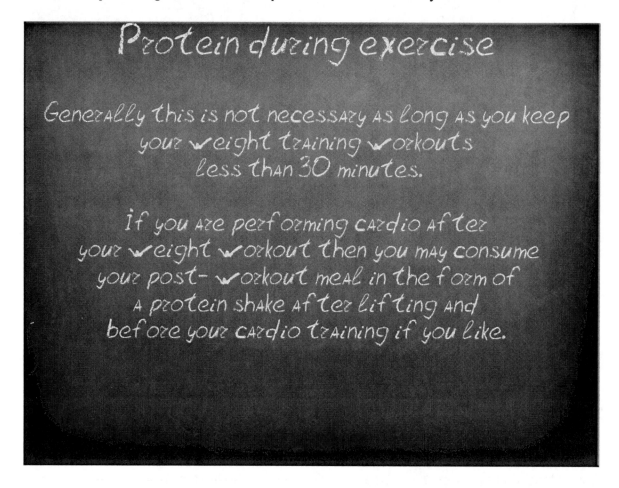

Protein after Exercise

Immediately following exercise, there is an elevation in protein synthesis by up to 100 percent of resting values lasting for about forty-eight hours.[48] There is also an increase in muscle breakdown lasting a similar period that *exceeds* the increase in synthesis. Therefore, in the absence of adequate post-exercise protein, the net result of exercise is a *loss* in lean muscle mass. It, therefore, becomes crucial that a ready pool of necessary amino acids is available to take advantage of this increased protein synthesis in the hours *immediately* following intense exercise. Studies looking at weight-training athletes who consumed a protein supplement either immediately or two to three hours after training have clearly shown the benefit of immediate post-workout protein ingestion. The longer the delay in post-workout protein ingestion, the lower the increased amount of protein synthesis and the lower the increase in added muscle tissue over time. If one provides a pool of high-quality amino acids for use after exercise, the body's net protein synthesis can be increased by up to 250 percent above that experienced with weight-training alone.[49] Most of the studies demonstrating this effect have used relatively small amounts of protein (usually between three and ten grams). Obviously, most athletes consume much greater amounts. The optimal amount of protein

48   MacDougall, J.D. et al. (1995). "The Time Course for Elevated Muscle Protein Synthesis Following Heavy Resistance Exercise."
Canadian Journal of Applied Physiology. 20: 480–486. 269:E309–315.
49   Ivy, John, and Robert Portman (2004). Nutrient Timing: The Future of Sports Nutrition USA: Basic Health Publications.

to ingest post-exercise has not been determined. As a general rule, consume as much protein as you would normally ingest during a typical meal while on one of the three Program diets. For most of you, this will be approximately twenty-five to thirty grams of protein. Both your pre-workout and post-workout meals/supplements should consist primarily of "fast" proteins like whey or essential amino acid tablets. This will allow you to take advantage of the increased blood flow to your muscles both during and immediately after training. Therefore, every effort should be made to consume a high-quality "fast" protein (either whey or EAA tablets) within the first hour after finishing your workout. Ideally, it should happen immediately after you finish training.

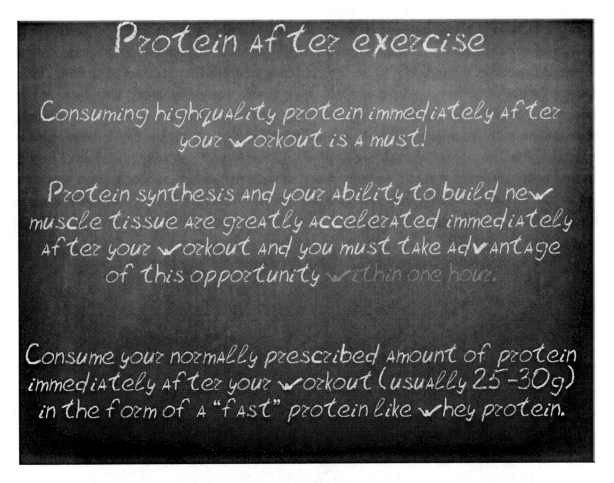

Protein at Bedtime

A myriad of hormonal and metabolic changes occur during sleep. A complete review of this subject is well beyond the scope of this book, but there are some important changes in terms of protein synthesis that are worth reviewing. During the first few hours of sleep, your body is absorbing and processing the nutrients you consumed from your last meal. After that meal has been digested and absorbed, the body enters a period where protein breakdown exceeds protein synthesis, often referred to as *nocturnal post-absorptive catabolism* (NPAC). The time it takes to enter this state varies depending on individual metabolic rate, time since last meal, the speed of digestion, and the type of meal ingested.

If your goal is to build (or keep) as much muscle mass as possible, then shortening your NPAC is clearly advantageous. NPAC can be minimized using two different strategies. The first is to consume a meal consisting of slow-digesting proteins like casein or egg protein immediately before bed. This could take the form of a regular meal or a protein shake. The goal in this case would be to provide the body with a steady supply of slowly absorbed protein through most of the night, thus minimizing the amount of time during which protein breakdown exceeds the synthesis of new protein. The other option is to set your alarm, wake up during the night, and consume a fast-acting protein to boost protein synthesis for the remainder of the night. With optimal timing, just as your body finished processing this meal, you would be waking up and preparing to eat breakfast.

For those of you looking to gain as much weight as possible while on the Ectomorphic Diet, nocturnal feeding might be advantageous. In that case, the additional calories would probably be beneficial as long as your daytime performance isn't impaired too much. My personal preference is to consume a low-carbohydrate egg protein shake immediately before bed consisting of around forty grams of protein. This slowly absorbed protein provides a steady supply of amino acids during most of the night. There may be a two- to three-hour period of NPAC just before waking, but the amount of protein lost is negligible as long as you consume a protein meal immediately on waking and don't skip meals during the day. Extreme hard-gainers on the Ectomorphic Diet may want to set their alarm clocks and consume an additional dose of slow protein three to four hours before they would normally wake up and then go back to sleep. They would then eat breakfast at the usual time to completely eliminate their NPAC.. This time frame coincides with the body's natural early morning insulin spike and will help ensure positive nitrogen balance throughout the night.

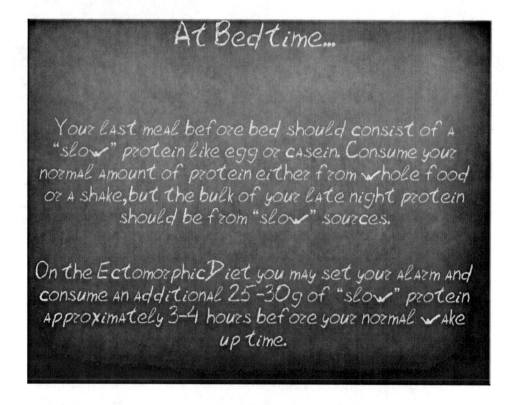

At Bedtime...

Your last meal before bed should consist of a "slow" protein like egg or casein. Consume your normal amount of protein either from whole food or a shake, but the bulk of your late night protein should be from "slow" sources.

On the Ectomorphic Diet you may set your alarm and consume an additional 25-30g of "slow" protein approximately 3-4 hours before your normal wake up time.

Glutamine

Glutamine is the simplest amino acid and constitutes the major energy source for specific body tissues like the intestines. It is worth discussing briefly because glutamine is often discussed in bodybuilding and athletic circles as a potential performance-enhancing substance or as an aid to building lean body mass. Under normal circumstances, glutamine is not considered an essential amino acid. Your body can produce it from other substances, like various keto-acids, in adequate amounts to meet its needs under normal circumstances. Glutamine is often referred to as a "conditionally essential" amino acid because under conditions of extreme stress or nutritional deprivation, the body may not synthesize adequate amounts. In that case, a dietary source must be found to meet these needs.

There has been a great deal of research in the critical care medical field regarding the supplementation of glutamine to severely ill and injured patients. During an extreme physical stress, such as severe burns or overwhelming infection, or during recovery from major surgery, the body may quickly deplete its stores of glutamine and may be receiving inadequate nutrition to make more. In these situations, supplemental glutamine has been shown to improve the function of the immune system, speed wound healing, and help patients retain lean body mass.[50]

Unfortunately, the data with healthy athletes has been far less promising. The majority of studies show no significant benefit with glutamine supplementation beyond what occurs naturally in the diet or in quality protein supplements. Glutamine has been studied to see if strength, lean body mass, fat loss, and muscle recovery could be improved by supplementation. Consistently, glutamine has been a disappointment. Therefore, unless you are a critically ill patient in an intensive care unit, I can't recommend that you spend extra money on glutamine supplementation. If you are following the dietary advice contained within this book, your body will be making and your protein supplementation will be providing more than enough glutamine to meet your needs.

Rating Protein Quality

There are a number of different ways to rank the quality of protein from a given source. Most of these scoring systems take into account the amount of essential amino acids present, the digestibility, and the bioavailability of protein. You will notice that, with a few exceptions, all the methods described rate egg, whey, and other milk-based proteins as well as animal sources near the top and various vegetable/plant-based proteins toward the bottom in terms of quality. Therefore, it is not essential that you completely understand all the intricacies of each system, as you will be consuming the bulk of your protein from these higher-quality sources anyway. However, it is likely that you will run into these terms at some point. I include them here so you can refer to them when needed. The most commonly used ranking systems are summarized in the following paragraphs.

Biological Value

The biological value (BV) is one of the older, but still very commonly used systems to measure protein quality. The BV measures how well the body uses protein from a given source to build new tissue. It is expressed as a ratio of the nitrogen used for tissue formation divided by the nitrogen absorbed from a

---

50   Buchman AL. Glutamine: commercially essential or conditionally essential? A critical appraisal of the human data. Am J Clin Nutr. 2001;74(1):25–32.

specific protein source. Generally, the higher the content of essential amino acids in a protein, the higher its BV. Therefore, animal protein sources generally rank higher than vegetable sources in terms of BV. Most of the time, BV is measured relative to a standard protein source. Usually, this is egg protein, which is given a standard BV of 100. Therefore, it is possible to have a BV greater than 100, as in the case of whey protein, which has a BV of 104. You will also occasionally see BV measured as a true percentage of utilization in which case 100 percent (meaning complete utilization of all the ingested protein) would be the highest possible value. The use of these two systems makes understanding the BV a little bit confusing but generally doesn't alter the ranking of different proteins. For example, no matter which way BV is measured, whey protein will always have a higher BV than protein from peanuts or legumes. The way in which a protein is prepared can influence its BV. Cooking or preparation with high heat (140 degrees) can denature many of the proteins thereby lowering their BV.

Biological Value

Whey Protein	104
Egg	100
Milk	91
Beef	80
Casein	77
Soy Protein	74
Wheat Gluten	64

Protein Efficiency Ratio (PER)

Protein efficiency ratios (PER) measure how well a particular protein promotes growth in animals. To measure the PER, rats are fed a given number of grams of a protein and then the amount of weight they gain per gram of ingested protein is measured. Casein has been arbitrarily chosen as the standard protein when comparing PERs. It has a value of 2.7. Anything greater than 2.7 is considered an excellent source of protein. This particular way to measure protein quality has fallen out of favor because of its limited applicability to humans, though you may occasionally encounter it. Its use is more widespread in agricultural circles.

Protein Efficiency Ratio

Egg	3.9
Whey Protein	3.2
Beef	2.9
Casein	2.7
Milk	2.5
Peanuts	1.8
Wheat Gluten	0.8

Protein Digestibility Corrected Amino Acid Score (PDCAAS)

The PDCAAS is the currently used and preferred method for measuring protein quality for the World Health Organization. It assesses protein quality by comparing the content of the first limiting essential amino acid in a given protein with the content of the same amino acid in a reference pattern of essential amino acids. The reference pattern is based on the estimated essential amino acid requirements of young children ages two to five years. This particular age group was used because they have the highest demands for essential amino acids due to the rapid growth that occurs in this stage of development. Proteins that provide 100 percent or more of all the essential amino acids needed for this group are given a value of 1.0.

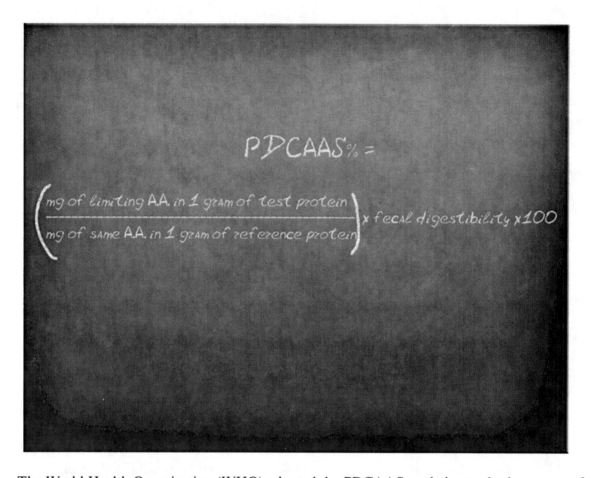

$$PDCAAS\% = \left(\frac{\text{mg of limiting A.A. in 1 gram of test protein}}{\text{mg of same A.A. in 1 gram of reference protein}} \right) \times \text{fecal digestibility} \times 100$$

The World Health Organization (WHO) adopted the PDCAAS as their standard measure of protein quality for a number of reasons, the primary one being that it is based on a human model, whereas other measurement techniques relied primarily on animal data. Like other methods for measuring protein quality, there are a number of sources of potential error when using the PDCAAS. Its use of young children as a standard reference obviously makes application to hard-training strength athletes as well as older adults questionable. Also, its reliance on measurements of "fecal true digestibility" doesn't take into account the absorption of amino acids by colonic bacteria. This may result in overestimations of the amount of essential amino acids actually absorbed into the body. Regardless of these flaws, the WHO and a variety of other organizations have adopted the PDCAAS as the standard measure of protein quality; therefore, you are likely to run into it eventually.

PDCAAS of common foods

Whey	1.0
Egg white	1.0
Casein	1.0
Milk	1.0
Soy Protein Isolate	1.0
Beef	0.92
Soybean	0.91
Black Beans	0.75
Kidney Beans	0.68
Rye	0.68
Whole Wheat	0.54
Lentils	0.52
Peanuts	0.52
Wheat Gluten	0.25

Adapted from U.S Dairy Export Council, Reference Manual for U.S. Whey Products 2nd Edition, 1999 and Sarwar, 1997.

How Much Protein Do You Really Need?

There has been considerable controversy over the years regarding how much, if any, additional protein is required by athletes to promote optimal performance, recovery, and muscle growth. It has generally been assumed that individuals engaged in high-intensity or prolonged bouts of lower-intensity exercise require more protein than sedentary individuals. A number of well-designed studies have indeed shown that athletes do seem to benefit from higher levels of protein intake. Unfortunately, some misguided individuals have interpreted these findings as meaning they should take in massive quantities of protein, far in excess of the needs of even the most elite athletes. As we will discuss later, this approach not only is not helpful but in some cases can be potentially harmful.

During high-intensity weight-training regimens, such as that found in The Program, increased protein requirements result from a number of different factors. During exercise itself, the free amino acid pool (the amino acids dissolved in the blood) is decreased in several ways. Amino acids are lost in both sweat and urine. Depending on the length and intensity of the exercise being performed, they may also be metabolized to create additional glucose or fatty acids for energy production. During periods of low protein intake, amino acids may be released into the blood via the breakdown of muscle tissue. Immediately after intense resistance exercise, there is a period of recovery where protein synthesis is significantly increased. During this period of time, the body is not only trying to repair the microscopic damage to its muscle fibers, but also trying to super-compensate (i.e., create more muscle tissue than was present previously) as a means to adapt to further training sessions. Several studies have shown that favorable changes, not only in protein synthesis, but also in protein breakdown can occur when protein intake is increased. Therefore, it is crucial for those looking for maximal gains in lean muscle mass to provide the body with a steady supply of high-quality protein, during periods of rest and recovery, but also, as we will discuss later, during key "windows of opportunity" before, during, and after training.

The current recommended daily allowance (RDA) for protein is 0.8 grams per kilogram of body weight per day. This level of intake is generally considered to be adequate to maintain lean body mass in relatively healthy, sedentary individuals. Obviously, individuals vary and so there may be those who require perhaps a little more or a little less. This rarely becomes an in issue in the Western world, especially in the United States, where most people consume well in excess of this number.

Athletes engaged in heavy resistance exercise will experience elevated levels of protein synthesis after training. In the case of untrained athletes who are new to this type of training, this period can last up to forty-eight hours. During this time, the body's need for additional protein must be met in order to secure optimal gains in lean muscle mass. Protein intake that falls short of these increased demands, while not dangerous, will likely result in suboptimal gains in lean muscle mass over the long term.

A review of multiple studies demonstrates an average recommended protein intake for weight-training athletes of between 1.6 to 2.0 grams per kilogram per day.[51] This amount may vary based on the quality of protein ingested, the degree of intensity and the volume of training, and the amount of additional calories from carbohydrates and fats. While on The Program, the recommendation will be to aim for a protein intake toward the higher end of this range. This will ensure that you are providing the body with adequate amounts of protein, not only for recovery from your intense workouts, but also for optimal muscle growth. Additionally, the added protein will provide needed calories that will replace those lost from carbohydrate restriction while on the Endomorphic Diet. While on this diet, as well as the Mesomorphic and Ectomorphic Diets, you should have very little difficulty reaching your goal of about 2.0 grams of protein per kilogram of body weight. Most foods that are rich in healthy fats are also high in quality protein. If anything, you may find yourself exceeding this amount, in which case you should scale back your protein intake. There is no benefit to be had by increasing your protein intake much beyond this level.[52] There appears to be a plateau effect in terms of increased protein synthesis when it comes to dietary protein. Consuming additional protein will provide a benefit only up to a certain point, after which excess protein merely increases urea production as your body attempts to eliminate the extra or convert the unnecessary calories into fats for long-term storage.[53]

The optimal amount of protein to be consumed for a given individual per meal is largely unknown. One study showed that when more than forty grams of pure essential amino acids were administered to healthy volunteers, there was not a significant increase in protein synthesis beyond that achieved with

51   KD Tipton, OC Witard. 2007. Protein requirements and recommendations for athletes: Relevance of ivory tower arguments for practical recommendations, Clinics in Sports Medicine, 26, 1, 17–36.
52   Lemon PW, Tarnopolsky MA, MacDougall JD, Atkinson SA: Protein requirements and muscle mass/strength changes during intensive training in novice bodybuilders. J Appl Physiol 1992, 73(2):767–77535.
53   Phillips SM. Protein requirements and supplementation in strength sports. Nutrition 2004; 20:689–95.

twenty grams.[54] How this translates to persons undergoing an intense resistance-training program who are consuming both whole-food protein sources and supplemental protein is unknown. There is very likely to be significant variation between individuals based on body weight as well as gender, but unfortunately, at this time, there is very little hard data from which we can make solid recommendations. There is no evidence that consuming more than forty grams of protein in a sitting is harmful, so I wouldn't be too concerned. In most cases, your average meals and your protein supplements will provide around forty grams of protein or less. It is unlikely that there is a benefit to consuming much more than this at a single sitting.

Using our goal of about 2.0 grams of protein per kilogram of body weight, a 220-pound (100 kilogram) male engaged in high-intensity weight training would have a goal intake of approximately two hundred grams of protein per twenty-four hours. Divided between six small meals, this yields a goal of about thirty-three grams of protein per meal. When looked at in this manner, it becomes apparent just how little this is in comparison to the huge quantities recommended in some bodybuilding magazines.

Protein: How Much Is Too Much?

While consumption of high-quality protein is essential in The Program, you can definitely go overboard. I have occasionally run into people who consume massive amounts of protein (sometimes over four hundred grams per day!) in the hopes of boosting their gains in lean muscle. As we learned previously, the liver performs the process of deamination whereby nitrogen groups ($NH2$) are cleaved off amino acids and transformed into the waste product urea. It turns out that the liver has a maximum amount of urea that it can synthesize in a twenty-four-hour period. The upper limit of this process is called the maximum rate of urea synthesis (MRUS). The MRUS varies with body weight with larger individuals having higher MRUS values. There is also individual variation (likely hereditary) in the efficiency of this process that affects the MRUS. For most individuals, the MRUS varies between fifty-five and seventy-five milligrams of urea synthesized per hour per kilogram of lean body weight ($N/h/kg^{-0.75}$). For our estimates, we will use the mean of 65 $N/h/kg^{-0.75}$ as an average MRUS for most healthy adults. When the amount of protein consumed exceeds the liver's ability to perform deamination, buildup of precursor substances occurs. This phenomenon may have caused the symptoms of so-called "rabbit starvation," a term coined by early American explorers for the nausea, diarrhea, headaches, general malaise, and in some cases death that occurred when their diets consisted almost exclusively of lean meats, such as those found in rabbits.

---

54   Tipton, KD, Gurkin BE, Matin S, and Wolfe RR. Nonessential amino acids are not necessary to stimulate net muscle protein synthesis in healthy volunteers. J Nutr Biochem 1999, 10: 89–95.

The average MRUS
for most individuals is about
65 mg/hr/kg.

Based on your body weight
from the chart below do not
exceed this amount of protein
(in grams) per day.

Maximum Daily Protein intake
for 60–110 kg individuals

MRUS	Weight in Kg					
	60	70	80	90	100	110
55	226	256	285	313	341	368
60	242	274	305	335	365	394
65	258	292	325	357	388	419
70	274	310	345	379	412	445
75	291	328	365	401	436	470

DiFulco, J.T. Galambos, R.B. 3rd Smith, A.A. Salam, and W.D. Warren. Maximal rates of excretion and synthesis of urea in normal and cirrhotic subjects. J.Clin Invest. 52:2241-2249, 1973.

The table above plots out the estimated maximal protein intake for individuals weighing between 60 and 110 kilograms. For example, a 90-kilogram athlete's liver could process between 313 and 401 grams of protein per day. Using a mean of sixty-five for the MRUS gives us an upper limit of about 357 grams per day for that individual. Calculating your specific MRUS is impractical without the assistance of a well-stocked university research lab. Therefore, we are stuck using the mean MRUS of sixty-five. If you want to choose a higher MRUS for yourself, then feel free. If you start to feel ill, then decrease your protein intake to correlate with an MRUS of sixty-five or less and reevaluate how you feel. Fortunately, while on the diets presented in The Program, you should not be in danger of exceeding this value. All three Program diets are considered high-protein diets when compared to the average American diet, but the requirement to meet specific ratios of fats, protein, and carbohydrate while maintaining a caloric intake that is not too far off from maintenance will ensure that you stay well below your liver's maximal ability to handle nitrogenous waste.

Different Types of Protein

Whey Protein

Whey is the clear liquid portion of milk that remains after the manufacturing of cheese. Whey, along with casein, is one of the two major protein sources found in cow's milk. Whey protein contains high levels of both essential and branched chain amino acids in addition to being rich in vitamins and minerals. Whey protein in its various forms has become the most popular source of supplemental protein consumed by athletes.

Whey Protein Powder

Whey protein powder is the crudest form of whey protein available on the market. It is used as an additive in a variety of foods, such as snack foods, dairy products, infant formulas, et cetera. Whey protein powder in its simplest form is composed of approximately 11 to 15 percent protein, 63 to 75 percent lactose, and about 1 to 1.5 percent milk fat.

Whey Protein Concentrate

Further processing of whey protein forms whey protein concentrate. This processing removes much of the water, lactose, ash, and some minerals found in raw whey. As a result, whey protein concentrate has a greater degree of bioavailability than standard whey protein. It is composed of approximately 25 to 89 percent protein, 10 to 55 percent lactose, and 2 to 10 percent milk fat.

Whey Protein Isolate

Whey protein isolate is the purest available form of whey protein. During the processing of whey protein isolate, almost all the lactose is removed and very little milk fat remains. Whey protein isolate is over 90 percent protein with less than 0.5 percent of its composition coming from lactose and milk fat. This makes whey protein isolate ideal for individuals with lactose intolerance.

Casein

Almost 80 percent of the protein found in milk comes from casein. Casein is considered a complete protein as it contains all the essential amino acids. Casein tends to clot and form clumps in the stomach. It is this property that gives casein its relatively slow absorption when compared to whey protein. An interesting property of casein is that during digestion, it can be broken down into small protein fragments known as casomorphins. Casomorphins have opioid-like activity, and in humans, they may have a histamine-releasing effect. This may be responsible for the flushing and itching that some people experience when consuming large amounts of casein.

Bovine Colostrum

The pre-milk liquid secreted by female mammals during the first few days of nursing is known as colostrum. Bovine (cow) colostrum is rich in infection-fighting antibodies and various growth factors, protein, and other nutrients essential for the early growth of their offspring. There have been a number of studies looking at the potential benefits of bovine colostrum in treating a variety of medical conditions as well as its effects on athletic performance.

Bovine colostrum has been shown to provide some degree of protection to critically ill patients who are at risk for developing sepsis. It is thought that various components in colostrum neutralize bacterial toxins in the gut.[55] In infants, this can speed recovery from E coli infections and reduce its most serious complications. Colostrum has also shown some benefit in treating diarrhea in immune-suppressed patients, including AIDS patients.[56] In athletes, the data supporting bovine colostrum's performance-enhancing abilities is a bit less solid. Some studies have shown that athletes supplementing with colostrum had elevated levels of IGF-1[57]; other studies have refuted this.[58] Similarly, some studies have shown improvement in the performance of endurance and sprint athletes, while other studies have shown no significant benefit. Unfortunately, most of the studies looking at improvements in athletic performance and/or body composition were limited by a small number of test subjects or poor methodology. This is clearly an area where more quality research is needed.

I have no experience with bovine colostrum, so I cannot share any personal anecdotes. I know there are well-educated authors who swear by it and others who say it is of little to no benefit. I certainly cannot think of a reason to persuade you not to try colostrum if it interests you. There are a variety of companies that provide purified colostrum in both tablet and powder form.

---

55 MTT Agrifood Research Finland (2008, September 17). Bovine Colostrum And Fermented Cabbage Can Help Restrict Infections. ScienceDaily. Retrieved October 25, 2008, from http://www.sciencedaily.com /releases/2008/09/080915083721.htm.

56 Struff WG, Sprotte G. Bovine colostrum as a biologic in clinical medicine: a review—Part II: clinical studies. J Clin Pharmacol Ther. 2008 May;46(5):211–25.

57 Mero A, Miikkulainen H, Riski J, Pakkanen R, Aalto J, Takala T. (1997) Effects of bovine colostrum supplementation on serum IGF-1, IgG, hormone, and saliva IgA during training. Journal of Applied Physiology 83(4):1144–51.

58 Kuipers H, van Breda E, Verlaan G, Smeets R. (2002) Effects of oral bovine colostrum supplementation on serum insulin-like growth factor-I levels. Nutrition 18(7-8):566–7.

Vegetable Protein

Vegetable proteins are generally considered of lower quality than animal sources because they may be low in one or more essential amino acids. Unfortunately, this has led many athletes and bodybuilders to avoid making vegetables a solid staple in their diet. While it is true that individual plant sources may be low in one or more amino acids, this is really of little consequence because other food sources can make up for the deficiency. It has generally been recommended that vegetarians attempt to combine various plant protein sources together with each meal in an attempt to create a meal that provides a complete protein profile. Multiple studies have shown that this is not necessary. As long as adequate amounts of all the essential amino acids are consumed throughout the day, positive nitrogen balance can be maintained and muscle growth can occur. Vegetable protein sources are also rich in vitamins, minerals, and antioxidants. Diets rich in vegetables are associated with lower risk for cardiovascular disease as well as various cancers. Regardless of which eating plan you choose while on The Program, be sure to include plenty of vegetables in your diet.

There are a number of professional and amateur bodybuilders who have built outstanding physiques while avoiding meat. Many of them, however, still consume protein from egg and dairy sources. In this situation, protein from eggs, dairy sources like whey, and plant sources like soy can more than make up for a lack of meat in the diet. Things start to get a bit more complicated when vegetarians cut out the egg and dairy all together. This scenario creates reliance on soy products and a broader range of vegetable sources to ensure adequate essential amino acid intake. Again, I'm not saying it cannot be done, but you have to be a very well-informed individual when following this sort of diet. The most obvious difficulty with following a strictly vegetarian diet while on The Program will be meeting the roughly two grams per kilogram protein requirement while keeping your carbohydrate intake under control on the Endomorphic and Mesomorphic Diets. Additionally, given the bulk and fiber content of most vegetable proteins, the volume of food you will be eating at each meal to meet this protein requirement will also be large. You may find that you simply don't have room to stuff all that food down at each meal. Strict vegetarian diets can also leave you deficient in two key nutrients: iron and B12. The iron found in vegetable sources generally is of lower bioavailability than that found in meats. This is partially offset by the increased dietary vitamin C consumed on a vegetarian diet. (Vitamin C improves the absorption of iron in the gut.) This is not as big an issue for men, but for menstruating or pregnant women, an iron supplement may be necessary. B12 is generally found in low concentrations in plant sources, and supplementation is often needed. Fortunately, there are many B12-fortified vegetarian foods on the market today including fortified soymilk and meat analogues. Nutritional yeast can also be purchased and included in the diet as a good source of B12.

My intention is not to dissuade those of you who wish to pursue a strictly vegetarian diet but rather to encourage you to become as knowledgeable as you possibly can be before embarking on this sort of diet. Vegetarian diets can be very healthy, and you can build muscle while following one.

Animal Protein

Generally speaking, protein from animal sources is very high-quality protein. Meats contain all the essential amino acids and are easily digestible Meats from all sources are excellent, low-carbohydrate sources of protein and, unless you have moral, religious, or other reasons for avoiding it, at least a portion of your daily protein intake should come from meat. Perhaps the biggest knock on regular meat consumption is its generally high saturated-fat and cholesterol content. Fortunately, for a little extra money, you can usually find very lean cuts of beef or simply buy turkey and chicken, which are much lower in both saturated fat and cholesterol. Beef protein isolate powder is also available and has amino acid profile that compares favorably to whey protein.

Soy Protein

Soybeans are relatively high in protein. They are the one of the few "complete" vegetable proteins available. This means that it contains all the essential amino acids. Soy protein is found in various forms in all sorts of packaged and processed foods. It is used to add protein, flavor, and texture to beef, chicken, and fish products as well as various "meat substitutes."

Soy Concentrate

When soybeans are de-hulled and most of their water-soluble carbohydrate is removed, you end up with soy concentrate. Soy protein concentrate is about 70 percent soy protein with the remainder being mostly insoluble fiber. You will see soy protein concentrate added to a variety of foods including pet foods, livestock feed, and a variety of processed meat products.

Soy Isolate

Soy isolate is the purest form of soy protein. Soybeans are defatted and nearly all other ingredients removed to produce an approximately 90 percent protein product. Soy isolate can be purchased in powder form but is also commonly included in a variety of protein bars, drinks, and various meat products to increase protein content and provide texture.

Soy Isoflavones

Most of the claims and controversy surrounding soy revolve around its high concentration of isoflavones. Isoflavones are a type of plant-based compound with estrogen-like activity. While isoflavones can be found in a variety of foods, they are found in highest concentration in the soybean. Soy isoflavones are known to have a weak estrogen effect in cells with estrogen receptors. This causes them to both express similar effects to that of endogenous estrogen but also to partially block estrogen from binding to these cells. As a result, there has been a great deal of interest in examining what effects, if any, regular consumption of soy isoflavones has a on a variety of cancers, cardiovascular disease, and endogenous hormones. There has also been a great deal of concern expressed among male athletes that consuming soy could potentially lower testosterone levels and impair athletic performance.

The FDA, after being petitioned by the soy industry, now allows soy manufacturers to claim that regular consumption of soy foods can lower the risk of heart disease. Take a look at just about any soy product in the grocery store, and you will see that they have wasted no time in plastering that claim all over the place. That claim comes from a variety of studies, which have shown that regular consumption of fairly large amounts of soy protein (twenty-five to fifty grams per day) can lower serum LDL levels somewhere between 3 and 10 percent. Considering this very modest effect, as well as the not entirely clear relationship between cholesterol levels and heart disease, I personally don't get too excited about soy protein's chances of helping anyone avoid heart disease.

Soy is often touted for its cancer-fighting properties. Unfortunately, these claims are largely over-stated. At this time, there is very little compelling evidence that soy isoflavones actually reduce the risk of any form of cancer in human beings, including breast, endometrial, or prostate cancer. Most studies showing potential benefits involve animals (usually rats) and are not supported by human trials. The same can be said for its ability to fight osteoporosis in postmenopausal females. There is a great deal of contra-dictory data. There is some data that a diet heavy in soy isoflavones may have some bone-sparing effects in women who already have osteoporosis.[59] The question of whether or not a soy-heavy diet actually prevents osteoporosis or actually prevents fractures has not been answered satisfactorily at this time. It is my suspicion that if any effect is found, it is likely to be very small and not of any practical significance.

A number of rat studies have raised the question of whether or not soy isoflavones can lower testoster-one levels. There does seem to be some evidence that in animal models, there may be some adverse hormonal effects. There is a lack of human studies to answer this question adequately. The few human studies seem to demonstrate that there isn't any significant effect on testosterone levels, though admittedly these studies are of very poor quality and have used very small numbers of subjects. One study of note supplemented the diets of twenty weight-training athletes with fifty grams per day of soy concentrate or soy isolate and compared their serum testosterone levels after twelve weeks to a similar group that was given an equal amount of whey protein. There were no significant differences in serum testosterone levels between the groups as well as no difference in the amount of lean mass gained.[60,61] It seems unlikely that regular consumption of soy protein in reasonable amounts will have much of an effect on body composition or testosterone levels in males. It is possible that ingesting larger amounts could have an effect, but no studies exist to evaluate this.

59   Lydeking-Olsen E, Beck-Jensen JE, Setchell KD, Holm-Jensen T. Soymilk or progesterone for prevention of bone loss—a 2 year randomized, placebo-controlled trial. Eur J Nutr. 2004;43(4):246–257.

60   Kalman D, et al. Effect of protein source and resistance training on body composition and sex hormones. Journal of the International Society of Sports Nutrition 2007, 4:4 23 July 2007.

61   Divi RL, Chang HC, Doerge DR. Anti-thyroid isoflavones from soybean: isolation, characterization, and mechanisms of action. Biochem Pharmacol. 1997; 54(10):1087–1096.

Isoflavones per 100g serving

Soy Protein Isolate	97.43 mg
Soy Protein Concentrate	102.07 mg
Miso	42.55 mg
Soy Milk	9.65 mg
Tofu (pressed, raw)	29.50 mg
Dry Roasted Soybeans	128.35 mg
Soy Flour	131.19 mg

(Adapted from USDA-Iowa State University Database on the Isoflavone Content of Foods - 1999)

Soy isoflavones have also been linked to thyroid dysfunction in a number of studies. They have been found to inhibit the activity of thyroid peroxidase, an enzyme required for thyroid hormone synthesis. There have been case reports of infants developing hypothyroidism from prolonged use of soy formula,[62] but this is generally considered to be only a factor for individuals who do not consume sufficient quantities of iodine. Since iodine deficiency is almost unheard of in the Western world, this really isn't a problem for most people.[63]

Hemp Protein

A plant-based protein that is increasing in popularity is hemp protein. Hemp you say? Isn't that marijuana? Well, yes and no. Hemp is the name used to describe all plants from the Cannabis genus. Marijuana typically refers to the unfertilized female cannabis plant, while hemp is usually meant to describe the male plant used for industrial and commercial purposes. THC (delta-9 tetrahydrocannabinol) is the psychoactive compound found to some degree in all cannabis plants. The THC content of hemp is negligible while, obviously, the content in marijuana can be quite high. Hemp has a long and distinguished history in this country and around the world and is used for a myriad of purposes, from making rope and paper to biofuels. Both George Washington and Thomas Jefferson were hemp farmers, and the Declaration of Independence was written on hemp paper.

---

62   Chorazy PA, Himelhoch S, Hopwood NJ, Greger NG, Postellon DC. Persistent hypothyroidism in an infant receiving a soy formula: case report and review of the literature. Pediatrics. 1995; 96 (1 Pt 1):148–150.

63   .Bruce B, Messina M, Spiller GA. Isoflavone supplements do not affect thyroid function in iodine-replete postmenopausal women. J Med Food. 2003; 6(4): 309–316.

In addition to its many commercial properties, hemp processed for human consumption is a good source of protein, fiber, and essential fatty acids as well as vitamins and minerals. In several respects, hemp protein is superior to soy. It undergoes significantly less chemical processing to arrive at the finished product. Additionally, there is no evidence that hemp protein has any of the potential complications associated with soy isoflavones. Hemp proteins' primary component is a globular protein known as edestin. Hemp protein also has more fiber than perhaps any available protein powder with average counts ranging from four to ten or more grams per serving. Since its primary carbohydrate content is in the form of insoluble fiber, hemp protein is perfect for low-carbohydrate dieters. Another benefit of hemp is its high concentration of essential fatty acids. Hemp contains omega-3 and omega-6 fatty acids in an approximately 1:3 ratio. Its omega-3 content comes primarily from ALA (15 to 25 percent) while its omega-6 content is primarily from LA (linoleic acid, 50 to 70 percent). While this is a good thing, hemp protein still falls short of flaxseed oil in terms of omega-3 content. As discussed in further detail in the chapter on fats, only a small percentage of ALA is actually converted into the more important DHA and EPA. Therefore, I wouldn't recommend using hemp protein as your primary source of essential fatty acids. However, mixing some flaxseed oil into your hemp protein shake is a great way to boost its EFA content.

Hemp protein does have some drawbacks, however. It falls short of whey protein in a few important aspects. As discussed above, leucine is a particularly important amino acid for stimulating protein synthesis. As compared to whey protein, hemp is relatively low in leucine. Most hemp protein preparations contain between four hundred and eight hundred milligrams of leucine for a typical thirty-gram serving, while whey protein isolate, which is roughly 13 percent leucine, contains around 3900 milligrams for a similar serving size. How much of an issue this becomes is hard to say. If you are consuming a wide range of other leucine-containing proteins, then it's probably not an issue. If you are using hemp as your primary protein source, then you may have to consume significantly more. Hemp protein, at least for now, is also slightly more expensive than whey protein. US farmers are prohibited from growing hemp unless they possess a special license from the federal government. As a result, all hemp protein is imported from other countries, mostly Canada. This likely has a lot to do with its increased cost.

The other concern many folks have is the fear of having a positive drug test for THC after using hemp products. Many employers, including the military, routinely screen employees for illicit drug use, and a THC screen is almost universally used on a routine urine drug screen. The THC content in typical hemp supplements is minute, but a number of studies have shown that consumption of hemp-seed products in recommended amounts can result in a positive THC screening urinalysis. These studies have primarily involved consumption of hemp seed oil.[64] It is possible that the processing of hemp into commercial oil may increase its THC content. Studies looking at other products like plain seeds or hemp beer have shown contradictory results. A military study performed at the Forensic Toxicology Department of the Armed Forces Institute of Pathology showed that normal consumption of a hemp beer product (Hempen Ale) did not produce a positive test for cannabinoids in four of the commonly

---

64   Costantino A, et al. Hemp Oil Ingestion Causes Positive Urine D9-Tetrahydrocannabinol Carboxylic Acid. Journal of Analytical Toxicology, Volume 21, Number 6, October 1997, pp. 482–485.

used tests.[65] However, other studies looking at various products, like protein bars made with hemp protein, have resulted in positive drug screens in some cases.[66]

No studies to date have yet looked at whether or not hemp protein powder will trigger a positive drug screen. However, given the large quantities of protein consumed by most athletes and the rather large recommended serving size of roughly thirty grams, I have to assume that they would. I think it goes without saying that the miniscule amounts of THC have no detectable psychoactive effects. It is impossible to get high from hemp protein powder. In the military, several active duty personnel have successfully defended themselves from prosecution by claiming they ingested commercially available hemp food products. The bottom line on this is that if you are subject to random drug screening by your employer or anyone else, the safest approach is to avoid hemp protein. You may be able to beat the rap by quoting the above studies, but it's doubtful that the pain and aggravation would be worth your while. On the other hand, if testing is not a concern, then feel free to use hemp protein if you like. Overall, it's a decent protein source, especially if you are a strict vegetarian. It falls short of whey protein but still has its uses for those who are interested.

Egg Protein

Egg protein is a high-quality protein that is worth adding to your diet. Consumed whole or as a protein powder supplement, egg protein provides a very high-quality source of readily absorbable protein. In fact, egg protein is generally considered a close second only to whey protein in terms of its biological value, and given its lower price, may actually be preferable for some athletes. Egg protein is a good source of branched chain amino acids and is easy to cook with. Egg protein, especially when raw, differs from whey protein in that it is more slowly digested. Raw egg white, in particular, is very slowly absorbed and makes an excellent source of "slow protein" for your bedtime protein meal.

---

65   Gary W. Kunsman, et al. Letter to the Editor. Journal of Analytical Toxicology, Volume 23, Number 6, October 1999, pp.563–564.
66   Fortner N, et al. Positive Urine Test Results from Consumption of Hemp Seeds in Food Products. Journal of Analytical Toxicology, Volume 21, Number 6, October 1997, pp. 476–481.

FAT METABOLISM

Fat has gotten a bad rap over the years. Most nutritional authorities say we should limit our fat intake as much as possible, and unless you are a sumo wrestler, most people want to avoid packing on additional weight in the form of body fat. It's important to understand, however, that fats are absolutely vital for your survival. Fats perform a number of essential roles. They provide energy and are, gram for gram, the most calorically efficient macronutrient. They are a vital part of all your cell membranes and keep your body's cells functioning properly. Your brain is almost completely composed of fat. All the important signals that travel between your brain cells are conducted along fatty highways known as axons. Fat is also an important storage depot for fat-soluble vitamins like vitamins A, K, D, and E. Fats are also used to make hormones. If your fat intake isn't adequate, you can shut down your body's production of a variety of important hormones including testosterone. Fat not only keeps us warm and helps regulate our body temperature, but the fat surrounding our internal organs provides energy and a protective cushion that holds them in place and helps prevent injury from sudden jarring as in falls or car accidents. Fats form vital parts of your cells' membranes. They also form the structural components to many hormones. So don't fear fat. You should learn how to use it to improve not only your health but your appearance as well. It's important to have a basic understanding of how your body digests, stores, and burns fat so you can better plan your diet and ensure you are getting the important nutrients you need to operate at peak efficiency.

Metabolism of fats is complex. It's not important that you understand every chemical step in the breakdown of the fats in your diet, but it is worthwhile having a "big picture" understanding of the process. Understanding how your body reacts to and utilizes different types of fats is also useful in deciding what you will include in your diet and what you can cut out.

Fats come in several different varieties, which we discuss later. They all enter the acidic environment of the stomach where they are emulsified. There is some minimal breakdown of fat in the stomach by the gastric lipase enzyme, but the bulk of digestion occurs in the small intestine, specifically the duodenum. Here, bile stored in your gallbladder breaks apart fat into smaller, more easily digestible units called micelles. Lipase pours in from the pancreas and breaks down these micelles into fatty acids and monoacylglycerol. There are three types of fatty acids: long-, medium-, and short- chain fatty acids. Short- and medium-chain fatty acids are small enough to enter the bloodstream directly. They are transported along with other nutrients directly to the liver. They are more easily oxidized and available for energy than long-chain fatty acids (more on this later). Long-chain fatty acids diffuse into the cells lining your small intestine and are transformed into triglycerides that are then packaged neatly with cholesterol and a few proteins into chylomicrons. Chylomicrons then leave the intestinal cells and move into small lymphatic vessels, which run adjacent to your blood vessels. They finally enter the bloodstream at the thoracic duct, which communicates with the left subclavian vein.

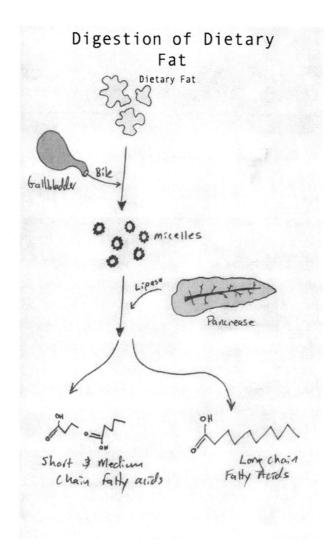

Once in the bloodstream, chylomicrons are transported throughout the body along with their fatty cargo. When they have reached their final destination, whether that is brain, muscle, liver, fat, or other tissue, another enzyme, lipoprotein lipase, frees the triglycerides for use as fuel or building blocks for other substances like cholesterol and hormones or to be stored in fat cells for later use.

It is important to emphasize again that it is insulin that is the primary "fat storage hormone." In a high-insulin environment, the body is in "storage mode," meaning that fatty acids will be preferentially shunted into fat cells for long-term storage. Most Westerners consume a diet rich in simple carbohydrates. This keeps insulin levels chronically elevated throughout most of the day and virtually guarantees that any co-ingested fats will be preferentially shipped off to the body's fat cells. While on the Endomorphic and Mesomorphic Diets, your insulin levels will be controlled. The relatively low intake of carbohydrate will lower insulin levels and raise the level of glucagon. This change in the yin-and-yang balance between insulin and glucagon will swing the pendulum of fat storage versus burning the other direction. In this environment, fat cells will be encouraged to give up their greasy cargo for use as fuel. The low levels of insulin will make it difficult for fat cells to take up and store additional fat, and the net effect will be a decrease in the size of your fat cells and ultimately a favorable change in your body composition.

Burning Fat

In times of perceived energy deficiency, the body resorts to its fat stores for fuel. In your fat cells, fatty acids are stored as triacylglycerols. In response to the body's energy demands, these triacylglycerols are broken back down into fatty acids in a complex chemical cascade powered by a key fat-burning enzyme: *hormone sensitive lipase* (HSL). HSL, as its name implies, is triggered by several body hormones: glucagon from the pancreas, epinephrine from the adrenal glands, and b-corticotropin from the pituitary gland in the brain. These hormones enter the bloodstream and bind to the surface of fat cells, which in turn triggers another series of chemical steps leading to the increased production of another key chemical messenger, cyclic adenosine mono phosphate (cAMP). This chemical activates HSL, which begins stimulating the release of fatty acids from your fat cells into your bloodstream. Once in the blood, these fatty acids travel to various tissues and enter cells to be used as energy.

The hormones that trigger HSL (glucagon, epinephrine, and b-corticotropin) are up-regulated in perceived starvation states. In times of starvation, very little glucose is available for fuel, so the body turns to its fat and protein stores for fuel. Low-carbohydrate diets work in a way by "tricking" the body into thinking it is in a starvation state by greatly limiting the carbohydrate available for fuel. The body then has no choice but to activate these hormones and use HSL to break down its fat stores. It will do this even though in reality you are not starving and are actually eating plenty of calories to sustain yourself. The other reason to limit your carbohydrate intake for maximum fat loss is that HSL is sensitive to insulin. But rather than activate it, insulin shuts down HSL and prevents it from releasing the fatty acids in your cells. The key in the Endomorphic Diet, and to a lesser extent the Mesomorphic Diet, is to kick HSL into high gear and keep it there. As long as HSL is active, you will be breaking down your fat stores and using them as energy.

Once inside a cell, free fatty acids enter cellular power plants known as mitochondria and undergo an even more complex process called beta-oxidation. I'll spare you the painful biochemical details, but the end result of this process is the long carbon chains on these fats are systematically cleaved off to produce multiple molecules of acetyl-CoA, which then enter a series of even more complex chemical steps known as the Krebs cycle followed by oxidative phosphorylation to ultimately produce the simple molecule that powers all life on earth: adenosine tri-phosphate (ATP).

A close look at this whole process yields one particularly important lesson: fats produce a lot more ATP (and therefore energy) than glucose does. The total number of ATP molecules generated from one molecule of glucose, from start to finish, through the whole energy cycle is about thirty-eight molecules of ATP. Not bad right? A 1:38 return on your investment sounds pretty good. Compared to what you get from metabolizing fats, that is chump change. The amount of ATP generated from a fatty acid depends on how long its carbon chain is. If we use a typical sixteen-carbon fatty acid (palmitate) and completely metabolize it, we end up with 131 molecules of ATP! There is a reason your body prefers to store most of its energy as fat rather than glycogen. Fat is the most compact form of stored energy available to your body. So, if you are overweight, don't complain that you don't have any energy. You are full of energy that is just waiting to be used!

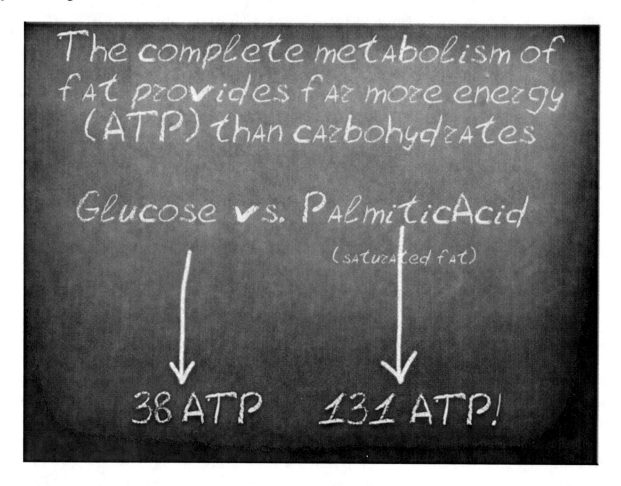

Where do ketones fit into all this? After all, during the Endomorphic Diet, you will be relying on ketones for much of your body's energy. During periods of carbohydrate restriction, acetyl-CoA has difficulty entering the Krebs Cycle. In order for it to be used as energy, the liver must convert it into the ketone bodies acetoacetate and b-hydroxybutyrate. These molecules can be used in various organs, including the heart and skeletal muscle, to produce ATP. The brain is also perfectly capable of running indefinitely on ketones for fuel. The commonly repeated statement that the brain can only use glucose for fuel is a myth. True, given equal availability, the brain will use glucose over ketones as its primary energy source, but when the glucose supply dries up, the brain easily switches to using ketones.

Types of Fat: Good Fats/Bad Fats

Dietary fats are essential for life. They not only form vital structures in all living cells but are important energy sources as well. In all phases of The Program, you will be consuming fats of different types in various quantities. It is important that you have some basic knowledge regarding fats so that you can ensure adequate intake and optimize your results.

Saturated Fats

Saturated fats are fats in which all available carbon bonds are occupied by a hydrogen atom. They are solid at room temperature. They are linear molecules and therefore can stack one on top of the other, and form a solid structure. Saturated fats are found in most animal products, including dairy as well as a few plant sources like coconut. The human body can also manufacture saturated fats from carbohydrate and protein.

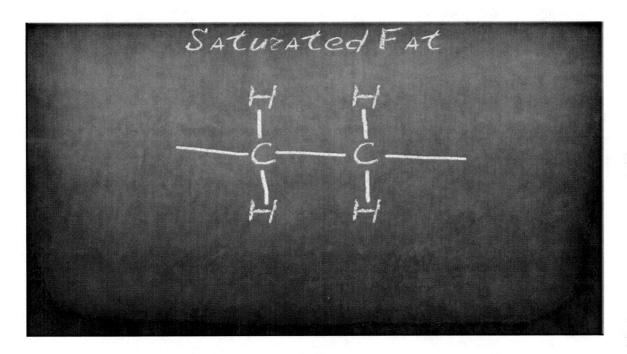

The three primary saturated fats found in human diets are stearic acid, palmitic acid, and lauric acid. Stearic acid is a highly stable eighteen-carbon (C18) fat used commonly for frying. It is also used in margarines, other spreads, and shortening and as a creme base in baked products. It is also found in high concentrations in chocolate.

Stearic acid appears to lower both LDL (bad) and HDL (good) cholesterol. Its HDL-lowering properties seem to be more pronounced in women.[67] In the gut, stearic acid is absorbed and carried to the liver where it is converted to the unsaturated fat oleic acid, which is then released back into the bloodstream. Oleic acid is considered neutral in terms of its effects on cholesterol. Despite its relatively benign effects on cholesterol, stearic acid in large amounts is associated with a slight increase in risk for cardiovascular disease, probably due to its HDL-lowering and pro-thrombotic effects.[68]

---

67   Aro A, Jauhiainen M, Partanen R, Salminen I, Mutanen M: Stearic acid, trans fatty acids, and dairy fat: effects on serum and lipoprotein lipids, apolipoproteins, lipoprotein(a), and lipid transfer proteins in healthy subjects. Am J Clin Nutr 65: 1491–1426, 1997.

68   Hu FB, Stampfer MJ, Manson JE, et al. Dietary saturated fats and their food sources in relation to the risk of coronary heart disease in women. Am J Clin Nutr 1999;70:1001–8.

Palmitic acid (C16) and lauric acid (C12) are saturated fats found commonly in coconut and palm kernel oil. Both these fats raise LDL cholesterol levels, but this is largely offset by their tendency to also elevate HDL levels.

There continues to be debate on how important saturated fat intake is in terms of the progression and incidence of cardiovascular disease. Some studies show a direct link between high levels of saturated fat intake and heart disease while others do not. Over the past half-century, national dietary recommendations have emphasized the need to cut down on total dietary fat intake as a means for preventing heart disease and obesity. The USDA has been surveying US households for over forty years and recording their dietary habits. From 1965 to 1995, total energy from dietary fat decreased from 43.7 percent to 33.1 percent. Saturated fat intake has similarly declined from 13.3 percent to 11.3 percent from 1985 to 1995.[69] Yet, despite these reductions, the prevalence of coronary artery disease has continued to climb, as has the epidemic of obesity and diabetes. The diets in The Program all have relatively high total fat content, but saturated fat is not the primary source of this fat. Your saturated fat intake should not exceed approximately one-third of your total fat calories and should come from natural sources like eggs, lean meats, poultry, and dairy products. The remainder of your fat calories should come from unsaturated and polyunsaturated sources, as we will discuss next.

---

69   Eileen T. Kennedy, Shanthy A. Bowman, and Renee Powell. Dietary-Fat Intake in the US Population. J. Am. Coll. Nutr. 1999 18: 207–212.

Food	Lauric acid	Palmitic acid	Stearic acid
Coconut oil	47%	9%	3%
Salmon	0%	29%	3%
Soybean oil	0%	11%	4%
Cashews	2%	10%	7%
Eggs	0%	27%	10%
Butter	3%	29%	13%
Ground beef	0%	26%	15%
Dark chocolate	0%	34%	43%

Trans Fats

Trans fats, also known as partially hydrogenated vegetable oil, are common additives in a variety of foods. They occur naturally in very small amounts in many animal-based foods, like dairy and meats, but the vast majority of trans fats in our diet are manmade. Artificial trans fats for human consumption were first synthesized in the early 1900s. The process was applied to a variety of oils like olive, fish, palm, and cottonseed to produce more solid and more stable fats. These new fats had much longer shelf lives, were easy to bake with, and were relatively easy and cheap to produce. As a result, their use has become rampant in the fast-food, baking, and fried-food industry. In fact, one of the first widely used products to rely heavily on trans fats was Crisco, which entered the market in 1911.

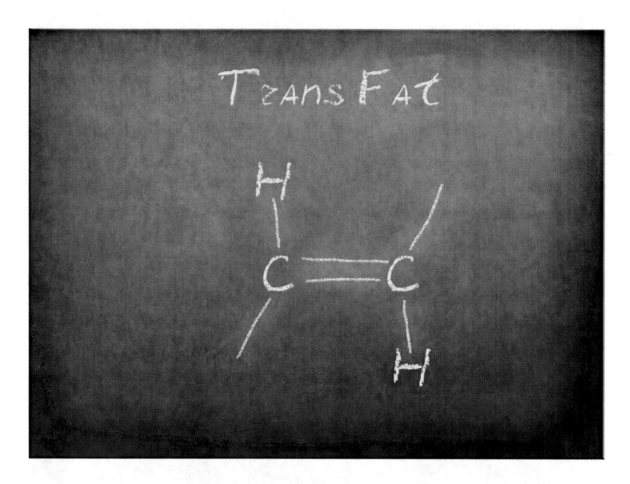

Recent research has shown a very strong link between intake of synthetic trans fats and a variety of diseases, with coronary heart disease being the most prominent. Even at low levels, intake of trans fats is associated with increased risk of heart disease. A recent study in the *New England Journal of Medicine* estimated that up to one hundred thousand deaths per year could be linked to regular consumption of trans fats.[70] Trans fats also have remarkably negative effects on blood cholesterol profiles, which likely contribute to its role in cardiovascular deaths. The effects of trans fats on cholesterol are universally negative. They raise LDL (bad) cholesterol and lower HDL (good) cholesterol, and they do so to a far greater extent than saturated fats. If that weren't bad enough, a number of animal studies have demonstrated that high intake of trans fats can lower healthy sperm counts and unfavorably alter breast milk leading to changes in offspring's brains that persist into adulthood.[71] Trans fats remain in the bloodstream longer than other fats and, therefore, are more likely to be deposited into artery-clogging plaques. Because of their relative scarcity in nature, lipase, the major enzyme used to break down fats, did not evolve the ability to effectively break down Trans fats as it does other types of fats. The body, therefore, deals with them as best it can. They are processed and readily incorporated into cell membranes and adversely affect the synthesis of a variety of essential substances, including essential fatty acids and cholesterol. If that weren't bad enough, trans fats also contribute to insulin resistance. When incorporated into the lipid bilayer that forms the wall

70   Mozaffarian D, Katan MB, Ascherio A, Stampfer MJ, Willett WC (April 2006). "Trans Fatty Acids and Cardiovascular Disease". New England Journal of Medicine 354 (15): 1601–1613.
71   Albuquerque KT, Sardinha FL, Telles MM, Watanabe RL, Nascimento CM, Tavares do Carmo MG, Ribeiro EB. Intake of trans fatty acid-rich hydrogenated fat during pregnancy and lactation inhibits the hypophagic effect of central insulin in the adult offspring. Nutrition. 2006 Jul-Aug;22(7-8):820–9.

surrounding all your cells, they alter the function of insulin receptors thereby decreasing the cells' sensitivity to insulin. This is precisely the opposite of what you want to occur.

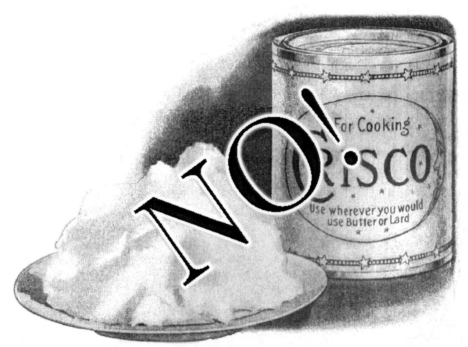

Crisco—Better than butter for cooking

Trans fats serve no biological purpose in the human body. They are neither essential nor helpful in any metabolic process. Their presence constitutes a purely negative influence in all cases; therefore, they should be completely avoided. Fortunately, most of the high trans fats foods available on the market are off-limits on The Program for other reasons, usually excess carbohydrate content, so you won't be eating them anyway. Given their thoroughly negative effects, avoiding them altogether, even on your "junk food" days, would be a good idea. Having said that, there is some evidence that the trans fats found in nature, primarily from animal sources, may not be as bad for you as synthetic trans fats. It appears that natural trans fats, while still raising total cholesterol, may not lower HDL to the degree that synthetic trans fats do.[72] More research is needed before any firm guidelines can be given. For now, it's probably best to limit your synthetic trans fat intake to as close to zero as possible and try to keep your natural trans fat intake to an absolute minimum.

Trans Fats and the Law

In 2003, the FDA passed regulations requiring food manufacturers to list the trans fat content on foods sold in the United States. Prior to 2003, the trans fat content of a given food item would have to be estimated or could be inferred by looking at the ingredient list and identifying the words "partially hydrogenated vegetable oil" buried somewhere within it. While this legislation is certainly helpful, there is one

---

72   Motard-Belanger A, Study of the effect of *trans* fatty acids from ruminants on blood lipids and other risk factors for cardiovascular disease. *The American Journal of Clinical Nutrition*, 2008; vol 87: pp 593–599.

caveat that you must keep in mind when reading these labels. The law requires that the amount of trans fat be documented if it equals or exceeds 0.5 grams *per serving*. If less than 0.5 grams, then the manufacturer is allowed to list the trans-fat content of a single serving as zero. The loophole here is obvious. If you are a food manufacturer and you want to make it seem like your product is trans fat free, then simply decrease the listed serving size until the trans-fat content is less than 0.5 grams per serving and you can legally claim your product has "zero trans fat per serving." Since most products packaged in this way contain multiple serving sizes and people rarely eat just one serving, it is still possible to be duped into consuming a large amount of trans fat. Therefore, you still have to read labels. Look for the phrase *"partially hydro-genated…"* in the list of ingredients. If you see that ingredient in your food, then simply do not eat it. You would be surprised by the number of foods whose labels claim zero trans fats per serving that still contain partially hydrogenated oils in their ingredient lists.

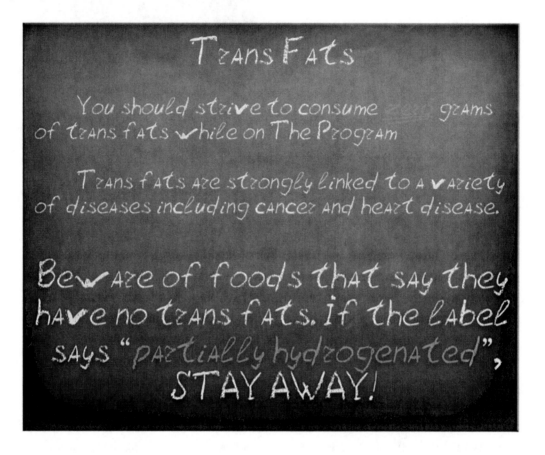

The push against trans fats by a number of consumer groups has led various cities and counties to ban their use altogether. Tiburon, California, became the first US city to voluntarily ban trans fats in all eighteen of its restaurants. In 2006, New York became the first major city to ban use of trans fats for frying foods in its restaurants. Philadelphia has followed suit, and its restaurants and eateries must discontinue using trans fats for frying foods. In 2008, California became the first state to ban trans fats from its restaurants. Many more cities, counties, and states are considering similar legislation. A reasonably up-to-date list can be found here: http://www.bantransfats.com/.

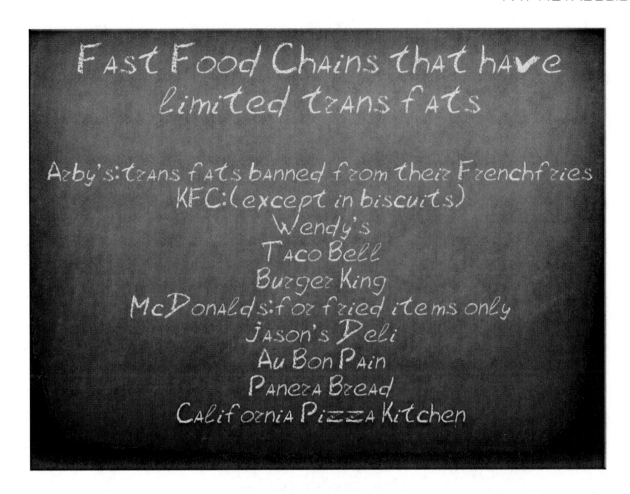

Fast Food Chains that have limited trans fats

Arby's: trans fats banned from their Frenchfries
KFC: (except in biscuits)
Wendy's
Taco Bell
Burger King
McDonalds: for fried items only
Jason's Deli
Au Bon Pain
Panera Bread
California Pizza Kitchen

In response to the anti-trans-fat bandwagon, a number of American fast-food chains have instituted voluntary bans on trans fats in a their restaurants. Many are switching to canola oil for use in their fryers.

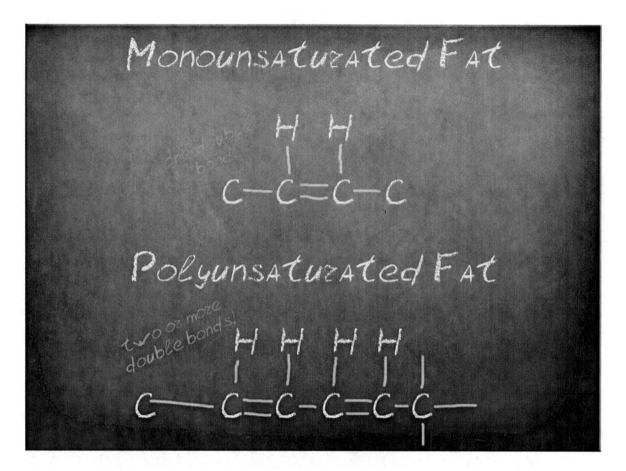

Monounsaturated Fats

Monounsaturated fats contain a single double bond in their carbon chain. They are found in a variety of foods, including almonds, pecans, peanuts, and cashews. They are also common in vegetable foods like avocados and in various oils, such as olive oil, sunflower oil, and safflower oil. The human body can also produce monounsaturated fats from saturated fat. The single double bond found in monounsaturated fats gives the molecule a distinctive "kink" or bend at the position of the double bond. This makes it difficult for them to stack neatly on top of each other like saturated fats do. As a result, monounsaturated fats are usually in liquid form at room temperature as compared to saturated fats, which are largely solid. Two common monounsaturated fats found in various foods are oleic acid and erucic acid. These are also sometimes referred to as omega-9 fatty acids. Like other monounsaturated fats, the omega-9 fatty acids are not considered essential because during times of dietary deficiency, they can be synthesized by the body from omega-3 and omega-6 fatty acids.

Monounsaturated fats are found in natural foods, such as nuts and avocados, and are the main component of tea seed oil and olive oil (oleic acid). Canola oil is 57 to 60 percent monounsaturated fat (erucic acid), olive oil is about 75 percent monounsaturated fat, and tea seed oil is commonly over 80 percent monounsaturated fat. Other sources include rapeseed oil, ground nut oil, peanut oil, flaxseed oil, sesame oil, corn oil, popcorn, whole grain wheat, cereal, oatmeal, safflower oil, sunflower oil, and the tea oil Camellia.

Monounsaturated fats have a number of beneficial properties. Like polyunsaturated fats, regular consumption can lower blood pressure, LDL cholesterol, and overall risk for cardiovascular disease.[73] A number of studies in which calories from carbohydrate were replaced with calories from monounsaturated fats have shown similar benefits.

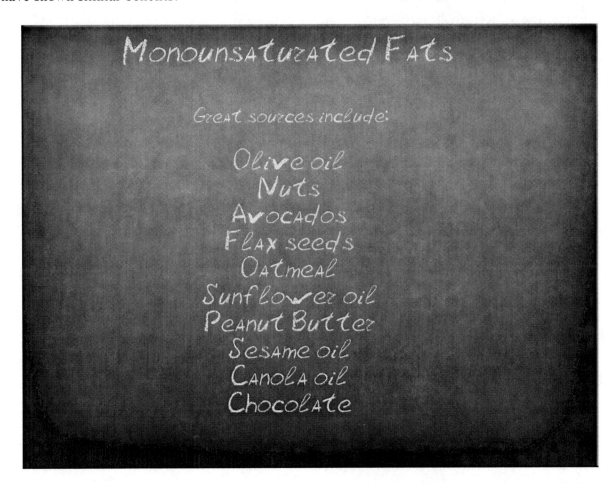

Interest in monounsaturated fats began to increase as epidemiological studies showed that populations in Europe that consumed a so-called "Mediterranean Diet" had much lower rates of heart disease than other Westerners. This was despite the fact that the traditional Mediterranean diet contained up to 40 percent of its calories from fats. This type of diet involved consumption of relatively large amounts of olive, canola, and sunflower oils, all of which are rich in oleic acid.[74] Oleic acid is an eighteen-carbon-chain fatty acid and is the most commonly known monounsaturated fatty acid. Olive oil contains approximately 75 percent oleic acid. In addition to its beneficial effects on cholesterol levels, consumption of oleic acid is also associated with decreased insulin resistance. This property alone should make food sources rich in oleic acid a primary staple of your diet no matter which eating plan you choose. You should attempt to obtain at least one-third of your total fat calories from monounsaturated sources while on The Program. Fortunately, this is quite easy since a variety of snack foods like peanuts are high in monounsaturated fats. Try adding olive oil to your recipes for additional flavor and a healthy dose of oleic acid.

73   Appel LJ, Sacks FM, Carey VJ, et al. Effects of protein, monounsaturated fat, and carbohydrate intake on blood pressure and serum lipids: results of the OmniHeart randomized trial. JAMA. 2005; 294:2455–64.
74   B E McDonald. Fatty acids and heart health. CMAJ. 1991 September 1; 145(5): 473.

As an interesting medical side note, oleic acid is one of the primary ingredients in Lorenzo's oil. Lorenzo's oil, which is composed of four parts oleic acid and one part erucic acid, is used in the treatment of the rare genetic disease known as adrenoleukodystrophy (ALD). Lorenzo was a young boy who suffered from this disease, which was, at the time, an untreatable condition. His parents, unwilling to accept their doctors' grim prognosis, scoured the medical literature and eventually formulated this blend of monounsaturated fatty acids, which, while not a cure, was able to greatly slow the progression of this terrible disease.

Polyunsaturated Fats

Polyunsaturated fatty acids, as the name implies, have more than one pair of double bonds. Polyunsaturated fats are also termed "essential" fats because, unlike other fats, the human body cannot manufacture them. They must be obtained through the diet. Polyunsaturated fats come in two basic varieties: Omega-6 and Omega-3. They are named based on the position of the last double bond in relation to the last carbon in the molecule (omega meaning "last" in Greek). For example, in omega-6 acids, the double bond is six carbon atoms from the end of the molecule. In omega-3 fatty acids, it is three carbon atoms from the end.

Polyunsaturated fat molecules, like monounsaturated fats, have numerous kinks or twists in their structure. This makes them prefer a liquid state, even when refrigerated. Unfortunately, the unpaired electrons in their double bonds also make unsaturated fats highly reactive with other compounds and thus they spoil easily in heat or when exposed to sunlight. For this reason, these fats are often stored in dark bottles and should not be used for cooking. Like monounsaturated fats, polyunsaturated fats have a very favorable cardiovascular profile. They raise HDL, lower LDL, improve insulin sensitivity, and will help you lose body fat while dieting. Polyunsaturated fats should be a major portion of your fat calories.

Omega-3 and omega-6 fatty acids are the precursors to a wide variety of compounds known as eicosanoids. Eicosanoids are twenty-carbon molecules that mediate a myriad of bodily functions. Eicosanoids both activate and suppress the immune system and cause smooth muscles in the gut, uterus, and bronchi to contract or relax. They can alter the blood's ability to clot as well as modulate the perception of pain. Eicosanoids are considered by many scientists to be the most important signaling molecules in the body. As a result, there is intense ongoing research into their roles in both preventing and exacerbating chronic diseases like rheumatoid arthritis, asthma, coronary disease, and many others.

The body attempts to maintain a delicate balance between competing metabolic processes. In the blood, for example, there are numerous biochemical reactions (many influenced by eicosanoids) that promote blood clotting. Obviously, the blood's ability to form clots is absolutely vital for survival. Any defect in the complex pathways that lead to blood clotting can leave a person vulnerable to life-threatening hemorrhage from even minor trauma (as often occurred in hemophiliacs before the widespread availability of synthetic clotting factors). The tendency of blood to clot, while helpful during times of injury, can be detrimental at other times. In order to navigate the tiny capillaries, blood must flow smoothly and not become too viscous. Therefore, there are competing chemical processes that inhibit blood clotting and promote the smooth flow of blood through even the tiniest blood vessels. The body constantly attempts to maintain a balance between these two competing tendencies. This sort of yin versus yang balance is known as homeostasis, i.e., the maintenance of an optimal environment in which the body is able to operate. Eicosanoids play a crucial role in maintaining homeostasis. In general, eicosanoids derived from omega-6 sources promote inflammation, smooth muscle constriction, cell proliferation, and blood clotting. Omega-3 derived eicosanoids do just the opposite. Therefore, maintaining as near an equal ratio of omega-3 to omega-6 fats in the diet is ideal. The current Western diet greatly exceeds the required amount of omega-6 fatty acids while generally being low in omega-3 fatty acids. In some regions, the ratio of omega-6 to omega-3 is as high as 20:1. This imbalance has been linked to numerous chronic disease states. Several studies have shown that as this ratio is lowered in favor of greater omega-3 intake, rates of chronic disease decline. In studies looking at the prevention of cardiovascular disease in patients who already had heart disease, decreasing the omega-6 to omega-3 ratio to 4:1 was associated with a 70 percent decrease in total mortality. A ratio of 2.5:1, reduced rectal cell proliferation in patients with colorectal cancer. A lower omega-6 to omega-3 ratio in women at risk for breast cancer may decrease the rate of malignancy. A ratio of 2–3:1 suppressed inflammation in patients with rheumatoid arthritis, and a ratio of 5:1 had a beneficial effect on patients with asthma, whereas a ratio of 10:1 actually worsened symptoms.[75]

Ever since mankind's transition from a hunter-gatherer existence to a more pastoral, farming existence, the amount of omega-6 fatty acids in the diet have increased while the amount of omega-3 fatty acids has decreased. Hunter-gatherers who consumed foraged nuts, vegetables, fruits, and hunted wild game had a near equal ratio of omega-6 to omega-3 fatty acids in their diets. As populations became more agricultural, they replaced much of their meat intake with cereals and grains. The meat they did consume was often from domesticated animals that were fed vastly different diets than their wild counterparts. Wild game has nearly equal levels of omega-3 and omega-6 fatty acids.[76] The meat you buy at the supermarket today has very likely been fattened up on a high-calorie grain-based diet. This has resulted in a marked increase in the omega-6 fatty acid content. Similarly, farm-raised fish have greater amounts of omega-6 fats than their wild counterparts.

On all three eating plans presented in The Program, you should attempt to consume as close to equal parts omega-6 and omega-3 fatty acids as possible. This can be difficult (but not impossible) to do without some sort of supplementation program. Fish oil capsules as well as flaxseed oil are two sources of omega-3 fatty acids that are readily available. I like to add flaxseed oil to my protein shakes. I find that it mixes fairly well and is far more palatable when combined with other ingredients. Both flaxseed oil and fish oil spoil rather quickly when exposed to air and sunlight. Be sure to purchase products that are packaged in air-tight, opaque containers. Both should be refrigerated to help prolong their shelf life and prevent spoiling.

Omega-6 Fatty Acids

The omega-6 fatty acids include linoleic acid (LA), arachadonic acid (AA), gamma linoleic acid (GLA), and dihomogamma linoleic acid (DGLA). The primary source of omega-6 fatty acids in the diet is LA. Using various enzymes, the human body converts LA into GLA and then into DGLA. DGLA is then converted to AA. LA is found in high concentrations in sunflower, safflower, and corn oils as well as avocados. Evening primrose oil and borage oil are also high in both LA and GLA.

---

75   Simopoulos AP. The importance of the ratio of omega-6/omega-3 essential fatty acids. Biomed Pharmacother. 2002 Oct; 56(8):365–79.

76   Medeiro, L.C. 2002. Nutritional content of game meat. B-920R. College of Agriculture, University of Wyoming USDA Nutrient Database.

AA is converted via various enzymes into a host of biologically active molecules known as prostaglandins. These molecules are largely responsible for a variety of pro-inflammatory processes. When you take ibuprofen or aspirin, you are inhibiting one of these enzymes and preventing the production of prostaglandins that lead to swelling, pain, and other inflammatory changes. It is theorized that excessive consumption of omega-6 fatty acids in relation to omega-3 fatty acids can shift the balance in favor of a pro-inflammatory state. LA and the omega-3 fatty acid alpha linolenic acid (ALA) both compete for the same two enzymes that lead to the formation of longer-chain fatty acids. These enzymes (elastase and desaturase) prefer ALA to LA. When both substances are consumed in roughly equal proportion, the net result is to keep inflammation in check. When large amounts of LA are consumed, however, this preference is negated and the amount of LA converted to AA is increased relative to the conversion of ALA.[77]

Chronic inflammation is increasingly being recognized as playing a role in a wide variety of diseases, including atherosclerosis, rheumatoid arthritis, stroke, and certain cancers.[78] It is known that supplementing both human and animal diets with arachadonic acid increases its levels in the cell membranes of inflammatory white blood cells. Therefore, while omega-6 fatty acids are essential for survival, excessive consumption could potentially lead to a variety of disease states. Given the abundance of omega-6 fatty acids available in the modern diet, it is rare that one would require specific supplementation of LA.

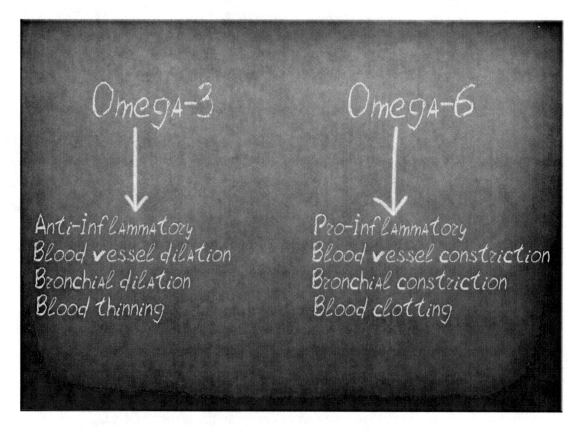

77   Burdge G. Alpha-linolenic acid metabolism in men and women: nutritional and biological implications. Curr Opin Clin Nutr Metab Care. 2004;7(2):137–144.
78   Calder, Philip C. (June 2006). "n–3 polyunsaturated fatty acids, inflammation, and inflammatory diseases." American Journal of Clinical Nutrition 83 (6, supplement): 1505S–1519S.

Omega-3 Fatty Acids

Omega-3 fatty acids have received a lot of scientific and media attention lately for their purported health benefits. Like omega-6 fatty acids, the omega-3 fatty acids are derived from a parent compound that cannot be synthesized by the human body and must be obtained from dietary sources. The most common omega-3 fatty acids encountered in the Western diet are alpha-linolenic acid (ALA), docosapentaenoic acid (DPA), eicosapentaenoic acid (EPA), and docosahexaenoic acid (DHA). ALA is found in high concentrations in green leaves, linseed, and flaxseed oils and meat from wild game. ALA can be considered a "parent-compound" because the human body, through a variety of enzymatic steps, can convert ALA into DPA and DHA. DPA, DHA, and EPA are found mostly in various fish oils as well as in algae. DHA can also be created in the human body from EPA.

Omega-3 fatty acids, like their omega-6 cousins, are involved in the production of various prostaglandins. Unlike omega-6 fatty acids, however, omega-3 fatty acids promote a net anti-inflammatory state and, therefore, help keep inflammation stimulated by omega-6 fatty acids in check.

There has been a large body of medical research showing a variety of health benefits associated with consumption of omega-3 fatty acids. Most studies have looked at supplementation with DPA and DHA or with fish consumption. In a large study of over forty-five thousand men followed for fourteen years, each one-gram-per-day increase in dietary ALA intake was associated with a 16 percent reduction in the risk of coronary heart disease.[79] The bulk of the scientific data on EPA and DHA shows that these compounds lower the risk of heart disease through a variety of different mechanisms. Both are able to lower blood triglyceride levels. At dosages of two to four grams per day and higher, blood triglycerides can be lowered by up to 30 percent. EPA and DHA also decrease the risk of blood clot formation and can slow the growth of cholesterol plaques in the arteries. Supplementation also improves the ability of blood vessels to contract and relax and lowers blood pressure. It can even prevent abnormal and potentially dangerous heart rhythms. DHA is heavily incorporated into the cells of the retina and plays an important role in developing and maintaining vision. Both DHA and EPA are crucial ingredients in the development of the human brain both in utero and in early childhood. All omega-3 fatty acid supplements are better absorbed when taken with meals and typically should be divided into two to three times daily routines to avoid some of the unpleasant taste and gastrointestinal effects of a single large dose.

One of the concerns raised about increasing intake of omega-3 fatty acids is that fish sources may be contaminated with various pollutants like methylmercury. This has caused some people, with good reason, to shy away from exclusively using cooked fish as their sole source of DHA and EPA. Fortunately, a number of independent laboratory studies of various US-manufactured fish oil capsules have shown that they are methylmercury free. Methylmercury and other toxins tend to accumulate in the muscle tissue preferentially. Since fish oil is derived from fatty tissue, it is virtually methylmercury free.[80]

---

79   Mozaffarian D, Ascherio A, Hu FB, et al. Interplay between different polyunsaturated fatty acids and risk of coronary heart disease in men. Circulation. 2005;111(2):157–164.
80   Fish or pills? Consumer Reports. 2003;68(7):30–32.

Good Sources of Polyunsaturated Fatty Acids

Food	% Polyunsaturated Fatty Acids
Safflower oil	74%
Walnut oil	70%
Sunflower oil	63%
Corn oil	51%
Vegetable oil	48%
Walnuts	47%
Sesame oil	44%
Mayonnaise	44%
Sunflower margarine	37%
Low fat spread	10%

There has been some controversy regarding whether consuming ALA from flax and other sources is just as good as consuming DHA and EPA directly in the form of fish oil capsules or in cod liver oil. As discussed, ALA is converted through a variety of enzymatic steps into DHA and EPA. Unfortunately, the conversion is not terribly efficient. In men, approximately 8 percent of dietary ALA is converted to EPA and up to 4 percent is converted to DHA. Women are actually more efficient at this process than men, and they convert about 21 percent of ALA to EPA and 9 percent to DHA.[81] In most cases, there is no significant difference between these two sources. As long as you are otherwise healthy, consuming either source will be beneficial. As we will discuss in the following section, there are a few instances when consuming EPA and DHA directly might be more advantageous. If you are really trying to cut calories on the Endomorphic Diet, you can consume a much smaller amount of fish oil for a given amount of EPA/DHA as compared to flaxseed oil. Some people just can't stand the taste of flaxseed oil, and for them, using fish oil capsules or perhaps cod liver oil is the way to go.

---

81 . Burdge GC, Jones AE, Wootton SA. Eicosapentaenoic and docosapentaenoic acids are the principal products of alpha-linolenic acid metabolism in young men*. Br J Nutr. 2002;88(4):355–364.

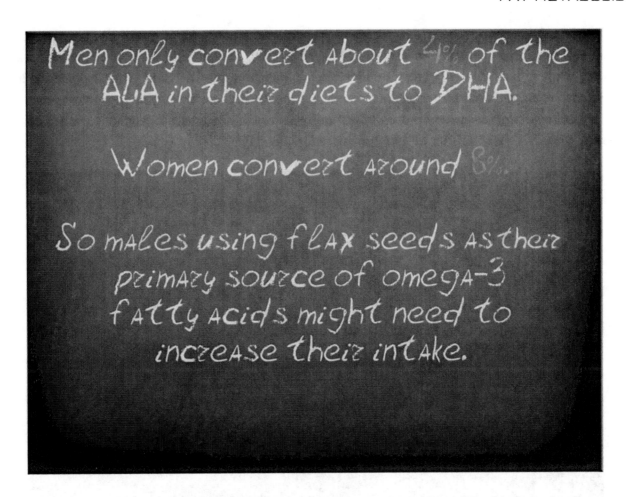

Men only convert about 4% of the ALA in their diets to DHA.

Women convert around 8%.

So males using flax seeds as their primary source of omega-3 fatty acids might need to increase their intake.

So how much EPA and DHA should you take in every day? The World Health Organization recommends between 0.3 to 0.5 grams of EPA+DHA per day for healthy adults. The American Heart Association doesn't provide specific recommendations for healthy adults other than to suggest that you eat some sort of fatty fish twice a week and that you use oils that are high in ALA like flax, canola, and soybean oils. Reviewing the medical literature allows us to make somewhat more specific recommendations, however. There have been a number of trials looking at how DHA and EPA supplementation affects the growth of cholesterol plaques in patients with heart disease. It is these plaques that ultimately lead to the narrowing of the heart's blood vessels, choking off the supply of blood and eventually leading to heart attacks. A procedure known as cardiac catheterization allows doctors to directly measure the degree of narrowing in patients' blood vessels caused by atherosclerotic plaques. With repeated procedures, the growth of these plaques can be measured and the results of various interventions to slow or even reverse their growth can be evaluated. In one particularly interesting study, patients with heart disease were given three grams total of DHA+EPA supplements for three months and then 1.5 grams for an additional twenty-one months.[82] When compared to patients receiving a placebo, the patients getting omega-3 fatty acids had less progression of their plaque size and tended to actually reduce the size of their plaques. As a result of this study and several others like it, while on The Program, the recommendation will be to consume a minimum of two grams per day total of DHA and EPA. You should consider consuming more if you have very high triglyceride levels on your cholesterol panel. Higher doses in the range of three to five grams per day can

---

82   Von Schacky C, Angerer P, Kothny W, et al. The effect of dietary omega-3 fatty acids on coronary atherosclerosis: a randomized, double-blind, placebo-controlled trial. Ann Intern Med. 1999; 130:554–562.

lower blood triglyceride levels by 25 percent to 30 percent.[83] That level of intake can also bump your LDL cholesterol 5 to 10 percent and minimally raise your HDL as well. This level of intake isn't usually necessary while you are following the Endomorphic or Mesomorphic Diet since your triglyceride levels will plummet from carbohydrate restriction and intense training alone. However, if you have a genetic tendency toward high triglyceride levels or a strong family history of heart disease, you may want to consider increasing your DHA+EPA closer to four grams or more per day.

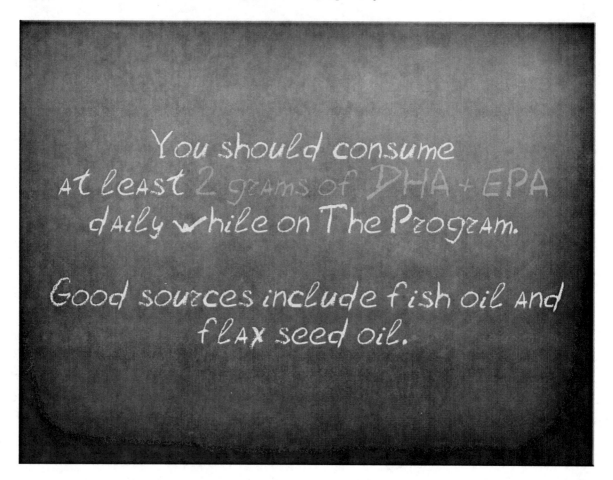

The average DHA+EPA content in commercially available fish oil capsules varies. Most have around 180 to 500 milligrams of EPA and 120 to 300 milligrams of DHA per capsule. There are more concentrated varieties available, however, that contain over 1000 milligrams of EPA and 700 milligrams of DHA. This is probably the easiest way to meet your daily goal for omega-3 intake. Be sure to purchase your capsules in sealed plastic or dark glass containers. Both light and air can rapidly cause fish oil to become rancid. You should periodically chew one of your capsules to be sure they are fresh. If you get a rancid one, you will know it! If that happens, I'd recommend throwing the rest of the bottle out and switching brands.

If swallowing fish oil capsules just isn't for you, then consider supplementing with flaxseed oil. I actually like the taste of flax and find that it mixes easily into the protein shakes I have for breakfast each morning. The relatively low conversion of ALA will mean that you will have to add a fair amount of flaxseed oil to your diet to meet the two-gram-per-day of DHA+EPA goal, but if divided throughout the day,

---

83   Harris WS. n-3 Fatty acids and serum lipoproteins: human studies. Am J Clin Nutr. 1997; 65(5 Suppl):1645S–1654S.

this is fairly tolerable for most individuals. Most flaxseed oils contain about 7.5 grams of ALA per tablespoon (15 milliliters). For a healthy male, one tablespoon of flaxseed oil would then be converted to about 600 milligrams of EPA and 300 milligrams of DHA. Women, being more efficient at this conversion, will get about 1575 milligrams of EPA and 675 milligrams of DHA per tablespoon of flaxseed oil. Therefore, only approximately 2.2 tablespoons of flax per day for men and just over 1 tablespoon for women will be enough to meet the goal of a combined DHA+EPA daily intake of two grams.

Most flaxseed oil preparations also contain ground flaxseed. Ground flax has high concentrations of other important compounds known as lignans (also referred to as phytoestrogens). Lignans can also be found in high concentration in legumes and whole grains. Plant lignans are converted in the intestines by bacteria into the mammalian lignans known as enterodiol and enterolactone. The ability of these lignans to weakly bind to estrogen receptors and therefore potentially block some of the effects of endogenous estrogen has led to a number of research studies examining whether or not consuming lignans could have an effect on various hormone-sensitive cancers like breast and prostate cancer. It is also theorized that their weak estrogen-like effect could help maintain bone density in women as they age. Without going into all the details of these studies, there remains controversy over whether or not lignans have cancer-fighting benefits. There doesn't seem to be any evidence that lignans from plant sources are harmful. For those men out there concerned about consuming anything that is even remotely related to estrogen, don't worry. Studies looking at lignan intake have shown that they have no effect on serum testosterone or estrogen levels.[84]

If neither fish oil capsules nor flaxseed oil are your cup of tea, then cod liver oil is another option for boosting your DHA and EPA intake. Traditionally, cod liver oil has had a fishy taste that most people find unpalatable, but now a variety of both flavored and virtually flavorless preparations are available. Cod liver oil is rich in EPA and DHA. Most formulations contain about 400 milligrams of EPA and 625 milligrams of DHA per teaspoon (5 milliliters). Cod liver oil is also rich in vitamins A and D. The only potential problem with using cod liver oil to obtain high levels of omega-3 acids, especially if you plan on taking more than two grams per day, is the potential for excessive vitamin A intake. Vitamin A, though vital for a variety of processes, including healthy vision, is fat-soluble and therefore can build up in the body and cause toxicity. Read the label of your particular brand of cod liver oil carefully. Some preparations have as much as 1500 IU of vitamin A per teaspoon. The generally recommended upper limit of healthy intake is about 3000 IU for adults. Generally, toxicity is associated with much higher amounts (up to 25,000 IU per day), but it is not known if chronic ingestion of lower amounts could lead to problems. Vitamin A toxicity typically manifests in vague symptoms, such as hair loss, fatigue, nausea, dry skin, and dizziness. Don't let this dissuade you from using cod liver oil if you prefer it over fish oil capsules or flaxseed oil, just be cautious not to overdo it.

If you are serious fish lover, you could eschew fish oil capsules, flaxseed oil, and cod liver oil in favor of getting your daily dose DHA and EPA by eating fish. Not all species of fish have the same levels of DHA and EPA. Small, oily fish like sardines and anchovies, as well as larger fish like mackerel, bass,

---

84   Frishce, et al. Effect of Flaxseed and Wheat Bran on Serum Hormones and Lignan Excretion in Premenopausal Women. Journal of the American College of Nutrition, Vol 22, No.6, 550–554 (2003).

and herring are particularly rich in omega-3 fatty acids. Consult the included list of average DHA+EPA for various fish species to see which of your favorite fish you can include in your diet.

The primary concern with obtaining the bulk of your DHA+EPA from eating fish is the level of pollutants like methylmercury that can be found in wild fish. Large, long-lived predatory fish tend to have the highest levels of mercury. This makes sense since big fish get big by eating smaller fish, which over time concentrates more and more toxins in their tissues. The longer they live, the more opportunities they have to eat other fish contaminated with methylmercury. For this reason, the FDA recommends that people completely avoid eating shark, king mackerel, or tilefish (a.k.a. golden bass or golden snapper). These fish are particularly high in methylmercury. They recommend eating no more than twelve ounces of low-mercury fish like shrimp, canned light tuna, salmon, pollock, and catfish per week.[85] This works out to about two meals per week. The problem here is that if you stick to these guidelines, you will fall well short of the recommended two grams per day of EPA+DHA. Is there any way around this? The answer is yes. There is one particular fish that is both low in methylmercury and high in DHA and EPA. That fish is the sardine. Sardines have about 0.016 micrograms of methylmercury per gram.[86] There are various recommendations for the maximum safe daily amount of methylmercury that can be consumed. A conservative estimate is about thirty micrograms per day. Now, since the average can of sardines contains about one hundred grams of fish, this translates into only 1.6 micrograms of methylmercury per can. That same one-hundred-gram serving also contains 982 milligrams of DHA+EPA. Eating about two servings per day of sardines would get you pretty close to the required daily two-gram goal. Sardines aren't for everybody. For some, they just taste too "fishy," but for those of you who enjoy them, they are probably the safest way to get your daily DHA and EPA by eating fish.

---

85   www.fda.gov/oc/opacom/hottopics/mercury/backgrounder.html.
86   http://www.cfsan.fda.gov/~frf/sea-mehg.html.

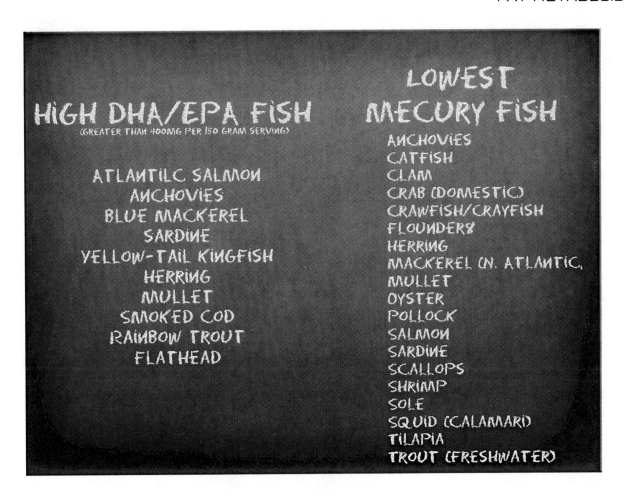

HIGH DHA/EPA FISH
(GREATER THAN 400MG PER 150 GRAM SERVING)

ATLANTILC SALMON
ANCHOVIES
BLUE MACKEREL
SARDINE
YELLOW-TAIL KINGFISH
HERRING
MULLET
SMOKED COD
RAINBOW TROUT
FLATHEAD

LOWEST MECURY FISH
ANCHOVIES
CATFISH
CLAM
CRAB (DOMESTIC)
CRAWFISH/CRAYFISH
FLOUNDER8
HERRING
MACKEREL (N. ATLANTIC,
MULLET
OYSTER
POLLOCK
SALMON
SARDINE
SCALLOPS
SHRIMP
SOLE
SQUID (CALAMARI)
TILAPIA
TROUT (FRESHWATER)

Chia Seeds

Chia (*Salvia hispanica* L.) seeds are an excellent source of both polyunsaturated fats as well as fiber. Chia was a main staple of the diet of Mesoamerican Indians in pre-Columbian times. Chia seeds contain the highest percentage of ALA (50 to 70 percent) and linoleic acid (17 to 26 percent) of any plant source. Like flax, they are high in both fiber and protein, but have a more neutral flavor. They incorporate very well into shakes, smoothies, yogurt, and baked goods. A typical 12-gram (1 tablespoon) serving of chia seeds contains 2.5 grams of polyunsaturated fats divided between linoleic and linolenic acid, 5 grams of fiber, 3 grams of protein, and virtually no net carbohydrates. Chia seeds, like flax, are a great addition to all the diets in The Program but particularly when you are trying to keep your carbohydrate intake low.

DIFFERENT TYPES OF BODY FAT

Adipose tissue serves a variety of functions. The most well-known adipose tissue functions to store energy in the form of triglycerides. Fat also has a myriad of other less well-known functions that include insulation and protection of the internal organs and the secretion of various hormones. When most of us think of fat, we think of relatively inert blobs of tissue that, if given the choice, we would mostly like to get rid of entirely. The truth is that fat tissue is far more metabolically active than once thought. Fat also comes in two distinct varieties: brown fat and white fat. White fat is the fat that most of us are familiar with. It makes up over 90 percent of adult fat stores and is widely distributed throughout the body, both directly under the skin and around our internal organs. Brown fat is a less well known type of fat that is found predominantly in young mammals. Its primary purpose is the generation of heat, and it has evolved as a key survival tool for infants to resist hypothermia.[87] Brown fat, as its name implies, has a brownish tinge owing to its increased vascularity and densely packed energy-producing mitochondria. Inside these mitochondria, there are special proteins that "uncouple" the normal process of oxidative phosphorylation so that instead of producing ATP, heat is generated instead. Rather than being widely distributed like white fat, brown fat is most dense in human infants in the area of the shoulders and upper back, the chest around the heart, and around the kidneys and adrenal glands.

For decades, it has been assumed that in humans, nearly all brown fat eventually atrophies and disappears in the first few years of life. Therefore, it has not been thought to play any significant role in heat generation or in the overall metabolism of human adults. Recent research, however, has shown that this may not be the case. Researchers looking for ways to image malignant tumors with PET scans stumbled across symmetric areas of increased metabolic activity in the upper shoulders and chest of study volunteers.[88] Since malignancies rarely grow symmetrically throughout the body, this increased activity must be originating from some yet undiscovered metabolically active tissue. Further study revealed that this tissue

---

87   Albright, A.L. and Stern, J.S. (1998). Adipose tissue. In: Encyclopedia of Sports Medicine and Science, T.D. Fahey (Editor). Internet Society for Sport Science: http://sportsci.org.

88   Belhocine T, Shastry A, Driedger A, Urbain JL. Detection of (99m)Tc-sestamibi uptake in brown adipose tissue with SPECT-CT. Eur J Nucl Med Mol Imaging 34: 149.

was indeed brown fat, and that in many adults this tissue, while greatly reduced in size as compared to what it was earlier, was still present and metabolically active, though not as active as it was during infancy.

Brown fat is stimulated through two basic mechanisms. The first is cold exposure. A drop in skin temperature signals the nervous system to begin producing more body heat. In adults, this is primarily achieved through shivering and stimulation of heat-conserving behaviors. Brown fat, however, still plays a role and has been shown to increase its metabolic activity in response to cold. The second way brown fat is stimulated is via stimulation from both endogenous and exogenous beta-receptor agonists. The human body produces a variety of these substances. Epinephrine and norepinephrine (often referred to as cat-echolamines) are the most well known. Brown fat is rich in beta-receptors of which there are three types: beta-1, beta-2, and beta-3. Brown fat contains all three types with beta-3 receptors predominating. In fact, beta-3 receptors are found almost exclusively in brown fat. When these receptors are stimulated, brown fat kicks into gear and begins burning fat and producing heat. It is beyond the scope of this chapter to go into all the details regarding the differences between the three receptor types and their effects. A simple but reasonable way to think of them is that beta-1 receptors are primarily responsible for cardiac effects, such as increased heart rate. Beta-2 receptors cause smooth muscle dilation and result in dilation of the bronchi as well as blood vessels, whereas beta-3 receptors, though not fully understood, appear to play a primary role in stimulating heat production from brown fat.

For some time now, athletes have been using various drugs that bind to the beta-receptor to stimulate fat loss. The most common of these drugs is ephedra, which is commonly taken in conjunction with caffeine and aspirin to potentiate its effects. A number of studies have shown that this combination of drugs can indeed stimulate thermogenesis and lead to increased fat loss. The problem with ephedra is that it is not particularly selective for the beta-3 receptor. There are prescription drugs like clenbuterol and various research drugs that better stimulate this receptor, but they are very difficult, if not impossible, to obtain in the United States legally. Ephedrine stimulates all three beta-receptors and therefore causes increased heart rate and blood pressure in addition to its fat-burning properties. As a result, many individuals experience side effects from ephedra use. Because of its nonselective beta receptor activity, there has even been some question about whether the fat lost stimulated by ephedra use is even a result of brown fat stimulation at all. One study in particular showed that ephedra did indeed stimulate brown fat thermogenesis but that its effects on skeletal muscle were significantly greater.[89] As it stands now, ephedra remains the only readily available agent to increase brown fat metabolism. Training in the cold will obviously stimulate your brown fat reserves as well, but it is very unlikely that this will result in significant enough weight loss to justify the increased risk of injury and general unpleasantness of prolonged exposure to cold.

---

89   A. Astrup, et al. Contribution of BAT and skeletal muscle to thermogenesis induced by ephedrine in man. Endocrinology and Metabolism, Vol 248, Issue 5 507–E515.

"Always rise
to an early meal,
but eat your fill before a feast.
If you're hungry
you have no time
to talk at the table".

- The Havamal

FOOD AND EXERCISE AS A DRUG: EFFECTS ON HORMONES

Most people recognize that drugs, both prescription and over the counter, can have significant effects on the human body. Anti-inflammatory drugs like ibuprofen work by inhibiting the creation of certain types of signaling chemicals known as prostaglandins. Antidepressants work by changing the levels of brain chemicals known as neurotransmitters. Most people are surprised to learn that food and exercise have equally, if not more, profound effects on the body's chemistry. Understanding this fact will change the way you look at food and exercise forever. Food becomes not just necessary fuel, not just something enjoyable, but something you can manipulate to create certain outcomes in the body. In the same way, exercise can be varied in intensity, duration, and timing to enact desirable changes in the body's chemistry as well.

It is widely accepted that a variety of hormones play key roles in the building of lean muscle tissue and the burning of fat. Nearly everyone is aware that professional athletes across a wide range of sports utilize anabolic steroids, which are all just synthetic variations of testosterone, to build muscle mass. Recent research has shown that both diet and exercise can also have effects on testosterone levels and potentially impact one's ability to build lean muscle. Many other hormones are similarly influenced by the way one chooses to exercise and diet. Knowing this, we can then design a diet and exercise regimen that helps create an environment within the body that is optimized for the building of lean muscle and the burning of fat.

Cortisol

Cortisol, also referred to as hydrocortisone, is one of the body's primary stress hormones. Cortisol has gotten a bad rap lately, primarily to due to outright fraudulent advertising for various nutritional supplements that claim to "regulate" cortisol. Cortisol has been blamed for every sort of malady from fatigue to abdominal weight gain. The truth is that cortisol plays crucial roles in helping the body adapt to both physical and emotional stressors. Without cortisol, even minor illnesses or injuries could often be fatal. Cortisol helps stimulate the production of glucose in the liver, raises blood glucose levels, increases the oxidation of fatty acids, and elevates blood levels of amino acids. Cortisol also has potent anti-inflammatory properties. Except in a few specific diseases, the body tightly controls the production and release of cortisol into the bloodstream. Precisely the right amount is produced to help you adapt to the stresses your body is undergoing. Rather than being a deleterious substance, as the hawkers of certain bogus supplements would like you to believe, cortisol is a vital, life-saving hormone that is essential for your survival.

It has been known for some time that exercise is a potent stimulus for the secretion of cortisol. This makes sense as exercise presents the body with a physiologic form of stress. Cortisol aids in both the short-term and long-term adaption to repetitive bouts of exercise.

Both low-intensity, aerobic exercise as well as high-intensity exercise stimulate the release of cortisol. Not surprisingly, high-intensity exercise, like what you will be performing while on The Program, produces a greater cortisol response than lower-intensity exercise. In fact, anaerobic exercise, like weight-lifting and sprinting, produces a greater cortisol response than aerobic exercise of a similar duration.[90] It is also interesting to note that the amount of cortisol secreted during exercise is independent of one's fitness level. You don't secrete less or more as you get in better shape. Older athletes do tend to secrete less cortisol in response to heavy-resistance exercise than younger athletes do. This has implications for recovery ability and may partially explain why older athletes need to take additional rest days or decrease the volume of their training relative to their younger counterparts.[91] Surprisingly, there doesn't appear to be much difference between men and women in terms of cortisol levels in response to intense exercise. Men and women appear to secrete similar levels for a given amount and intensity of exercise.[92]

As cortisol rises in response to exercise, it eventually returns to baseline levels during the recovery period. In a chronically overtrained state, however, cortisol levels remain high. Additionally, the body's ability to respond to additional stress by further elevating cortisol levels appears reduced.[93] Thus, in an overtrained state, athletes may be relatively cortisol deficient despite having elevated baseline cortisol levels. This may partially explain the chronic fatigue, frequent minor illnesses, inability to maintain

90   Hackney AC, Premo MC, McMurray RG: Influence of aerobic versus anaerobic exercise on the relationship between reproductive hormones in men. *J Sports Sci* 1995; 13:305–311.

91   Häkkinen K, Pakarinen A: Acute hormonal responses to heavy resistance exercise in men and women at different ages. *Int J Sports Med* 1995; 16:507–513.

92   Davis SN, Galassetti P, Wasserman DH, et al: Effects of gender on neuroendocrine and metabolic counterregulatory responses to exercise in normal man. *J Clin Endocrinol Metab* 2000; 85:224–230.

93   Uusitalo AL, Huttunen P, Hanin Y, et al: Hormonal responses to endurance training and overtraining in female athletes. Clin J Sport Med 1998:8(3);178–186.

previous training loads, overall poor performance, and higher risk of injury associated with the overtraining syndrome.

While one is consuming a very low carbohydrate ketogenic diet, cortisol levels will generally be slightly higher than when consuming a more balanced diet. This adaptation is part of the normal mechanisms that keep blood sugar constant throughout the day. Ketogenic diets appear to inhibit the amounts of cortisol lost in the urine as well as decrease its breakdown in the body[94].

Growth Hormone

Growth hormone (GH) is a 191-amino-acid-long peptide hormone secreted by the anterior pituitary gland in the brain. It has potent growth-stimulating properties. GH has its most profound effects during puberty, when it stimulates the growth of cartilage in the growth plates of long bones. A person's final adult height is greatly determined by the amount of growth hormone produced during the teenage years. Growth hormone also increases bone density, stimulates protein synthesis, and promotes the burning of fat stores. Excess GH, however, can lead to a number of serious problems. The most well known is gigantism or acromegaly. This is usually caused by a pituitary-secreting tumor that produces very high growth hormone levels. Acromegalics often reach the extremes of human height and develop characteristic large jaws and brow ridges and enlarged internal organs and often die prematurely from diabetes or heart or kidney failure. GH exerts most of its effects through specific mediators known as somatomedins, the best known of which is IGF-1. GH stimulates the synthesis and release of these hormones both in the bloodstream and local tissues.

GH use has been popular among athletes as a performance-enhancing agent as well. Unfortunately for them, GH remains extremely expensive and is not terribly effective in terms of improving athletic ability or promoting rapid gains in muscle mass. GH is also becoming popular in the anti-aging community. A number of high-profile individuals, such as Sylvester Stallone, have made comments that GH supplementation has greatly improved their quality of life. Medical GH therapy is well beyond the scope of this book. However, it is important to understand how you can adjust your training and diet to maximize your own endogenous production of GH.

Exercise is a potent stimulator of GH secretion and can raise levels up to one hundred times above baseline. Generally speaking, the more intense the exercise, the greater the amount of GH secreted. Weight-training sessions using moderate weights and a relatively high number of repetitions (eight to fifteen) appear to be more effective at stimulating GH release than those using very heavy weights and low repetitions.[95] GH stimulation generally occurs with exercise lasting at least seven to ten minutes. Most studies show that even very intense exercise lasting less than seven to ten minutes is not sufficiently long to produce significant elevations in GH. Exercise-induced GH spikes tend to peak at around twenty-five

94   Stimson R, et al. Dietary Macronutrient Content Alters Cortisol Metabolism Independently of Body Weight Changes in Obese Men. Journal of Clinical Endocrinology Metabolism, doi:10.1210/jc.2007-0692.
95   Cuneo RC, Wallace JD: Growth hormone, insulin-like growth factors and sport. *Endocrinol Metab* 1994; 1:3–13.

to thirty minutes into exercise.[96] While on The Program, your training regimen will be optimal for stimulating GH release. Your workouts will be very intense and last approximately twenty to thirty minutes. Therefore, your GH levels will just be peaking at the conclusion of your workout. This will provide a perfect opportunity to consume a high-quality protein source while your GH levels are peaking. This influx of amino acids will provide a ready pool from which GH can stimulate further muscle growth.

The other important stimulant of GH release is sleep. GH is secreted in a pulsatile fashion throughout the night, but the amount tends to be highest around midnight. The highest levels occur during so-called slow-wave sleep. Slow-wave sleep is the deepest form of sleep in your sleep cycle. This is yet another reason why getting adequate sleep is so important. Your goal should be for a minimum of eight hours of uninterrupted sleep per night. Avoiding alcohol and big meals just before bed will also help maximize your nocturnal GH output.

Another factor influencing GH secretion is proper hydration. Exercising while dehydrated will blunt GH secretion.[97] High-fat meals as well as training in cold environments can also potentially decrease GH release during exercise. Obesity in and of itself tends to blunt GH release during exercise. So, if possible, try to train in a warm environment and keep yourself well hydrated.

It is not clear if low-carbohydrate ketogenic diets have any effect on GH levels. Some short-term studies (seven days) have shown that GH secretion really doesn't change much while on such a diet.[98] The high protein content of these diets, however, provides ample substrate for GH-induced muscle growth. GH, along with glucagon and cortisol, helps maintain stable blood sugar levels while one is on a low-carbohydrate diet.

A number of amino acids have been shown in clinical studies to stimulate the release of growth hormone. Arginine, valine, methionine, and various other amino acids have been shown to raise growth hormone levels when infused intravenously.[99] Oral administration of these same substances has, with some exceptions, also been demonstrated to raise GH levels in a number of laboratory studies. Unfortunately, the dosages required (often in excess of thirty grams), combined with their notoriously foul taste, led to high rates of stomach upset, nausea, and diarrhea. Additionally, no studies have shown that the exercise-induced spike in GH can be augmented by taking oral amino acids beforehand. Furthermore, no evidence exists that ingesting these substances leads to any further increase in muscle mass or strength or reduction in body fat than exercise alone.

96   Felsing NE, Brasel JA, Cooper DM: Effect of low and high intensity exercise on circulating growth hormone in men. *J Clin Endocrinol Metab* 1992; 75:157–162.
97   . Peyreigne C, Bouix D, Fedou C, et al: Effect of hydration on exercise-induced growth hormone response. *Eur J Endocrinol* 2001; 145:445–450.
98   Harber MP, Schenk S, Barkan AL, Horowitz JF: Effects of dietary carbohydrate restriction with high protein intake on protein metabolism and the somatotropic axis. J Clin Endocrinol Metab 2005, 90(9):5175–81.
99   Isidori A, Lo Monaco A, Cappa M. A study of growth hormone release in men after administration of amino acids. Curr Med Res Opin 1981;7:475–81.

IGF-1

Insulin-like growth factor (IGF-1), also known as somatomedin C, is the most well-known intermediary by which growth hormone exerts its effects on body tissues. Growth hormone triggers the liver and some other body tissues to synthesize and secrete IGF-1, which then mediates the growth-promoting effects of growth hormone. IGF-1, as its name implies, also has the ability to lower blood glucose levels similar to insulin. It has been a common misconception that growth hormone itself is responsible for the increase in height and muscle mass that occurs during puberty when in fact it is IGF-1 and other somatomedins that have a far greater effect. Growth hormone itself is secreted in short duration pulses and only has a half-life in the blood of around twenty minutes before it is taken up by the tissues. IGF-1, however, has a much longer half-life of up to twenty hours and thus leads to prolonged growth-promoting effects. A good example in nature of the need for IGF-1 to promote normal growth is African pygmy populations. Pigmies have normal to high levels of growth hormone production. They remain short-statured, however, because of a genetic mutation that leads to low levels of IGF-1.

On the surface, it may appear that IGF-1 would be a prime candidate for use by athletes to augment muscle mass and sports performance. Unfortunately, studies looking at supplemental IGF-1 injection in both elderly and healthy young subjects have been disappointing. In most studies, additional IGF-1 did not lead to significant increases in protein synthesis or muscle strength.[100] Side effects of IGF-1 supplementation include hypoglycemia and a shift to preferential carbohydrate use for energy at the expense of fat oxidation. Additionally, it has been theorized that high circulating levels of IGF-1 may be associated with increased risk for breast, colon, and prostate cancer.

Nevertheless, IGF-1 has an important role in adaption to exercise. Bouts of intense exercise lead to spikes in GH release and sustained elevations in IGF-1. Local muscles up-regulate IGF-1 receptors as well as their own production of IGF-1 in response to exercise. This stimulates adjacent satellite cells (dormant cells that lie between muscle cells) to fuse with and increase the size of surrounding muscle cells.[101]

There is little to no data available on the effects of low carbohydrate diets on IGF-1 levels. It is known that low blood sugar stimulates the release of GH, which in turn should elevate IGF-1. Low-carbohydrate diets, in some studies, do seem to increase skeletal muscle expression of IGF-I messenger RNA. Whether this is a direct result of carbohydrate restriction or the increased availability of dietary protein is unclear. What is clear is that even a marginal protein deficiency will lower GH and IGF-1 levels and lead to muscle fiber atrophy. This is essentially a nonissue since you will not be anywhere near protein deficient on any of the diets in The Program.

100   Yarasheski KE, Zachwieja JJ, Campbell JA, et al. Effect of growth hormone and resistance exercise on muscle growth and strength in older men. Am J Physiol 1995;268: E268–E276.
101   Adams GR, Role of insulin-like growth factor-I in the regulation of skeletal muscle adaptation to increased loading. J Nutr Health Aging. 2000; 4(2):85–90.

Thyroid Hormone

The thyroid gland is located in the neck and is responsible for secreting two hormones T4 (thyroxine) and T3 (triiodothyronine). Both these hormones have dramatic effects on nearly all of the body's tissues. They increase your ability to burn fat as fuel, increase both the rate and the strength of your heart's contractions, and increase motility of food through the digestive tract as well as myriad of other important functions. An improperly functioning thyroid gland, therefore, can result in a wide range of symptoms including weight gain, fatigue, depression, abnormal menstrual bleeding, heat or cold intolerance, and many others. The secretion of T3 and T4 is controlled primarily by thyroid-stimulating hormone (TSH). TSH is secreted by the pituitary gland and when taken up by the thyroid gland triggers the synthesis and release of T3 and T4.

Studies looking at high-intensity, short-duration exercise generally show an increase in TSH but not much of a change in T3 and T4. This is largely a result of the long delay in the production of T3 and T4 after TSH stimulation. It takes hours to days to see a noticeable effect from a spike in TSH. Similarly prolonged bouts of endurance exercise have shown mixed results in terms of T4 and T3 levels.[102] Training in cold weather does tend to raise TSH and T4 levels, however. Whether chronic cold weather training has any lasting effects on thyroid hormone levels is unknown.

Low-carbohydrate diets can have an effect on thyroid hormone levels. During very low carbohydrate intake (less than fifty grams per day), T3 levels decrease while TSH and T4 remain unchanged. It is possible that the decrease in T3 results from the suppression of the conversion of T4 to T3, but the exact mechanism underlying this decrease in T3 is unknown. A decrease in T3 appears to decrease the breakdown of protein and promote a general conservation of energy.[103] This may in part play a role in the observed protein-sparing effects of ketogenic diets.

Given the potential changes in thyroid hormones while ingesting a low-carbohydrate diet, you should consult with your physician if you have any preexisting thyroid disease or are taking thyroid hormone replacement medication for any reason.

Testosterone

Testosterone is perhaps the most well-known hormone in the male body. It is secreted in large quantities by cells in the testicles known as Leydig cells and, to a much lesser degree, cells in the adrenal glands. In males, the primary source of testosterone is the testes, while in females; the adrenal glands provide the bulk of the body's testosterone production. On average, females produce less than 10 percent of the testosterone typically found in a male. The primary function of testosterone is to trigger the development of male secondary sexual characteristics. These include the growth of facial hair, deepening of the voice,

---

102   Viru A. Plasma Hormones and Physical Exercise. Int J Sports Med 1992;13:201–209.
103   Hennemann G, et al. Causes and effects of the low T3 syndrome during caloric deprivation and non-thyroidal illness: an overview. Acta Med Austriaca. 1988;15 Suppl 1:42–5.

stimulation of muscle growth, increased oil production in the skin, strengthening of bones, enlargement of the genitals, and many more.

Testosterone is secreted from the testes when they are stimulated by luteinizing hormone (LH), which is produced by the pituitary gland in the brain. LH in turn is secreted when levels of gonadotropin-releasing hormone (GnRH), which arises in the hypothalamus, are elevated. The average human male secretes around four to ten milligrams of testosterone per day from the testes with the adrenal glands contributing perhaps around 500 micrograms.[104]

The majority of testosterone (98 percent) circulating in the bloodstream is bound by various proteins, the most well-known of which is steroid-hormone-binding globulin (SHBG). When bound to these proteins, testosterone is unable to interact with the body's tissues and for all practical purposes has no physiologic effects. It is only the free testosterone (FT) that is able to leave the bloodstream and enter into your cells to exert its effects.

Testosterone is not secreted at steady levels throughout the day but rather is produced in pulses. GnRH is released from the hypothalamus every one to three hours. The amount of GnRH secreted can vary and has a direct correlation with the amount of testosterone eventually produced. LH, when stimulated by GnRH is secreted in a similar pulsatile fashion, which in turn is passed on to the testes, which release short pulses of testosterone. Testosterone has a much longer half-life than its precursor signaling hormones, and so, despite its pulsatile release, there are not large swings in testosterone levels with each pulse of GnRH. There are variations in testosterone levels throughout the day, however. In general, testosterone levels are highest in the early morning and tend to fall in the afternoon and evening.

The secretion of testosterone can be influenced by environmental factors, such as diet and exercise. Dietary variations, not only in total calories, but in the composition of macronutrients (fat, protein, and carbohydrate) can have significant effects on testosterone levels. It is well documented that severe caloric restriction can greatly reduce testosterone levels. Army ranger students undergo an intense eight-week training course where they routinely have up to one-thousand-calorie-per-day deficits, sleep an average of 3.6 hours per night, and expend up to six thousand calories per day. Studies looking at their testosterone levels during this period show that they rapidly plummet to near castration levels.[105] Fortunately for them, their testosterone levels rapidly return to normal when they are allowed to consume calories freely. It is not clear at which point caloric restriction in humans begins to decrease testosterone levels. Studies with rats have shown declines with a 25 percent reduction of calories below maintenance levels while a 15 percent reduction in human males did not appear to lower testosterone levels significantly.[106,107] This should not be

104   Griffin JE. Ojeda SR, editors of: Textbook of Endocrine Physiology, 3rd edition. New York, Oxford University Press, 1996.
105   Mays M, et al. Acute Recovery of Physiological and Cognitive Function in US Army Ranger Students in a Multistressor Field Environment. Report at RTO HFM Workshop 3-5 April 1995.
106   Govic A, et al. Alterations in male sexual behaviour, attractiveness and testosterone levels induced by an adult-onset calorie restriction regimen. Behav Brain Res. 2008 Jun 26;190(1):140–6. Epub 2008 Feb 16.
107   Garrel DR. Todd KS. Pugeat MM. Calloway DH. Hormonal changes in normal men under marginally negative energy balance. American Journal of Clinical Nutrition. 39(6):930–6, 1984 Jun.

an issue on any of The Program diets, as none will require you to make such drastic cuts in your caloric intake.

Dietary protein intake can also influence testosterone levels though the research in this area is not entirely consistent. Studies looking at high-protein intakes (over 40 percent of total calories) have shown reductions in total testosterone of about 28 percent.[108] This drop in total testosterone, however, is usually associated with a drop in SHBG.[109] As you will recall, SHBG binds testosterone and eliminates it from the available pool of free testosterone. When SHBG levels drop, the amount of usable free testosterone usually increases. Therefore, it is possible that while total testosterone levels drop with increasing protein intake, this drop may be of little clinical consequence because there is a compensatory rise in free testosterone. Given the increases in muscle mass and strength documented in weight-training athletes who consume increased amounts of protein, it appears unlikely that this drop in total testosterone has any significant effect. There may also be an as yet undefined threshold beyond which increased protein intake leads to decreased testosterone production but below which there is no effect. One study in particular showed a general trend toward lower testosterone levels as protein intake increased, but the most significant drop occurred when protein intake exceeded about 30 percent of total calories.[110] BCAAs may also have some testosterone-sparing effects. One study showed that a BCAA supplement was able to blunt the drop in testosterone levels seen during overtraining and helped maintain serum testosterone and SHBG levels during intense exercise.[111]

The source of protein also appears to have some influence on testosterone levels. One study looking at male distance runners who consumed a meat-rich diet showed that their exercise-induced testosterone increases were blunted when they switched to a lacto-ovo vegetarian diet. This was despite the fact that total calories as well as the proportion of fat and carbohydrate did not change.[112] It is theorized that the increased amount of saturated fat found in meat may have been responsible for the higher testosterone levels in meat-eating athletes.

The effects of dietary fat on testosterone levels are also quite interesting. As mentioned above, some studies suggest that saturated fats can raise testosterone levels. Monounsaturated, but not polyunsaturated fats, also share this property. These findings have not been reported in all studies, but what data are available seem to show an association.[113] Ultimately, the clinical significance of these has yet to be determined. It is probably not necessary or useful to deliberately increase your saturated fat intake in an attempt to obtain a testosterone boost. There just isn't enough data at this time to show a clear benefit. All diets in The Program have a significant amount of monounsaturated fat, and saturated fat is consumed to a modest

---

108   Anderson KE. Rosner W. Khan MS. New MI. Pang SY. Wissel PS. Kappas A. Diet-hormone interactions: protein/carbohydrate ratio alters reciprocally the plasma levels of testosterone and cortisol and their respective binding globulins in man. Life Sciences. 40(18):1761–8, 1987 May 4.

109   Anderson K, et al. Diet-hormone interactions: Protein/carbohydrate ratio alters reciprocally the plasma levels of testosterone and cortisol and their respective binding globulins in man. Life Sciences Volume 40, Issue 18, 4 May 1987, Pages 1761–1768.

110   Volek J. Testosterone and cortisol in relationship to dietary nutrients and resistance exercise. Journal of Applied Physiology. Vol. 82, No. 1, pp. 49–54, January 1997.

111   Di Luigi L, Pigozzi F, Casini A, et al. Effects of prolonged amino acid supplementations on hormonal secretion in male athletes. Med Sport 1994;47:529–39.

112   Raben, A., B. Kiens, E. A. Ritchter, L. B. Rasmussen, B. Svenstrup, S. Micic, and P. Bennett. Serum sex hormones and endurance performance after a lacto-ovo vegetarian and a mixed diet. Med. Sci. Sports Exercise 24: 1290–1297, 1992.

113   Hamalainen E, H Adlercreutz, P Puska, et al. Diet and serum sex hormones in healthy men. Journal of Steroid Biochemistry. 20(1): 459–464, 1984 Jan.

extent on the Endomorphic Diet. If there is a testosterone-raising effect from these fats, you will likely get it while on The Program.

The macronutrient that appears most correlated with increased testosterone levels is carbohydrate. Studies looking at diets rich in carbohydrates show that those with higher intakes of carbohydrate relative to protein tend to be associated with higher total testosterone levels.[114] Most studies showing a boost in testosterone levels have had subjects consuming 50 to 70 percent of their calories from carbohydrates with varying amounts of fats and protein. As with the studies examining fat and protein intake, however, those looking at carbohydrate's effects on testosterone have not been entirely consistent and suffered from serious methodological flaws. There continues to be debate in scientific circles about just how much of an effect carbohydrate intake has on testosterone levels. Given this lack of rock solid data and the clearly demonstrated benefits of carbohydrate restriction for those looking to lose body fat, I don't think you should be too concerned about missing out on a potential testosterone boost by restricting carbohydrates while on the Endomorphic and Mesomorphic Diets. If there is indeed an effect, those looking to gain as much muscle as possible on the Ectomorphic Diet should receive it, as they will be consuming carbohydrates in similar quantities as the subjects in the previously mentioned studies.

Perhaps the most potent stimulus for endogenous testosterone production is intense exercise. A variety of studies have demonstrated that with high-intensity exercise, testosterone levels rise and peak around thirty to forty-five minutes after the initiation of exercise. This rise occurs with a variety of high-intensity exercises including weight-lifting, running, and cycling. Increases of more than 150 percent in total testosterone have been documented in some studies.[115] In particular, heavy compound movements like squats and deadlifts appear to be the most effective way to boost testosterone during resistance training. These powerful whole-body exercises tend to increase testosterone levels to a greater extent than more specific, isolation-type movements.[116] For this reason, your workouts should focus on these types of exercises when at all possible. A workout regimen built around core exercises lasting about thirty minutes should give you the most significant short-term boost in your testosterone levels. It is possible that this increase in testosterone has some role in the increased protein synthesis seen post-exercise. Since you will be completing your workout just as testosterone levels are peaking, take advantage of this anabolic hormonal environment by providing your body with a quality protein source immediately after your workout.

While acute high-intensity exercise appears to boost testosterone levels in the short term, prolonged resistance exercise, on the other hand, has been shown to acutely decrease testosterone levels. Exercise duration much beyond two hours has consistently been shown to elevate cortisol levels and decrease testosterone levels. The exact mechanism behind this phenomenon is unclear, but it may be due to direct suppression of testosterone synthesis by elevated cortisol levels. Similarly, endurance exercise has been demonstrated to lower testosterone levels as well. Long-distance runners, rowers, and cyclists tend to have

114   Anderson KE. Rosner W. Khan MS. New MI. Pang SY. Wissel PS. Kappas A. Diet-hormone interactions: protein/carbohydrate ratio alters reciprocally the plasma levels of testosterone and cortisol and their respective binding globulins in man. Life Sciences. 40(18):1761–8, 1987 May 4.

115   Kraemer WJ, Gordon SE, Fleck SJ, Marchitelli LJ, Mello R, Dziados JE, Friedl K, Harman E, Maresh C, Fry AC. Endogenous anabolic hormonal and growth factor responses to heavy resistance exercise in males and females. Int J Sports Med. 1991 Apr; 12(2):228–35.

116   Hakkinen K, Pakarinen A. Acute hormonal responses to two different fatiguing heavy-resistance protocols in male athletes. J Appl Physiol. 1993 Feb;74(2):882–7.

lower resting testosterone levels than their sedentary peers.[117] Therefore, unless you have a tremendous amount of body fat to lose or are training for a specific endurance event, it is not recommended that you engage in prolonged endurance exercise.

The effect of training on women's hormones, particularly testosterone, is not as well studied as it is in men. It does appear that testosterone, estrogen, growth hormone (GH), and cortisol all increase, to small degrees, with endurance exercise. High-intensity exercise does not appear to have much influence on testosterone levels but does still elevate GH, estrogen, and cortisol. Given that these changes, particularly in testosterone, are quite small, it is unlikely that they have much real-world effect.[118]

Testosterone deficiency in men is a widely unrecognized condition and one that increases in prevalence with age. Symptoms are generally non-specific and include fatigue, weight gain, loss of libido, depression, loss of muscle mass, and many others. I have been surprised at the number of men over age 40 who suffer from low testosterone. In many cases they attribute their symptoms to normal aging when in fact they are suffering from a real medical condition. Maintaining a normal, healthy testosterone level is essential to making the most out of The Program. I strongly recommend men over age 40, or any man that is experiencing the symptoms described above, have their testosterone level checked and, if low, discuss options for treatment with their doctor.

117   Dessypris, A. Hormonal response in long-term physical exercise, Psychiatria-Fennica, (Suppl.), 45–53, 1986.
118   Consitt LA, Copeland JL, Tremblay MS: Endogenous anabolic hormone responses to endurance versus resistance exercise and training in women. Sports Med 2002; 32:1–22.

If we could give every individual the right amount of nourishment and exercise, not too little and not too much, we would have found the safest way to health.

—Hippocrates

MICRONUTRIENTS

Vitamins and minerals are referred to as micronutrients (as opposed to protein, fats, and carbohydrates, which are termed *macro*nutrients) and are essential for a host of metabolic processes throughout the body. Of most importance to athletes are their roles in energy production as well as metabolism of proteins, fats, and carbohydrates. Most nutritionists state that when consuming a well-balanced diet, most individuals should receive an adequate supply of these nutrients. Surprisingly, however, studies looking at the nutritional profiles of even high-level athletes show that many are deficient in at least one micronutrient.[119] Micronutrient deficiency is shockingly common in the general population as well. In fact, micronutrient deficiency is now the norm amongst Americans. In certain populations, like the elderly and teenagers, these deficiencies are striking. Less than half the US population meets the EAR for magnesium but 78% of teenage boys and 91% of teenage girls consume less than the EAR[120]. The elderly don't fare much better. 81% of Americans over age 65 consume less than the EAR of magnesium.[121] The story is similar for vitamin D. In dark skinned individuals, those who get limited or no sun exposure, the obese, and breastfed infants rates of deficiency can exceed 40%[122]. Similar rates of deficiency are seen across the board when other important micronutrients like calcium, selenium, folate, B12, choline, niacin, and many others are examined.

Recommended intake of essential vitamins and minerals is expressed in a variety of ways. The most common is the RDA (recommended dietary allowance), which is the minimum intake that is considered adequate for 98 percent of the US population. The AI (adequate intake) value is an estimate of what is considered adequate for nutrients in which an RDA is not known. Also used is the EAR (estimated average requirement). The EAR estimates the average nutritional requirements of 50 percent of individuals within a certain group,

---

119   Beals KA. Eating behaviors, nutritional status, and menstrual function in elite female adolescent volleyball players. J Am Diet Assoc 2002;102(9):1293–6.

120   U.S. Department of Agriculture Agricultural Research Service. (1999) *Data Tables: Food and Nutrient Intakes by Income, 1994–96*

121   Vaquero MP *(2002) J Nutr Health Aging 6:147–153)*.

122   J. Nutr. **April 2006** vol. 136 no. 4 **1126-1129**

such as infants, breast-feeding mothers, et cetera. Applying these requirements to hard-training athletes, especially those cutting calories, is difficult. Very few studies are available that actually give clear-cut recommendations on micronutrient intake for athletes. Obviously, individual requirements can vary widely based on one's age; the intensity, duration, and frequency of training; and variations in individual metabolism.

Vitamin and mineral deficiencies, when severe and prolonged, generally manifest themselves in ways that make the diagnosis relatively straightforward for a physician trained to look for them. Subtle deficiencies, however, can be difficult to detect. In athletes, they can manifest simply as worsening performance or a slowdown in muscle recovery after stressful workouts and therefore may go undetected. Hard-training athletes, in particular, put themselves at risk for these subtle deficiencies by restricting calories, overtraining, and failure to include a wide variety of different foods in their diets.[123] In athletes without a preexisting deficiency, however, there is very little evidence to support that supplementation with either vitamins or minerals will improve performance or recovery.[124]

Despite the lack of concrete recommendations for vitamin and mineral intakes for hard-training athletes, there are some basic principles and general recommendations that should be followed. It makes sense that hard-training athletes would require greater amounts of some vitamins and minerals than those recommended by the RDA for sedentary individuals. Whether through increased consumption or through greater losses through sweat, it is likely that the athlete would be at higher risk for subtle deficiencies if consuming micronutrients at only RDA levels. Therefore, you should make every attempt to eat a wide variety of foods from fruit and vegetable sources. This is obviously not always easy given the hectic schedules many of us lead and may also be difficult when significantly cutting calories or carbohydrate intake. In this case, using a daily multivitamin and mineral supplement is probably a good idea. Indeed, given that it can be difficult to detect subtle deficiencies in these nutrients, taking a daily supplement can provide an inexpensive "insurance policy" that can help you avoid any unintended deficiencies. Megadoses of vitamins and minerals have not been proven to improve athletic performance and, in some cases, may be harmful. While there is likely little harm in supplementing with water-soluble vitamins, except in very high doses, use caution if you supplement with fat-soluble vitamins. Fat-soluble vitamins are not excreted as rapidly, and prolonged consumption of excessive amounts can lead to toxicity in some cases.

There is one important caveat to the above recommendations that specifically pertains to females. This involves calcium, vitamin D, and iron. Calcium is absolutely essential for the formation of strong bones and for the prevention of osteoporosis later in life. The bulk of a woman's bone mineral density is formed during the teenage years and peaks in her early thirties. Therefore, it is essential that an adequate amount of calcium is supplied during this crucial timeframe. Current recommendations are that women consume approximately 1500 milligrams of calcium daily. Unfortunately, only about half of all women meet this goal. If you do not regularly consume dairy products or other high-calcium foods, I would suggest that you consider adding a calcium supplement to your daily routine. Vitamin D is also essential for building and maintaining healthy bones. It is recommended that adults consume approximately 600 IU

123   Clarkson PM, Haymes EM: Exercise and mineral status of athletes: Calcium, magnesium, phosphorus, and iron. Med Sci Sports Exerc 27:831–843, 1995.
124   Oregon State University (2006, December 27). Poor Athletic Performance Linked To Vitamin Deficiency. ScienceDaily. Retrieved November 13, 2008, from http://www.sciencedaily.com /releases/2006/11/061116091853.htm.

per day either through dietary intake or supplementation.[125] However, more recent research indicates that larger amounts may be needed and indeed be optimal. Diets high in phosphorous (primarily found in sodas) can negatively impact calcium balance so try to limit your intake of these beverages.

Iron is of particular interest to women as well. Iron is essential for the normal development of red blood cells and the transport of oxygen to your tissues. A deficiency in iron can lead to anemia. Iron deficiency in women can result from a number of different factors. The most common is decreased intake. But iron loss resulting from heavy menstrual flow also can contribute. Additionally, a variety of factors can inhibit the absorption of iron from the diet. Chemicals known as tannates found in tea inhibit the absorption of iron as well as certain prescription medications used for acid reflux like proton-pump inhibitors and H2 blockers.[126] Very high fiber intake can also block the absorption of iron from the diet. Conversely, iron absorption can be improved by ingesting it with two hundred milligrams of vitamin C. Symptoms of iron deficiency anemia include fatigue, decreased exercise tolerance, pallor, and a variety of other non-specific complaints. If you are concerned you may be suffering from iron deficiency, a simple blood test can confirm the diagnosis. Treatment in most cases involves the addition of an iron supplement to the diet. Since only about 5 to 10 percent of ingested iron is normally absorbed in non-deficient individuals, you may need to consume a fairly large amount to build up significant stores. Discuss this with your physician before embarking on any iron supplementation program.

Vitamin A (Retinol)

Vitamin A is crucial for maintaining the integrity of a number of body tissues including those of the eye and the respiratory and intestinal tracts. Animal foods like liver, milk, and fish (particularly cod liver oil) and carrots are good sources of vitamin A. Most dietary sources of vitamin A are ingested as carotenes (such as beta carotene), which the body then safely converts to the active form of vitamin A-retinol.

Vitamin A deficiency is a common cause of blindness in the third world but is extremely rare elsewhere. The earliest signs of vitamin A deficiency are a drying of the eyes and decreased night vision. Even minimal deficiency in vitamin A can leave one more susceptible to common bacterial and viral infections. In non-immunized individuals, there appears to be a link between low vitamin A levels and increased risk for acquiring measles.

Since it is a fat-soluble vitamin, the body absorbs and stores retinol very efficiently but lacks the means to dispose of excess amounts. Retinol can build up in the system and lead to a number of adverse effects. The current RDA is 900 micrograms per day (3000 IU) for healthy, non-pregnant adults. The safe upper limit of Vitamin A intake is estimated to be around 3000 micrograms (9900 IU) per day. Daily ingestion of levels greater than this can lead to dry skin, eczema, conjunctivitis, and bone and muscle pain, as well as osteoporosis.[127] Toxicity from excess vitamin A occurs exclusively in individuals who take supplements. Toxicity from natural carotenes does not occur. You should examine your daily multivitamin

125   Osteoporosis prevention, diagnosis, and therapy. NIH Consens Statement 2000;17:1–45.
126   Killip, S et al. Iron Deficiency Anemia. American Family Physician Vol. 75/No. 5 March 1 2007.
127   Melhus H, Michaelsson K, Kindmark A, Bergstrom R, Holmberg L, Mallmin H, Wolk A, Ljunghall S. Excessive dietary intake of vitamin A is associated with reduced bone mineral density and increased fracture risk of hip fracture. Ann Intern Med. 1998; 129: 770–778.

closely as most have greater than the recommended levels of vitamin A. Recent studies have shown that supplementation with beta carotene has no beneficial health effects in people already receiving the recommended daily allowance from their diet and suggested that smokers in particular were at *increased* risk of lung cancer if they took beta carotene supplements. Therefore, I don't recommend you specifically supplement your diet with vitamin A. If you take a multivitamin and are following any of the diets in The Program, you will be getting more than enough vitamin A.

Vitamin D

For a long time, Vitamin D has received a lot of attention for its role in maintaining healthy bone mass in children and women. Recent research has shown that vitamin D also has several other important roles. Vitamin D deficiency may not only be more common than previously recognized but also linked to a number of disease states. In the United States alone, low vitamin D levels are present in over one-third of otherwise healthy young people. In older individuals, those with chronic medical problems, or those living in far northern latitudes, the number may be even higher. Given the high prevalence of vitamin D deficiency, obtaining a simple blood test from your physician to assess your vitamin D status, especially for females, would not be a bad idea.

The active form of vitamin D is known as *1,25 dihydroxyvitamin D* (1,25(OH)2D) or simply calcitriol. Calcitriol can be produced in your body from two different precursors: vitamin D3 (cholecalciferol) and vitamin D2 (ergocalciferol). Cholecalciferol is produced in the skin when it is exposed to ultraviolet light, and ergocalciferol comes from the diet, usually by ingesting various plants rich in the vitamin. After vitamin D is ingested from the diet or synthesized in the skin, it is metabolized in the liver to a biologically inactive *25-hydroxyvitamin D* [25(OH)D]. 25(OH)D is then converted to the biologically active calcitriol primarily in the kidney. If you go to your physician and have your vitamin D levels measured, it is the 25(OH)D level that the lab will check, not your actual calcitriol level, in most cases.

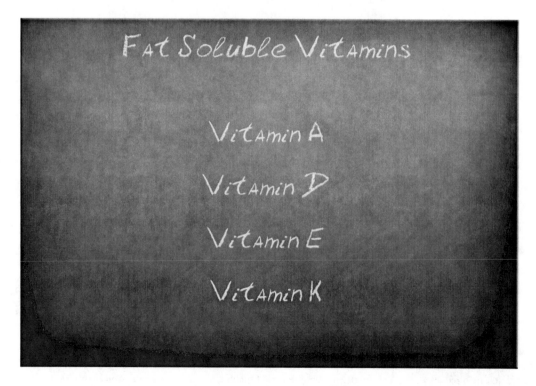

Vitamin D is well known for its association with healthy bone formation in both children and adults. Vitamin D is necessary for the normal calcification of growing bones in children as well as for the maintenance of bone density in adults. Without vitamin D, only about 10 percent of the calcium you ingest from your diet will be absorbed by your intestines.[128] Children who are vitamin D deficient develop the disease rickets while adults generally develop osteoporosis. Up to 50 percent of women and 25 percent of men over the age of fifty will experience a fracture as a result of osteoporosis at some point in their lives. Of older adults who experience a fracture from minimal trauma, like a ground-level fall, almost all have vitamin D levels lower than recommended.[129]

Low vitamin D levels are also associated with a number of autoimmune diseases, such as multiple sclerosis, lupus, rheumatoid arthritis, and many others. There is a significant amount of ongoing research in this area, and it remains to be seen exactly what role vitamin D plays in the prevention and treatment of these diseases. Vitamin D deficiency has also been linked to various cancers, a worse prognosis for patients with heart disease, and declining cognitive function in the elderly. Studies on vitamin D levels in athletes engaged in intense weight-training programs are limited, but it is safe to say that they are at as much risk, if not more, because of strict dieting in many cases, as the general population. Due to the nature of their training, they may actually have higher daily requirements because of increased bone remodeling and turnover.

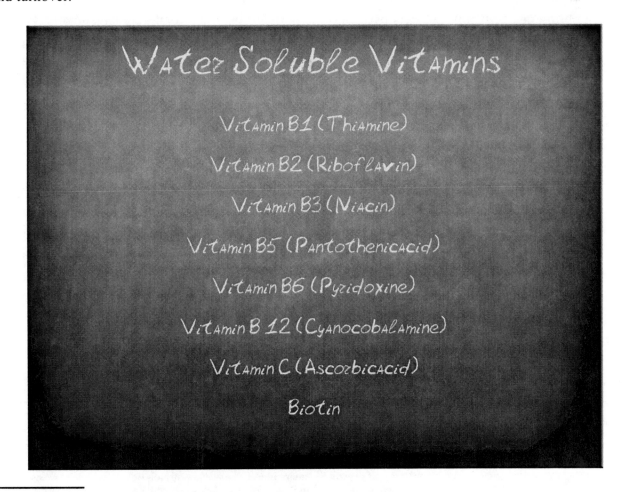

128   .Holick MF. Vitamin D deficiency. N Engl J Med. 2007;357:266–281.

129   Simonelli C, Weiss TW, Morancey J, et al. Prevalence of vitamin D inadequacy in a minimal trauma fracture population. *Curr Med Res Opin.* 2005;21:1069–1074.

A number of food products are fortified with vitamin D. These are primarily dairy products that are also high in calcium like milk, yogurt, and cheese. Oily fish like cod, mackerel, sardines, and tuna are also high in vitamin D. Cod liver oil, in addition to being very high in omega-3 fatty acids, also contains very high levels of vitamin D and provides an excellent way to supplement your diet with both nutrients.

The Institute of Medicine recommends that healthy children and adults up to age fifty with normal baseline vitamin D levels should take in a minimum of 200 IU of vitamin D per day to maintain those normal levels. After age fifty, up to 600 IU per day is recommended. Postmenopausal women, however, may require 1000 IU or more.[130]

These recommendations are controversial, however, and a number of scientists who study vitamin D argue that a significantly greater amount of vitamin D is required. Physicians at the Vitamin D Council recommend that most healthy people take at least 2000 IU per day during summer months and up to 5000 IU per day during the winter.

Keep in mind though that these recommendations are for otherwise healthy individuals who already have *normal* vitamin D levels (greater than thirty nanograms per milliliter). To correct deficiency, much higher doses are required and for long periods of time. In most cases, it can take more than three to four months to bring one's vitamin D levels back into the normal range with oral supplementation. For example, it is estimated that the daily ingestion of 1000 additional IUs of vitamin D can raise blood levels of 25(OH)D by about 10 nanograms per milliliter over three months.[131] Depending on your vitamin D level, you may need to supplement with much more than this. For significantly deficient patients, physicians often prescribe up to 50,000 IUs taken twice a week or even up to 500,000 IU given as an intramuscular injection. Before you consider supplementing with this much vitamin D, you should discuss your concerns with your physician and obtain a 25(OH)D level to determine your precise need for supplementation. There are individuals with certain medical conditions, like hyperparathyroidism, sarcoidosis, and certain cancers, who shouldn't supplement with additional vitamin D except under the care of a physician. If you have a chronic medical condition, consult with your doctor before adding vitamin D to your regimen.

A simple blood test can determine if you are vitamin D deficient. Though the definition of deficiency can vary in the medical literature, it is generally recognized that levels of 25(OH)D less than 20 nanograms per milliliter indicate outright deficiency. Levels between 21 and 29 nanograms per milliliter indicate inadequate intake, while those above 30 nanograms per milliliter are considered adequate for most people. Some physicians use a goal level of 35 to 40 nanograms per milliliter because of the inherent variability in the results of the most commonly used lab tests for vitamin D deficiency.[132] If you decide to supplement your vitamin D intake, keep in mind that vitamin D3 (cholecalciferol) is at least twice as effective at raising blood levels of 25(OH)D and therefore should be your preferred form for supplementation. There are prescription preparations of calcitriol, but these are expensive and unnecessary.

---

130   Standing Committee on the Scientific Evaluation of Dietary Reference Intakes, Food and Nutrition Board, Institute of Medicine. Dietary Reference Intakes for Calcium, Phosphorus, Magnesium, Vitamin D and Fluoride. Washington, DC: National Academy Press; 1999.

131   Cannell JJ, Hollis BW. Use of vitamin D in clinical practice. *Altern Med Rev.* 2008; 13:6–20.

132   Holick MF, Chen TC. Vitamin D deficiency: a worldwide problem with health consequences. *Am J Clin Nutr.* 2008;87:1080S–1086S.

Despite being a fat-soluble vitamin, toxicity from taking in more than the recommended amount of vitamin D is extremely rare. Keep in mind that with thirty minutes of full-body sun exposure, most light-skinned individuals produce approximately 10,000 units of vitamin D in their skin.[133] Toxic doses of Vitamin D are very difficult to achieve. Most animal studies indicate that it takes ingestion of over 20,000 IU per kilogram of bodyweight to achieve toxicity acutely (5000 standard 400 IU capsules!) and over 40,000 IU per day chronically.[134]

If you decide to supplement with vitamin D and are able to see a physician, then obtaining a baseline vitamin D level is worthwhile. If you are otherwise healthy and wish to supplement, then starting at 2000 to 5000 IU per day seems reasonable.

Vitamin E

Vitamin E is an essential fat-soluble vitamin found in all tissues. Its primary role in the body is as an antioxidant. Vitamin E prevents the oxidative breakdown of various essential fatty acids and fat-soluble vitamins. High levels are found in foods, such as leafy green vegetables, plant oils, eggs, nuts, seeds, and butter. The most common form of vitamin E found in foods and supplements is known as alpha-tocopherol. Alpha-tocopherol is the form found in highest concentration in the body's tissues and probably has the most nutritional significance. The adult RDA for alpha-tocopherol is 22.5 International Units (IU) per day.[135] Many foods, as well as some supplements, contain other versions of Vitamin E, such as beta-tocopherol, delta-tocopherol, and gamma-tocopherol. You may see the term "mixed " tocopherols on a bottle of Vitamin E tablets indicating that the product contains a variety of different Vitamin E types. There is no established RDA for these forms of vitamin E. The exact role and benefit, if any, of these other forms of Vitamin E are unknown at this time. There is some evidence that gamma-tocopherol (which tends to be found in higher amounts than alpha-tocopherol in some foods) may have important cardio-protective and anticancer benefits. Unfortunately, there isn't enough research at this point to say anything conclusive about these other vitamin E types. They may or may not have health benefits.

Vitamin E deficiency is very rare. Individuals with severe gastrointestinal disorders that limit their ability to absorb fats from their diets are potentially at risk. It is sometimes seen in very premature infants as well. People suffering from vitamin E deficiency typically have a variety of neurological symptoms, such as pain and tingling in the extremities.

Because of its powerful antioxidant properties, vitamin E has been studied extensively for its role in preventing heart disease and cancer. Some early studies linked higher intakes of vitamin E with decreased mortality from heart attack. Unfortunately, more recent studies specifically looking at heart disease prevention in those at high risk for heart attack have generally failed to show any benefit from supplementation with alpha-tocopherol either alone or in combination with other antioxidants, such as vitamin C and

133   Holick MF. Environmental factors that influence cutaneous production of vitamin D. Am J Clin Nutr. 1995 Mar;61(3 Suppl):638S–645S.

134   Vieth R. Vitamin D supplementation, 25-hydroxyvitamin D concentration and safety. Am J Clin Nutr. 1999;69:842–856.

135   Food and Nutrition Board, Institute of Medicine. Vitamin E. Dietary reference intakes for vitamin C, vitamin E, selenium, and carotenoids. Washington DC: National Academy Press; 2000:186–283.

beta-carotene. The HDL-Atherosclerosis Treatment Study actually showed a worsening of artery block-ages in patients taking antioxidants in combination with prescription cholesterol-lowering drugs.[136] As a result, most physicians recommend that you not take additional vitamin C and E supplements if you are on cholesterol-lowering medication unless specifically advised by your physician.

The data for cancer prevention have been mixed but generally disappointing. There have been con-flicting data from a wide variety of studies. In general, it does not appear that supplementation with vita-min E from synthetic or natural sources has much overall impact on the rates of various cancers.[137]

Based on this data, I don't recommend that most people take additional vitamin E supplements at this time. Obviously, there is ongoing research in this area that may change that in the future. There is no evidence that taking vitamin E supplements is harmful. Very high doses (greater than 1000 to 1500 IU/day) could potentially increase the risk of bleeding due to vitamin E's effect on blood platelet function, but intake at levels lower than this is not associated with any known problems. All three diets in The Program are designed to be rich in natural vitamin E. It may be that the combination of various forms of vitamin E along with a number of phytochemicals found in whole foods is what really provides long-term benefit in terms of heart disease and cancer prevention. Until there is compelling research indicating that supple-mental vitamin E is beneficial, it seems more reasonable to rely on whole, natural foods to provide what your body needs.

Vitamin K

Vitamin K is actually a group of related compounds that are primarily involved in providing the building blocks for proper blood clotting. There are two primary types of vitamin K: vitamin K1 and vi-tamin K2. K1 is the form that primarily comes from various foods like green leafy vegetables, liver, and legumes. Normal, healthy bacteria in your intestines produce K2. Your liver uses both forms to synthesize the clotting factors your body requires.

Vitamin K deficiency is very rare in healthy adults. Even with extremely low dietary intake, suffi-cient K2 is produced by intestinal bacteria to prevent the development of deficiency. The only exception to this general rule is with individuals who are on long-term antibiotics (which kill off the healthy K2-producing bacteria in your gut) and also have poor dietary intake. Therefore, dietary supplementation with vitamin K is unnecessary for the vast majority of healthy individuals. While on The Program diets, you should be taking in plenty of leafy green vegetables and therefore, even if you were on antibiotics for a period of time due to illness, vitamin K deficiency should not become an issue.

---

136   Brown BG, Zhao XQ, Chait A, Fisher LD, Cheung MC, Morse JS, Dowdy AA, Marino EK, Bolson EL, Alaupovic P, Frohlich J, Albers JJ. Simvastatin and niacin, antioxidant vitamins, or the combination for the prevention of coronary disease. N Engl J Med. 2001; 345: 1583–1592.
137   I-Min Lee, MBBS, ScD; Nancy R. Cook, ScD; J. Michael Gaziano, MD; David Gordon, MA; Paul M Ridker, MD; JoAnn E. Man-son, MD, DrPH; Charles H. Hennekens, MD, DrPH; Julie E. Buring, ScD. Vitamin E in the Primary Prevention of Cardiovascular Disease and Cancer. The Women's Health Study: A Randomized Controlled Trial. 2005;294:56–65.

Vitamin B1 (Thiamine)

Thiamine is a water-soluble vitamin that works as a cofactor for a number of energy-producing enzymes. Thiamine is found in a variety of foods, such as cereals, yeast, pork, lentils, wheat germ, and peas. Most bread and cereal products in the United States are fortified with thiamine, making deficiency in this country rare. Thiamine is a fairly heat-sensitive molecule so cooking and baking can destroy the thiamine found in some foods.

Thiamine deficiency manifests itself as a condition known as beriberi (wet, dry, or cerebral) and can cause neurological symptoms and heart failure, as well as a condition known as the Wernicke-Korsakoff syndrome seen mostly in chronically malnourished alcoholics. Most cases of thiamine deficiency occur in low-income, malnourished populations whose diet consists of low-nutrient, processed carbohydrates. Strenuous physical exercise and chronic illness can increase the body's requirement for thiamine. Healthy adult males need about 2 milligrams of thiamine per day, and females require about 1.2 milligrams. Most adults eating a regular diet meet this minimum but adults over the age of sixty tend to ingest somewhat less than this.[138] Thiamine deficiency will not be an issue while on The Program, as you will be consuming more than enough dietary thiamine. Most multivitamins contain ample thiamine as well, ensuring you will not become deficient.

Vitamin B2 (Riboflavin)

Riboflavin is necessary for proper tissue growth of mucous membranes and organs. Milk and dairy products, eggs, meat, and dark-green vegetables are good sources of riboflavin. Riboflavin deficiency in the United States is extremely rare since most cereal and bread products are fortified. Symptoms of riboflavin deficiency, as with most of the B vitamins, are nonspecific. Sufferers may experience skin rashes, inflammation of the tongue, painful drying and cracking of the lips and corners of the mouth, dry eyes, and irritation. The recommended daily intake for riboflavin is approximately 1.5 milligrams per day, which is easily achieved from dietary sources, making additional supplementation unnecessary for most. Riboflavin supplementation is very safe, and even very high levels are not associated with toxicity.

Vitamin B3 (Niacin)

Niacin, also known as nicotinic acid, is a water-soluble vitamin also involved in a number of energy-producing chemical reactions. Nicotinamide is a derivative of niacin that is used to create a number of important coenzymes (NAD and NADP). Foods high in niacin include chicken, turkey, beef, and salmon. Some cereals in the United States are also fortified with niacin to prevent deficiency. The body is able to use niacin absorbed from the diet as well as convert the amino acid tryptophan to niacin to meet its needs. The average person can convert sixty milligrams of tryptophan into one milligram of niacin.

---

138   Food and Nutrition Board, Institute of Medicine. Thiamine. Dietary Reference Intakes: Thiamine, Riboflavin, Niacine, Vitamin B6, Vitamin B12, Pantothenic Acid, Biotin, and Choline. Washington DC: National Academy Press; 1998:58–86.

Niacin deficiency, known as pellagra, used to be endemic in the southwestern United States in the 1800s due to the reliance on corn, which is low in both niacin and tryptophan, as a primary dietary staple. Pellagra, which means "raw skin," affects all body tissues and typically manifests with weakness, diarrhea, and a burning sensation involving the limbs. Long-term pellagra causes chronic diarrhea, skin irritation, and cognitive problems.

Niacin in both immediate- and sustained-release preparations is commonly used to treat high cholesterol and is particularly effective at lowering triglyceride levels and improving HDL (good cholesterol) levels.

There is no known toxicity associated with ingesting large amounts of niacin from food. However, niacin taken as a supplement or as a prescription drug can cause intense skin flushing, itching, and tingling. Long-term ingestion of excess niacin from supplements or prescription medications can cause liver injury. The RDA for niacin is about twenty milligrams per day but as little as thirty-five milligrams may cause a flushing sensation. In general, you will easily meet the RDA for niacin while on any of the diets in The Program and supplementation is not required.

Vitamin B6 (Pyridoxine)

Vitamin B6 is another one of the water-soluble B vitamins. Like other B vitamins, it plays a key role in a wide array of enzymatic processes. Vitamin B6, however, has some unique properties that set it apart from other B vitamins. It is required for the conversion of tryptophan to niacin, and therefore, vitamin B6 deficiency can lead to a secondary deficiency of niacin in the setting of inadequate niacin intake. It is also required for the transformation of stored glycogen into glucose, something of vital importance on a low-carbohydrate diet.

Most Americans eating a regular diet easily meet the minimum RDA for B6 of approximately 1.3 milligrams per day. Foods such as bananas, chicken, turkey, and salmon are good sources of vitamin B6, and many cereals in the United States are fortified as well. As a result, B6 deficiency in the Western world is very rare. Symptoms of deficiency include seizures in infants, mood changes, generalized weakness, oral ulcers, and skin rashes. People at risk for deficiency in this country are those eating very restrictive vegetarian diets and those taking certain medications for tuberculosis (isoniazid) and certain drugs used for Parkinson's disease.

Toxicity from B6 never occurs when its source is food. It's only when extremely high doses of oral B6 supplements are ingested over a long period of time. The development of toxicity manifested by neurological symptoms like numbness, burning, and altered sensation has been reported with chronic ingestions ranging from five hundred milligrams to one thousand milligrams a day.

Given the ease of achieving the required intake of vitamin B6 with diet alone, supplementation in healthy individuals is rarely needed. Like for the other B vitamins, the diets in The Program will provide more than adequate levels for optimum athletic performance and muscle growth.

Folic Acid

Folate is yet another of the water-soluble B vitamins. Folate in various forms is found in abundance in leafy green vegetables, orange juice, lentils, and since 1998 has been added to all cereal grain products in the United States. Folic acid is the form of folate commonly found in vitamin supplements and rarely occurs in natural foods. Folic acid has gotten a lot of publicity for its role in preventing neural tube defects during pregnancy. As a result, all pregnant women are recommended to supplement with folic acid.

Most non-pregnant adults need between two hundred and four hundred micrograms per day. Folate is required for the synthesis of DNA. It is also required, along with B12, for the synthesis of the amino acid methionine. When folate deficiency occurs (usually as a result of an inadequate diet), it typically manifests as weakness, fatigue, and anemia. Folate is vital for the proper formation of red blood cells in the bone marrow. Deficiency often results in an overabundance of large, immature red blood cells but a deficiency of healthy, mature red blood cells. Folate deficiency almost always occurs as a result of a diet that is poor in leafy green vegetables and other sources of folate, but sometimes people with chronic medical conditions like cancer or alcoholism or those on powerful drugs like methotrexate, certain drugs for malaria prevention, and anti-seizure medications may develop a deficiency. Large doses of anti-inflammatory medications like ibuprofen, aspirin, and naproxen can interfere with your body's ability to metabolize folate as well. If you have any of these problems, discuss your need for additional folic acid with your doctor. Folate is easily destroyed by heat, so make sure that you eat plenty of raw, leafy vegetables and other non-cooked sources to avoid losing out on your dietary folate. Most vitamin supplements contain folic acid in varying quantities as well.

There is no known toxicity from the intake of large amounts of folate from dietary sources. Large amounts of folic acid appear to be well tolerated as well since the body simply excretes excess folic acid in the urine. Theoretically, large amounts of folic acid could mask an underlying B12 deficiency (since both cause a megaloblastic anemia), but in most healthy individuals, this is unlikely. There is no known benefit to supplementing with large doses of folic acid. Aim for between 400-800mcg daily from your diet and a multivitamin. Taking additional folic acid supplements is not recommended.

Vitamin B12

Vitamin B12 (cyanocobalamin) is probably one of most well-known water-soluble B vitamins. It is a common ingredient in almost all multivitamins and is often included in various "energy supplements." B12 works with folate to help your body synthesize the amino acid methionine from homocysteine. It is also used in the production of succinyl-CoA, which plays a role in the production of energy (ATP) in your cells. This is probably where B12 got its label as an "energy" vitamin. To be clear, vitamin B12 doesn't give you added energy. In the absence of deficiency, taking extra B12 does not improve either cognitive or athletic performance.

Unlike other B vitamins, the only natural source of B12 is bacteria. It is found in various animal products, particularly chicken, turkey, fish, clams, mussels, and crab meat. Plant products, which tend to be high in B vitamins, are typically rather low in B12, which can be a problem for vegetarians. Most healthy adults need about 2.4 milligrams of vitamin B12 per day. For most, this is easily achieved with a balanced diet. Unfortunately, certain populations, specifically the elderly, strict vegetarians, and those with medical problems involving the stomach, small intestine, and pancreas can have high rates of deficiency relative to the general population. Certain medications like proton-pump inhibitors (Prilosec, Nexium, Aciphex, et cetera) can reduce blood levels of B12 if used long term (over three years).[139] The diabetes drug metformin can also decrease B12 absorption in the stomach by binding up the calcium needed for proper B12 absorption. Supplementing with calcium or taking metformin with a high-calcium food like milk, cheese, or yogurt can offset this particular effect.

B12 deficiency can manifest itself in a number of ways. Like with folate, deficiency can result in anemia and produce fatigue and weakness. B12 deficiency also affects the nerves, and symptoms can include numbness, tingling, and burning sensations of the arms and legs. If you experience these symptoms and feel you may be at risk for vitamin B12 deficiency, a simple blood test can be performed to measure your B12 levels and treatment with B12 via oral or injectable routes initiated if needed.

Excess vitamin B12 is efficiently excreted in the urine, and even ingestion of extremely large amounts is not associated with any known toxicity. In conclusion, following any of the diets in The Program will provide you with sufficient amounts of B12. The addition of a multivitamin will even more certainly prevent deficiency. Unless you have a known deficiency or are directed to take additional B12 by your doctor for a medical condition, ingestion of greater amounts of B12 are unnecessary and provide no benefit.

Vitamin B5 (Pantothenic Acid)

Vitamin B5 is a water-soluble B vitamin that is essential for a wide range of metabolic reactions. In the body, pantothenic acid is converted to its usable form, coenzyme A (CoA). CoA is vital for the proper metabolism of fats, carbohydrates, and proteins into energy. It is also involved in a myriad of other vital functions from the synthesis of hormones and neurotransmitters to the replication of DNA. Pantothenic acid is absolutely vital for life, not just in humans but in virtually all organisms.

Vitamin B5 is widely available in nature from a wide range of plant and animal foods. Most meat, like fish and chicken, is high in pantothenic acid. Dairy products, legumes, and whole grains are also good sources. The processing of grains as well as freezing or canning, however, can deplete pantothenic acid levels so good sources of this vital nutrient should be consumed with as little processing as possible.

Most healthy adults require about five milligrams of vitamin B6 daily. Pregnant and breast-feeding women may need slightly more. Fortunately, given the wide range of foods containing pantothenic acid, deficiency is exceedingly rare. As a result, there is very little data on symptoms of deficiency in humans. Animal studies showed that animals with pantothenic acid deficiency developed a whole range of problems affecting almost all major organ systems.

---

139   Kasper H. Vitamin absorption in the elderly. Int J Vitam Nutr Res. 1999;69(3):169–172.

Pantothenic acid does have one unique property that sets it apart from the other B-vitamins and makes it more attractive as a supplement for some individuals. Pantethine, which is a derivative of pantothenic acid, is used in Asia and Europe as an effective cholesterol-lowering agent. Doses in the four-hundred- to nine-hundred-milligram range appear to be effective in reducing triglycerides as well as LDL cholesterol when taken in divided doses throughout the day.[140] Side effects of pantethine as well as pantothenic acid are virtually nonexistent. There is no known toxicity from even very large doses of pantothenic acid.

In conclusion, for most individuals without a preexisting cholesterol problem, supplementation with vitamin B5, as with many of the B vitamins, is unnecessary. However, if you are looking for a safe, effective, and inexpensive way to naturally reduce your cholesterol levels beyond those achieved with diet and exercise, then you may want to discuss a trial of pantethine with your doctor. More studies need to be done with pantethine before I can give it my full endorsement, but it certainly looks promising and there appears to be little downside to trying it.

Vitamin C

Vitamin C, also known as ascorbic acid, is an essential water-soluble vitamin. It is found in abundance in most fresh citrus fruits and vegetables, such as broccoli, green peppers, tomatoes, and cabbage. Humans cannot make their own vitamin C and must obtain it from their diet or through supplementation. Vitamin C is crucial for a host of bodily functions including tissue repair, proper immune function, iron absorption, proper endocrine function, and many others. Vitamin C also acts as a potent antioxidant and is excreted primarily through the kidneys. Deficiency of Vitamin C can cause the disease known as scurvy. Symptoms included bleeding, weakness, loosening of teeth, poor wound healing, and, in later stages, jaundice, seizures, and death. Scurvy once caused a significant amount of morbidity among British sailors until it was discovered that lime juice (which is naturally high in vitamin C) could cure those afflicted. Today, vitamin C deficiency is rare in the Western world. The most at-risk populations are infants fed only cow's milk during the first year of life, chronic alcoholics, and elderly individuals with restricted diets. The recommended daily intake of vitamin C is approximately 80 to 120 milligrams daily. However, certain individuals may require greater amounts. Smoking greatly increases the oxidative stresses placed on the body and lowers vitamin C absorption while increasing its metabolism. Pregnant and nursing mothers require increased amounts to sustain their needs and those of their infant. Hard-training athletes also require increased vitamin C intake to aid in recovery between workouts and to build new muscle mass.

There has been considerable debate about the need to supplement vitamin C to a diet that already contains moderate or high levels of the vitamin. The Nobel Prize–winning physicist Linus Pauling was the first to promote mega-doses of vitamin C. He reportedly consumed ten thousand milligrams daily and was known to increase his intake to up to forty thousand milligrams at the first signs of a cold or other illness. His popular book *Vitamin C and the Common Cold* encouraged people to supplement their diets with at least a thousand milligrams daily to prevent and treat the common cold. He made similar claims for higher doses in regards to the treatment and prevention of cancer. Unfortunately, extensive study of mega-doses of vitamin C intake has failed to confirm Dr. Pauling's findings. Multiple well-done trials have

---

140   Horváth Z. Current medical aspects of pantethine. Sz - 30-JUL-2009; 62(7-8): 220–9.

shown no reduction in the frequency of colds among subjects taking mega-doses of vitamin C.[141] Some studies have shown a small reduction in cold symptoms with high intake of vitamin C, but it is uncertain if this represents an actual effect of vitamin C on the body's ability to fight the cold virus or whether it is an effect of vitamin C's natural antihistamine properties. Similarly, studies looking at vitamin C's ability to fight cancer have been disappointing.[142] Despite the apparent lack of benefit in taking mega-doses of vitamin C, there appears to be little evidence that it is harmful.[143] Vitamin C in excess of bodily requirements is simply excreted. Very high intake may cause gastrointestinal upset and may theoretically increase the risk of certain types of kidney stones, but these have rarely been reported. So how much vitamin C should you take while following The Program? It would be a good idea to supplement with around one thousand milligrams in divided doses daily especially while on the Endomorphic Diet, as your intake of citrus fruits will be limited. This should more than cover your body's requirements as well as provide adequate levels for repair and growth of muscle and connective tissue.

141   Marshall CB. Vitamin C: Do High Doses Prevent Colds? Quackwatch, Oct 3, 1999.
142   Creagan ET and others. Failure of high-dose vitamin C (ascorbic acid) therapy to benefit patients with advanced cancer. A controlled trial. New England Journal of Medicine 301:687–690, 1979.
143   John N Hathcock, et al. Vitamins E and C are safe across a broad range of intakes. American Journal of Clinical Nutrition, Vol. 81, No. 4, 736–745, April 2005.

"The three most harmful addictions are heroin, carbohydrates, and a monthly salary."

—Nassim Nicholas Taleb

SWEETENERS

One of the primary complaints of low- or moderate-carb dieters is that they have to miss out on all the delicious, sweet foods they were accustomed to eating. Fortunately, today, there are a variety of sugar substitutes on the market that provide the same (or greater) degree of sweetness found in regular sugar. A preference for the sensation of sweetness is hardwired in human beings. In nature, sweetness is generally a sensory cue for foods that are rich in nutrients. Unfortunately, many processed foods are loaded with additional sugar to enhance flavor but provide very little in the way of valuable nutrition. As you know, these types of foods are off-limits for those of you trying to shed unwanted body fat. If you crave sweet foods, artificial sweeteners will make sticking to both the Endomorphic and Mesomorphic Diets much easier. You don't have to abandon the sensation of sweetness just because you are on a carbohydrate-restricted diet. Artificial sweeteners can allow you to indulge your sweet tooth without blowing your diet.

There are a variety of sweeteners on the market, and more are being added on a regular basis. In general, they can be divided into two categories: nutritive sweeteners and non-nutritive sweeteners. These two classes have important differences, and understanding this will allow you to choose wisely between them. Nutritive sweeteners usually have between one and four kilocalories per gram (regular sugar or glucose has four kilocalories per gram). These include sugar alcohols and polyols. They are partially absorbed by the intestines but generally have a minimal effect on blood sugar. If you look at the ingredients of most low-carb protein bars or other foods, you will see one or more of these compounds listed in their ingredients. They not only provide sweetness but also texture and act as a binding agent to hold foods together.

The bulk of these agents are passed through the intestines without significant absorption into the bloodstream. This is beneficial for those trying to maintain ketosis since insulin levels are not significantly affected when these sweeteners are consumed in normal doses. The downside to this lack of absorption is a potent laxative effect when these substances are consumed in excess. Additionally, bacteria in the colon are able to digest some of these compounds leading to the formation of gas. Most of these foods carry a warning label stating, *"Excess consumption may have a laxative effect."* I can state from personal experience that if you overindulge in low-carb treats, you can expect to be spending a significant part of your day in the bathroom! Also, though sugar alcohols are lower in calories, gram for gram, than sugar, they are not calorie free. If consumed in excess, their calories can add up and should be factored into your overall calorie intake.

Common Nutritive Sweeteners

	kcal/gram
1. Sorbitol:	2.6
2. Maltitol:	2.1
3. Lactitol:	2.0
4. Xylitol:	2.4
5. Erythritol:	0.2
6. HSH (hydrogenated starch hydrosylates)	3.0
7. Isomalt	2.0

Nonnutritive sweeteners, also referred to as high-intensity sweeteners, have no calories and generally are perceived by your brain as hundreds of times sweeter than sugar. As a result, very little is needed to get a significant sweetening effect. They have little to no effect on blood sugar, but some can raise insulin levels, though the degree to which this occurs is small and likely of little consequence when they are consumed in reasonable amounts. Because so little sweetener is needed to provide a pleasurable sensation, most of them are combined with some other agent, usually maltodextran or polydextrose, to provide some bulk to the product and modify its taste. This is a key fact to be aware of. While the sweetener itself may have no significant effect on glucose or insulin levels, the other ingredients it is mixed with can. Maltodextran, for example, is a simple sugar that is rapidly absorbed, provides a full four kilocalories per gram, and stimulates a significant amount of insulin secretion. While the overall effect of, say a packet of Equal, may be less than a similar amount of refined sugar, its effect should not be ignored and in large quantities could still adversely affect your diet.

Recently, there has been speculation sparked by several studies that the consumption of artificial sweeteners may actually lead to weight gain.[144] The theory is that the intense sweetness of these substances combined with their lack of calories will lead users to consume more calories than they ordinarily would. Some researchers speculate that artificial sweeteners actually increase cravings for sugar so you end up eating more calories later in the day. This hypothesis, to date, has not been consistently demonstrated in subsequent studies. Indeed, the bulk of the data shows that the replacement of sugar with artificial

---

144   Blundell, J.E. and A.J. Hill, *Paradoxical effects of an intense sweetener (aspartame) on appetite*. Lancet, 1986. 1(8489): p. 1092–3.

sweeteners can lead to weight loss and improved blood sugar control in diabetic patients.[145] More studies are needed to determine if this phenomenon is real.

There are currently six nonnutritive sweeteners approved by the FDA as food additives. They are:

1. **Saccharin**—Brand names: Sweet and Low, Sweet Twin, Necta Sweet
2. **Aspartame**—Brand names: NutraSweet, Equal, Sugar Twin
3. **Acesulfame-K**—Brand names: Sunett, Sweet & Safe, Sweet One
4. **Sucralose**—Brand names: Splenda
5. **Neotame**—Brand names: none yet
6. **Rebaudioside A**—Brand name: Rebiana, Truvia

Saccharin (Benzoic Sulfilimine)

Saccharin was first discovered in 1878 and became popular as a sugar substitute during World War I. For decades, it was the only commercially available artificial sweetener. Beginning in the early 1900s, there were concerns raised that saccharin may have a number of deleterious effects. Several studies in rats suggested that it might be responsible for inducing bladder cancer. As a result, saccharin-containing products were required to carry a warning label. A number of subsequent studies have failed to show evidence of negative health effects in humans, and laws requiring this labeling have now been withdrawn.[146] In a December 14, 2010, release, the EPA stated that saccharin is no longer considered a potential hazard to human health.[147] Ingestion of saccharin can cause a small elevation in insulin levels but does not appear to affect glucose levels.[148]

Aspartame

First discovered in 1965, aspartame has become one of the most widely used and most controversial artificial sweeteners on the market. Aspartame is created by combining the amino acids L-phenylalanine and L-aspartate and is approximately two hundred times sweeter than ordinary sugar (sucrose). Aspartame was given full approval by the FDA for general use in 1996. Upon digestion, aspartame breaks down into three components (aspartic acid, phenylalanine, and methanol) all of which are found naturally in a number of foods including fruits. The absolute upper limit of safe intake of aspartame, as determined by animal studies, is very high. The World Health Organization defines the acceptable upper limit of aspartame intake at forty milligrams per kilogram per day. This level of aspartame intake was found to have no adverse effects on lab rats.[149] To place this figure in more easily understood terms, that is equivalent to approximately twenty cans of diet soda or one hundred standard packets of sweetener for an average seventy-kilogram adult.

145   Renwick, AG. Intense sweeteners, food intake, and the weight of a body of evidence. Physiol. Behav. 1994. Jan:55(1):139–143.

146   Morrison, 1984. Morrison AS: Advances in the etiology of urothelial cancer. *Urol Clin North Am* 1984; 11:557.

147   Federal Register: December 17, 2010 (Volume 75, Number 242)] [Rules and Regulations] [Page 78918–78926].

148   Horowitz, DL. Response to single dose of aspartame or saccharin by NIDDM patients. Diabetes Care. Mar 1988. 11(3): 230–234.

149   Joint FAO/WHO Expert Committee on Food Additives, *Toxicological Evaluation of Certain Food Additives*. WHO Food Additives Series, 1983. 16.

Obviously, average daily intake, even for heavy users, is well under this. Aspartame itself does not appear to have any significant effect on blood glucose or insulin levels.[150] Keep in mind though that, particularly in artificial sweetener packets, aspartame and other sweeteners are often combined with simple sugars like maltodextran, which can definitely impact both insulin and glucose levels.

Despite a large amount of scientific literature demonstrating the safety of aspartame, there continues to be controversy regarding potential toxicity, and anecdotal reports of adverse effects are still somewhat common. Common complaints regarding aspartame are that it can trigger headaches or other neurological symptoms.[151] This has largely been blamed on its breakdown products: methanol, phenylalanine, and aspartic acid. In the body, methanol is metabolized in the liver to formaldehyde and then to the more toxic substance formic acid. In toxic methanol ingestions (moonshine ingestion, et cetera), it is formic acid that is largely responsible for the serious neurological symptoms and blindness that often occur. When the body metabolizes aspartame, about 10 percent of it is converted to methanol.

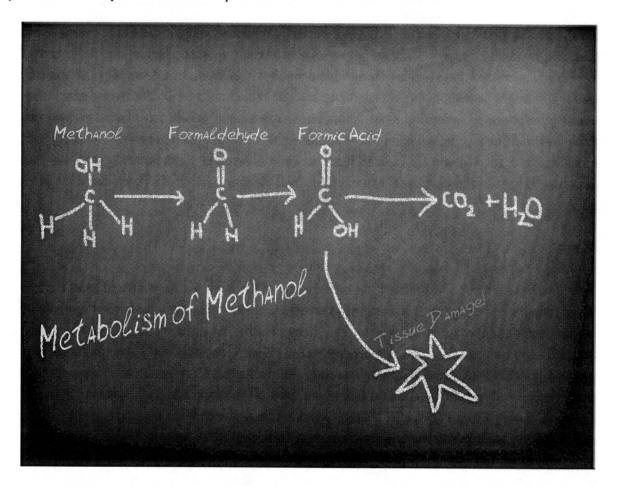

In the case of aspartame, however, the scientific data to date does not support the link between aspartame ingestion and any adverse effects when it is consumed in normal amounts.[152] While the thought

150   Shigeta H, Effects of aspartame on diabetic rats and diabetic patients.—no effect on blood glucose or insulin. J Nutr Sci Vitaminol (Tokyo). 1985 Oct;31(5):533–40.
151   Kroger, M., K. Meister, and R. Kava, *Low-calorie Sweeteners and Other Sugar Substitutes: A Review of the Safety Issues*. Comprehensive Reviews in Food Science and Food Safety, 2006. 5: p. 35–47.
152   Magnuson BA, Burdock GA, Doull J, *et al.* (2007). "Aspartame: a safety evaluation based on current use levels, regulations, and toxicological and epidemiological studies". *Critical Reviews in Toxicology* 37 (8): 629–727.

of ingesting a potential poison like methanol might seem frightening, keep in mind that many completely natural foods also contain methanol.

Some fruit juices contain up to 140 milligrams of methanol per liter. The methanol content of fresh orange juice is approximately 34 milligrams per liter while the average methanol produced from a typical diet soft drink produces approximately 56 milligrams of methanol per liter.[153, 154] The other breakdown product of aspartame is aspartic acid. Aspartic acid is an excitatory neurotransmitter in the brain. Several studies have shown that very high levels of aspartic acid can cause damage to neurons in lab animals. The human brain is protected from toxins circulating in the blood by a complex defensive barrier referred to as the blood-brain barrier. The blood-brain barrier effectively isolates the brain from a wide variety of ingested substances as well as infectious organisms that would ordinarily damage sensitive neurons. Aspartic acid in the bloodstream is effectively prevented from coming in contact with the brain via the blood-brain barrier.[155] Only extremely high levels of aspartic acid can overwhelm this barrier and cause toxicity. In studies where humans ingested very large amounts of aspartame (two hundred milligrams per kilogram of body weight), serum levels of aspartic acid still remained less than one-twentieth of the level needed to cause brain damage in infant mice.[156,157] It therefore seems unlikely that the aspartic acid produced when consuming average amounts of aspartame poses any significant hazard to the brain.

The final breakdown product of aspartame is the amino acid phenylalanine. Phenylalanine is a naturally occurring amino acid and poses no health risks. Only individuals with the rare genetic disorder phenylketonuria (PKU) should avoid aspartame for this reason. This is why all aspartame-containing products have a label warning patients with PKU to avoid their use.

Therefore, I think the data we have so far shows aspartame to be safe when consumed in moderation.[158] If more studies are brought forward showing otherwise, then clearly I would change my position on this substance. Obviously, if you are one of those individuals who experience headaches or other ill effects from aspartame, you should avoid it. Fortunately, there are now many other sweeteners you can choose from.

153   Lund ED, Kirkland CL, & Shaw PE (1981) Methanol, ethanol and acetaldehyde contents of citrus products. J Agric Food Chem, 29:361–366.

154   Kretchmer, Norman, and Clari B. Hollenbeck, ed., *Sugars and Sweeteners* (Boca Raton: CRC Press, 1991), pp. 151–167, 232–237.

155   Spiers, P.A., et al., *Aspartame: neuropsychologic and neurophysiologic evaluation of acute and chronic effects.* Am J Clin Nutr, 1998. 68(3): p. 531–7.

156   Stegink, L.D., L.J. Filer Jr., G.L. Baker, and J.E. McDonnell, "Effect of an Abuse Dose of Aspartame Upon Plasma and Erythrocyte Amino Acid Levels of Amino Acids in Phenylketonuric Heterozygous and Normal Adult Subjects," *Journal of Nutrition*, vol. 110 (1980), p. 2216.

157   Schomer, D.L., P. Spiers, and L. Sabounjian, *Evaluation of behavior cognition, mood, and electroencephalograms in normal adults and potentially vulnerable populations.*, in *The Clinical Evaluation of a Food Additive:* Assessment of Aspartame.1996, CRC Press: Boca Raton, FL. p. 217–233.

158   Magnuson BA, Burdock GA, Doull J, *et al.* (2007). "Aspartame: a safety evaluation based on current use levels, regulations, and toxicological and epidemiological studies". *Critical Reviews in Toxicology* 37 (8): 629–727.

Acesulfame-K

Acesulfame-K was discovered in 1967 and approved by the FDA for use in nonalcoholic beverages in 1998 and as a sweetener safe for general use in 2003. It is related to saccharine and usually combined with other sweeteners like aspartame to counteract its somewhat bitter aftertaste. It is used commonly in

Levels of aspartame in common consumer items

Product Category	Serving Size	Aspartame Content (mg)
Dry sweetener	1 packet	35 mg
Diet soft drink	12 oz	180 mg
Hot chocolate	6 oz	50 mg
Gelatin dessert	4 oz	95 mg
Instant pudding	4 oz	25 mg

Kretchmer, Norman, and Clara B. Hollenbeck, ed., Sugars and Sweeteners (Boca Raton: CRC Press, 1991), pp. 151-167, 232-237.

chewing gum, yogurt, and various sugar-free desserts, sauces, and candies. Acesulfame-K has not undergone quite the same rigorous evaluation for safety as aspartame and saccharine but is considered to be safe for general use. The primary concern raised by critics of acesulfame-K is that it may be a potential carcinogen. Studies to date looking at very large, chronic ingestions in mice, however, have not shown a statistically significant increase in malignancies.[159] A consensus report published by the US Department of Health and Human Services' National Toxicology Program in 2005 reviewed the available data on toxicity for acesulfame-K and concluded that evidence for carcinogenesis was lacking. Therefore, based on the available data, acesulfame-K appears to be a safe alternative nonnutritive sweetener.

Acesulfame-K does appear to significantly raise insulin levels. In fact, acesulfame-K elevates insulin as much as an equivalent amount of glucose.[160] However, since most food and beverages have relatively

---

159   Beems, G.S., and Williams, R.L. Carcinogenicity Study of Acesulfame-K in Mice. In *Acesulfame-K*, pp 59–70. 1991.
160   Liang Y, Steinbach G, Maier V, Pfeiffer EF. The effect of artificial sweetener on insulin secretion. 1. The effect of acesulfame K on insulin secretion in the rat (studies in vivo). *Horm Metab Res*. 1987 Jun;19(6):233–8.

low levels of acesulfame-K (most soft drinks have between 20 and 70mg), this effect on insulin secretion is not terribly significant.

Sucralose

Sucralose was first created in 1976 and has since experienced widespread use. Its high degree of sweetness (six hundred times sweeter than sucrose) and stability when exposed to high cooking temperatures has made sucralose a popular nonnutritive sweetener. Sucralose is actually made from ordinary sucrose through a series of simple chemical reactions. Despite being created from sucrose, sucralose cannot be metabolized by the human body. Most passes unabsorbed through the intestines and what little is absorbed into the bloodstream is excreted intact into the urine. Despite anecdotal reports of various side effects, the scientific literature to date has failed to show any adverse effects from regular consumption of sucralose.[161] Because the creation of sucralose involves the exchange of hydroxyl groups for chlorine atoms on a sucrose molecule, there has been some concern by various laypersons that it may have adverse effects similar to other chlorine-containing substances, such as hydrocarbons. Examination of the metabolism and chemical properties of sucralose has shown this to be untrue. Unlike chlorinated hydrocarbons, sucralose is water-soluble and does not have the ability to accumulate in body tissues. When consumed, less than 25 percent is absorbed from the intestines, and what is absorbed is excreted quickly in the urine.[162]

Sucralose itself does not appear to significantly raise insulin levels.[163] The primary problem with most sucralose formulations (and other sweeteners) is that they are composed of significant quantities of bulk fillers like maltodextran. These fillers are high-glycemic sugars that add up to four kilocalories per gram and significantly raise insulin and glucose levels. Current FDA regulations allow manufacturers to label any product that has less than five calories per serving as having "zero calories." Obviously, if you don't take these fillers into account, you can end up consuming much more carbohydrate and calories than you intend. If you add large amounts of powdered sucralose (Splenda) to your beverages or use it to cook with, it is definitely possible, especially on the Endomorphic Diet, to put yourself out of ketosis and sabotage your weight-loss efforts. Therefore, you should count each packet of sucralose and other sweeteners containing fillers as containing one gram of carbohydrate and factor that into your daily calorie and carbohydrate count.

Neotame

Neotame is one of the newest FDA-approved nonnutritive sweeteners. It received approval for general us in the United States in 2002. Since then, it has been included in a wide range of beverages and foods. Neotame is a very high-potency sweetener. It is about eight thousand times as sweet as sucrose. As a result, it typically is only used in small amounts or combined with other sweeteners. Neotame has no calories and does not influence insulin secretion. Neotame has a chemical structure similar to aspartame but does not break down in to phenylalanine. It does break down into very small amounts of methanol

161   "Which additives are safe? Which aren't?" Center for Science in the Public Interest.
162   Roberts, A., et al., *Sucralose metabolism and pharmacokinetics in man*. Food Chem Toxicol, 2000. 38 Suppl 2: p. S31–41.
163   N. H. Mezitis, C. A. Maggio, P. Koch, A. Quddoos, D. B. Allison and F. X. PiSunyer. Glycemic effect of a single high oral dose of the novel sweetener sucralose in patients with diabetes. *Diabetes Care*. September 1996 vol. 19 no. 9.

but still far less than most natural sugars and fruit juices.[164] Neotame has undergone extensive animal and human studies and has not been shown to have any adverse effects, even when consumed at hundreds of times its recommended intake.[165]

Stevia

Stevia is the common name for the flowering plant *Stevia rebaudiana*. Stevia is native to both North and South America and has been used for centuries as both a sweetener and food ingredient. Stevia is used widely in Japan but banned in other countries over potential safety concerns. The leaves of the stevia plant are about thirty to forty times as sweet as sucrose, but its most commonly used extracts, rebaudioside A (rebiana—brand name Truvia) and stevioside, are over three hundred times sweeter than sucrose.[166] In the United States, stevia is not approved for use as a sweetener per se. Instead, it is approved for use as a "dietary supplement." In practical terms, this doesn't have much impact on its availability. Rebaudioside A, which is patented by the Coca-Cola Company under the name Rebiana, is one of the active stevia glycosides responsible for its sweetness. It is, however, approved for use as a sweetener and found in various brand-name sweeteners like Only Sweet, PureVia, Reb-A, SweetLeaf, and Truvia. The stevia plant itself contains several dozen other compounds, which may have pharmacologic activity but have yet to be adequately studied to see what, if any, effects they have on human metabolism.

There is some controversy regarding stevia's ability to induce insulin secretion. Animal studies with genetically modified diabetic rodents and with isolated pancreas cells have shown that high doses of stevia extract can slightly lower blood glucose levels and stimulate insulin secretion.[167,168] Studies looking specifically at oral administration of pure stevioside and rebaudioside A in humans, however, do not appear to show much, if any, significant insulin-producing effects, even when subjects were given up to one thousand milligrams per day.[169] It may be possible that consuming an extract of whole stevia plants may have insulin-producing effects but purified extracts of its two most commonly used components do not. More research in this area would be helpful. In the meantime, it seems safe to use reasonable amounts of stevioside and rebaudioside A while on the Endomorphic Diet without sabotaging your weight loss efforts by unnecessarily raising your insulin levels.

Stevia was initially banned in the United States because of some early studies showing it may have cancer-inducing properties in certain bacteria and isolated rat liver cells. Since that time, multiple studies

---

164   World Health Organization, *Environmental health criteria 196: methanol*. Geneva, 1997. WHO.

165   American Dietetic Association. *Position of the American Dietetic Association: use of nutritive and nonnutritive sweeteners*. J Am Diet Assoc, 2004. 104(2):p. 255–75.

166   Geuns JM (2003). "Stevioside". *Phytochemistry* 64 (5): 913–21.

167   Jeppesen, P. B., et al. "Stevioside acts directly on pancreatic beta cells to secrete insulin: actions independent of cyclic adenosine monophosphate and adenosine triphosphate-sensitive K+-channel activity." Metabolism 2000; 49(2): 208–14.

168   Jeppesen PB, Gregersen S, Alstrup KK, Hermansen K. Stevioside induces antihyperglycaemic, insulinotropic and glucagonostatic effects in vivo: studies in the diabetic Goto-Kakizaki (GK) rats. Phytomedicine. 2002 Jan;9(1):9–14.

169   Maki, K.C., Curry, L.L., Reeves, M.S., Toth, P.D., McKenney, J.M., Farmer, M.V., Schwartz, S.L., Lubin, B.C., Boileau, A.C., Dicklin, M.R., Carakostas, M.C., Tarka, S.M., Chronic consumption of rebaudioside A, a steviol glycoside, in men and women with type 2 diabetes mellitus, Food and Chemical Toxicology (2008b).

have failed to replicate these lab findings in human or animal subjects.[170,171] The World Health Organization (WHO) issued a statement in 2006, after reviewing the available data on stevioside and rebaudioside A, that these substances and their metabolites are not carcinogenic and can be safely consumed without concern for the induction of cancer.[172]

Therefore, the commonly available extracts from the stevia plant, stevioside and rebaudioside A, appear to be safe for general use as sweeteners. Studies on whole stevia plant extracts are sparse, however, and it may be possible that some of the plant's other compounds have deleterious effects. There just isn't enough research at this time to say. It would seem prudent then, until more research becomes available, that if you want to use stevia, you should stick to products that use one of the two above substances.

170   A. Yamada, S. Ohgaki, T. Noda, and M. Shimizu. 1985. Chronic toxicity study of dietary stevia extracts in F344 rats. Journal of the Food Science and Hygiene Society of Japan 26, 169–183.
171   Kobylewski S, Eckhert C. Toxicology of Rebaudioside A: A Review. University of California, Los Angeles, 2008.
172   D. J. Benford, M. DiNovi, J. Schlatter, Safety Evaluation of Certain Food Additives: Steviol Glycosides, in WHO Food Additives Series, World Health Organization Joint FAO/WHO Expert Committee on Food Additives (JECFA) 2006, 54, 140.

Honesty pays, but it don't seem to pay enough to suit some people.

—Frank Mckinney Hubbard

NUTRITIONAL SUPPLEMENTS

The nutritional supplement industry has literally exploded in size over the past decade. With the Dietary Supplement Health and Education Act (DSHEA) of 1994 congressional legislation allowed supplement manufacturers to avoid many of the limitations placed on prescription drugs. Since then, the number of new products flooding the market has only increased. They vary from simple vitamin and mineral preparations to exotic herbal products. Take a look at your local nutritional foods store or the "health food" aisle at Walmart, and you'll see a dizzying array of these products.

The manufacturers of these products frequently claim that their product will speed weight loss, help build muscle, increase sex drive, et cetera. Like most of us, I believed these claims whenever a new bodybuilding supplement hit the market. I tried them all: DHEA, *androstenedione*, HMB, sterols, pro-hormones, CLA, creatine, vanadyl sulphate, and many more. For the most part, I was disappointed and quite a bit poorer. Nevertheless, I still held out hope that as science advanced, maybe the next big supplement to hit the market would actually work for me. Unfortunately, it took years of trial and error, quite a bit of money, and countless hours of research on my part to see through the lies and misinformation put forth by the makers of many nutritional supplements. With this book, I hope to make that process a lot easier for you. If you remember only one thing, remember this: *There is no magic pill that will transform your body over night!* It still takes hard work and discipline. Even the most potent muscle builders we know of (anabolic steroids) do *nothing* unless you exercise. For those of you looking for a magic bullet, I'm very sorry. Prepare to be disappointed.

Before we go into detail about specific supplements, I think it is worthwhile to explain the details of the DSHEA. This extremely important piece of legislation impacts the entire supplement industry. Understanding its key points is important as a consumer because it will assist you in critically evaluating the supplements you see sold all over this country. Before the DSHEA, nutritional supplements were regulated using the same guidelines and laws that governed foods and food additives. The Federal Food, Drug and Cosmetic Act of 1938 and the Food Additive Amendment of 1958 required manufacturers of foods and nutritional supplements to prove their products were safe prior to entering the market. The FDA was also authorized to inspect companies' manufacturing sites to ensure safety.

In the 1990s, the number of new nutritional supplements grew dramatically. With the growing HIV epidemic, increased public demand for "alternative" medical therapies, and growing research that dietary modifications could impact chronic diseases, it was clear that new legislation was required. After intense lobbying by the nutritional supplement industry and high pressure from the general public, Congress passed the DSHEA and President Clinton signed it into law in 1994.

The DHSEA redefined what the FDA considered a "nutritional supplement." They defined it as "a product taken by mouth that contains a dietary ingredient intended to supplement the diet." Vitamins, minerals, herbs, botanicals, amino acids, enzymes, organ tissues, glandulars, extracts, concentrates, and metabolites are included in this definition. They may be packaged as tablets, capsules, soft gels, gel caps, liquids, or powders. If a supplement is packaged as a bar or beverage, the label is not allowed to display the item as a conventional food. It must clearly state that it is a nutritional supplement. Supplements that use a transdermal delivery system are considered to use a "drug-like" delivery system and therefore are not allowed. This definition, obviously, includes a very wide range of substances.

The DSHEA also regulates how supplement manufacturers label and advertise their products. They are not allowed to make health claims related to specific diseases or claim that their product has drug-like properties. Specifically, they cannot state that their product is intended to treat any disease or medical condition. For example, the statement "Super-Vitamin Complex X fights heart disease and cancer" would not be allowed. However, the DSHEA does allow what is termed "statements of support." It is through this clause that many supplement companies insinuate or suggest that their product does, in fact, treat a medical condition without stating it explicitly. If you are not a savvy consumer, it is easy to be fooled by these sorts of statements, and that is exactly what the advertising executives who market many supplements are trying to do. "Statements of support" allow the following things:

1. **"Claim a benefit related to a classical nutrient deficiency disease"**—This clause relates to specific dietary supplements that are known to be required by the human body and in which deficiency causes a specific disease state. For example, it is well known that vitamin D deficiency can cause the disease known as rickets—a condition that leads to abnormal bone formation. Another example is Vitamin C deficiency leading to the disease scurvy or thiamine deficiency leading to a condition known as beri-beri. Under the DSHEA, companies that manufacture and sell these products can rightly claim that their product can prevent those specific conditions in individuals with inadequate dietary intake. These sorts of statements are not used frequently, at least in this country. The incidence of diseases specifically related to deficiency in vitamins, minerals, or other micronutrients are extremely low. Many of our foods are fortified with added vitamins and minerals already. Therefore, an ad campaign, for example, that encouraged consumers to buy a certain brand of Vitamin C in order to avoid scurvy, while legal under the DSHEA, probably wouldn't be very successful in terms of sales.

2. **"Describe how ingredients affect the structure or function of the human body"** and **"characterize the documented mechanism by which the ingredients act to maintain structure and function."** This clause is similar to that described above but allows for far more varied claims. For

example, the makers of a calcium supplement can state that "daily calcium intake is essential for healthy bones" or the makers of a protein bar can state that their product is "packed with muscle-building protein." This is where supplement companies really bend the rules and create the greatest amount of deception. Though they cannot make specific drug claims about their products, they are allowed to make statements related to specific bodily organs. For example, they can claim their product "supports healthy heart function," "promotes healthy vision," "enhances memory," "enhances weight loss," et cetera. Note that they don't claim their product improves heart function, improves sight, or treats obesity—those could be interpreted as drug claims intended to treat a specific disease or condition. However, many people are fooled into believing that if they take Product X, it will improve their failing vision, help them lose weight above and beyond normal means, or somehow improve how well their heart functions. As we will see later, supplement manufacturers are not required to demonstrate that their products have any effects whatsoever. This allows all sorts of misleading statements to be made when advertising these products.

3. **"Describe general well-being from consumption of the ingredients"**—Supplement manufacturers are allowed to advertise that their products can improve the consumers' overall well-being without making specific health claims. We have all seen these advertisements, and they are among the most effective in enticing consumers to purchase these products. Magazine and television ads show people laughing, enjoying life, and leading healthier, more active lifestyles after using Product X. The insinuation is that you can be like those people if you take this product.

Quality Concerns

The DSHEA has made bringing new supplements to the market relatively easy for nutritional companies. They are now no longer required to prove that their products are safe or that they actually do what they claim prior to entering the market. For new supplements, companies are required to provide written information to the FDA at least seventy-five days prior to the product's release in the market. This information only has to show the data the company has used to determine that their product is reasonably expected to be safe. I find this particularly troubling. The FDA has essentially abdicated its responsibility to protect the public and placed the onus of safety on companies whose primary concern is not necessarily the health and safety of the general public but rather their own profit margin.

There are also no requirements that supplement companies prove their products actually contain the ingredients listed on their labels. They are not held to any set standards regarding the purity of their ingredients, and there is no oversight of their manufacturing process. This means that there is no way to tell if the protein supplement you just purchased, which claims to have thirty grams of whey protein, in fact contains that much protein. It may have more, less, or none at all. Or quite possibly, the higher-quality whey protein was mixed with lower-quality (and cheaper) powdered-milk protein. Unfortunately, there is no way to tell by looking at a product's bottle exactly what is inside. Remember, this applies to *all* supplements from herbal preparations to multivitamins.

There are a few independent sources of information regarding supplement purity—*http://www.consumerlab.com/* is an excellent resource. They routinely test various popular supplements and compare their findings with what the manufacturers claim. I highly recommend you visit their website before purchasing any supplement. You will find that some companies have better track records than others. When you find a company that is reliable, stick with them. The problem of supplement purity will be very important in particular phases of The Program. If you have reduced your carbohydrate intake to the required levels on the Endomorphic Diet yet are still not in ketosis, one possibility is hidden carbohydrates in the supposedly low-carb supplements you are using. Many protein powders claim to be low carb but, in fact, have far more carbohydrate content than stated on their labels. These sorts of products can doom your diet from the beginning. If you find that you just are not achieving ketosis despite your best efforts, try changing supplement brands (preferably to one whose ingredients are independently verified) and see what happens. There are also several laboratories that can be found online that will be glad to test supplements for you. Of course, this service can be expensive and time-consuming, but it is available.

The potential discrepancies in supplement ingredients become particularly important when older patients mix in supplements with their prescription medication. While most supplements, when taken as directed, are safe to take with prescription medications, there are several potential interactions that consumers should be aware of. If you take anticoagulant medications (often referred to as "blood-thinners") like aspirin or Coumadin, there have been reports of bleeding complications with gingko, ginseng, garlic, and ginger. Those on anti-seizure medications, like phenytoin and phenobarbital, can have their blood levels decreased by kava kava and valerian. St John's Wort has been known to have mild antidepressant effects for some time. However, when combined with prescription antidepressants, there is potential of unpredictable side effects. The same can be said for ginseng and prescription antidepressants. People taking digoxin need to be aware that ginseng, liquorice, hawthorn, figwort, and mistletoe can alter digoxin blood levels significantly. There are numerous other documented potential interactions between supplements and prescription medications and many more that are not yet known. Obviously, if you are using a supplement whose exact ingredients are not known, the potential danger increases. I encourage you to speak directly and openly with your physician if you are using or planning to use any supplement in addition to your prescription medication. There is now a PDR (*Physician's Desk Reference*) for nutritional supplements that can be a valuable resource for both you and your doctor. The worst thing you can do is keep your supplement use a secret from your physician. While your doctor may not approve of or have much knowledge about your particular supplement plan, it is imperative that you keep an open dialogue so that you can both be on the lookout for potential problems.

It is not my intention to go into a comprehensive review of all the major nutritional supplements on the market. As I stated previously, I'm not a big proponent of nutritional supplements. I believe I've made the case for including a quality protein powder and fish oil into your daily routine. The benefits of these two items are self-evident. There are two other substances that you may want to consider using as well. When used properly, they are safe and can provide your workouts with an added boost. These two substances are caffeine and creatine monohydrate.

Caffeine

Caffeine is a naturally occurring compound found in over sixty plant species. It is most commonly found in teas, sodas, chocolates, and coffees. In tea and coffee form, it is extremely popular and, next to oil, is the second most commonly traded commodity worldwide. It is also the most popular stimulant drug in the world. It belongs to a family of chemicals known as methylxanthines, which have wide-ranging effects on the cardiovascular system, kidneys, and brain.

Athletes have known for some time that caffeine can improve performance in various athletic activities as well as improve concentration and memory. Caffeine's effects on alertness have been recognized for millennia. Ingestion of moderate amounts is known to improve memory and cognitive function in sleep-deprived test subjects. Reaction times, motor skills, and coordination are also improved.[173] Caffeine also has effects on other body systems. Shortly after ingestion, heart rate and blood pressure increase. These effects are sustained for several hours. Lung function is also improved with caffeine use. Both asthmatics and healthy subjects experience relaxation of bronchial muscles leading to dilation of their airways. Some studies have shown increased VO2 max (the maximal amount of oxygen the body can consume during intense exercise) in runners. This finding has not been consistent in all studies but may partially explain why endurance athletes seem to get a performance boost from caffeine use.[174] Caffeine is also well-known for its diuretic properties. Though this effect is generally mild, it can lead to dehydration if fluid losses are not properly replaced.

Ingestion of caffeine leads to an increase in fatty acids in the bloodstream. These fatty acids come from the breakdown of body fat. It is theorized that this may accelerate fat loss, but this has not been conclusively demonstrated at this time. What seems clear, however, is that caffeine impairs the body's ability to respond to insulin. Specifically, it appears to inhibit the uptake of glucose into muscles leading to increased insulin levels and insulin resistance.[175] This is precisely the opposite of what is desired when one is attempting to lose body fat. In fairness, it is not clear if this effect actually has real-world implications when it comes to weight loss, and it seems unlikely that the occasional use of caffeine would sabotage your fat-loss efforts. However, if you are a heavy user and find that you are having difficulty losing weight despite following The Program to the letter, consider eliminating or greatly reducing caffeine from your diet for a couple weeks and see what happens. Similarly, if you are following the Endomorphic Diet and having trouble staying in ketosis, try to reduce your caffeine intake and see if that helps.

Some recent research has added a twist to the notion of caffeine and insulin-resistance problems. A recent study showed women who consumed four or more cups of either caffeinated or decaffeinated coffee regularly had lower insulin levels than those who did not.[176] Those who consumed tea did not show the same reduction. The rate of type 2 diabetes also seems to be lower in heavy coffee drinkers (greater than seven cups per day).[177] It is likely that this apparent benefit is from one or more other substances in coffee and not related to its caffeine content.

173   Burke LM, Desbrow B, Minehan M. 2000. Chapter 17: Dietary supplements and nutritional ergogenic aids in sport. In: Burke L, Deakin V, Ed. Clinical Sports Nutrition. 2nd ed. Sydney: McGraw-Hill. p 472–77, 535–40.
174   Applegate E. Effective nutritional ergogenic aids. Int J Sport Nutr 1999;9(2):229–39.
175   H. Petrie, S. Chown, L. Belfie, et al. Caffeine ingestion increases the insulin response to an oral-glucose-tolerance test in obese men before and after weight loss. Am J Clin Nutr;80:22–28 (July, 2004).
176   Wu T, Willett WC, Hankinson SE, Giovannucci E. Caffeinated coffee, decaffeinated coffee, and caffeine in relation to plasma C-peptide levels, a marker of insulin secretion, in U.S. women. Diabetes Care. 2005 Jun;28(6):1390–6.
177   Van Dam RM, Feskens EJM. Coffee consumption and risk of type 2 diabetes mellitus. Lancet 2002; 360: 1477–8.

The greatest use for caffeine while on The Program is as a workout performance enhancer. Some studies have shown a positive effect in terms of muscle strength during both maximal and submaximal weight training.[178] It is thought that caffeine may help the brain recruit more motor units to increase the amount of force a muscle can generate as well as the amount of calcium in the muscle cell, which also aids muscle contraction.[179] Neither of these two theories has been proven conclusively, but they appear to be likely explanations. Endurance activities like running and cycling appear to benefit the most from caffeine use. Caffeine allows endurance athletes to perform longer and with less perceived effort. The increase in fatty acids in the blood may help spare the glycogen in the muscle for later use thereby increasing endurance during long bouts of exercise.

Despite its many benefits, there are obvious drawbacks to regular caffeine use. The first is dependence and withdrawal symptoms. Regular use of even small amounts (less than a hundred milligrams a day) followed by abrupt stoppage can lead to headaches, depressed mood, irritability, trouble concentrating, and a general feeling of malaise. Fortunately, for most, these symptoms are mild and resolve in under a week. High doses of caffeine are associated with agitation, palpitation, irregular (and possibly dangerous) heart rhythms, insomnia, and increased urination. Regular users tend to have blunted responses to some of these effects but not all.

A chemical commonly found in grapefruits seems to prolong the effects of caffeine. Naringenin slows the breakdown of caffeine in the liver thereby prolonging its half-life.[180] This may allow users to decrease their caffeine ingestion while maintaining the benefits of higher dosages.

In general, caffeine is a safe and well-tolerated substance. In coffee form, it does not appear to negatively impact your insulin sensitivity. If you choose to use caffeine as a performance-enhancing substance prior to your workouts, I recommend one hundred to two hundred milligrams about thirty to sixty minutes prior to exercise. Those of you on the Endomorphic Diet who use caffeine regularly should consider switching to coffee or lowering your dosage if you are having difficulty achieving or maintaining ketosis.

178   Woolf K, Bidwell WK, Carlson AG: The effect of caffeine as an ergogenic aid in anaerobic exercise. *Int J of Sport Nutr Exerc Meta* 2008, 18:412–29. .
179   Kalmar JM. The Influence of Caffeine on Voluntary Muscle Activation. Med Sci Sports Exerc. 2005 Dec;37(12):2113–9.
180   Fuhr, Inhibitory effect of grapefruit juice and its bitter principal, naringenin, on CYP1A2 dependent metabolism of caffeine in man. Br. J. Clin. Pharmac. 35:431–436, 1993.

Caffeine content of some common drinks and food items		
Drink or food	Serving size	Caffeine content
Brewed coffee	237 ml (8 oz)	60–100 mg
Instant coffee	237 ml	50–80 mg
Double espresso	60 ml (2 oz)	45–100 g
Decaffeinated coffee	237 ml	1–5 mg
Black tea	237 ml	30–100 mg
Green tea	237 ml	20 mg
Cocoa	150 ml (5 oz)	30–60 mg
Coca-cola	355 ml (12 oz)	34 mg
Diet Coke	355 ml	45 mg
Pepsi	355 ml	38 mg
Diet Pepsi	355 ml	36 mg
Pepsi One	355 ml	55 mg
Jolt cola	355 ml	72 mg
Dr. Pepper	355 ml	41 mg
Barq's root beer	355 ml	22 mg
Mountain Dew	355 ml	55 mg
Sunkist	355 ml	41 mg
Red Bull	245 ml (8.3 oz)	80 mg
Snapple	355 ml	32 mg
Nestea iced tea	355 ml	17 mg
Nestea sweetened iced tea	355 ml	27 mg
Milk chocolate	55 g (2 oz)	3–20 mg
Dark chocolate	55 g	40–50 mg

Data from www.coffeeteaabout.com. About coffee/tea. www.erowid.com. The vaults of erowid. Accessed November 10, 2004; www.druginfo.com.au. Drug info clearing house.

Creatine

Creatine monohydrate is one of the few, and perhaps the only, nutritional supplements with a proven track record of effectiveness and safety. Creatine is a naturally occurring substance produced in the liver, pancreas, and kidneys. It is formed from the amino acids L-arginine, L-methionine, and glycine. It is stored primarily in muscle tissue bound to a phosphate molecule (known as phosphocreatine). During bouts of high-intensity, short-duration activity, working muscles rely on immediately available pools of ATP (adenosine triphosphate) to provide needed energy. ATP is broken down to ADP (adenosine diphosphate) in a process that releases energy and powers muscle contraction. ADP is then recycled back into ATP by the addition of a phosphate molecule, and the cycle continues. When the available phosphate pool (phosphocreatine) is depleted in this manner, the muscle fatigues and high-intensity contractions can no longer be sustained. It has been theorized that loading the muscles with creatine will increase stores of phosphocreatine and thereby delay muscle fatigue. Multiple scientific studies have shown that both oral loading of creatine monohydrate (typically fifteen to thirty grams daily for five to seven days followed by maintenance intake of three to five grams daily) significantly raises muscle phosphocreatine levels by up to 40 percent.[181] It also appears that skipping the loading phase and ingesting three to five grams of creatine daily results in similar elevations of phosphocreatine but over a longer period of time.[182]

---

181   Balsom P, Söderlund K, Sjödin B, Ekblom B. Skeletal muscle metabolism during short duration high-intensity exercise: influence of creatine supplementation. Acta Physiol Scand 1995;1154:303–10.
182   Hultman E, Söderlund K, Timmons J, Cederblad G, Greenhaff P. Muscle creatine loading in man. J Appl Physiol 1996;81:232–7.

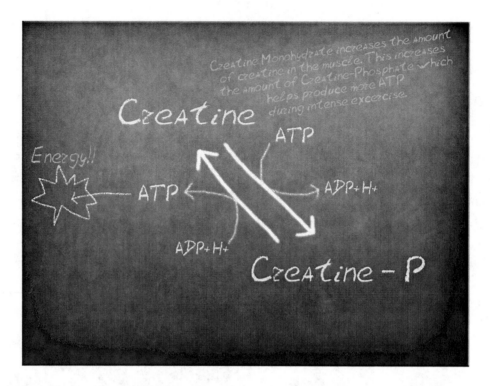

In the mid-1990s, the first widely available creatine supplements hit the market, though elite athletes had been using them for many years before that. Since that time, creatine has become one of the most widely studied nutritional supplements ever. The majority of studies demonstrate benefit in strength, muscular power, and during activities requiring multiple sets of maximal-effort muscle contractions. Creatine does not appear to be helpful in improving performance in longer, low-intensity, endurance-type activities like distance running. Creatine use is also clearly associated with gains in both fat-free mass (FFM) and muscle mass. FFM refers to bodyweight from all sources except fat and is composed mostly of water, but includes muscle, bone, and other body tissues. During the first week of creatine loading, there is typically a weight gain of one to three pounds or more. This is thought to be primarily due to water retention. As creatine enters skeletal muscle, it draws water along with it, expanding the volume of individual muscle fibers and increasing their diameter. Longer-term use, however, does appear to be related to gains in muscle mass. It has been theorized that since creatine seems to allow athletes to work harder, they may be able to generate more muscle mass through more intense training stimuli. Some researchers have also suggested that the increased water retention and resulting expansion of muscle fibers stimulates increased protein synthesis which leads to increases in muscle mass. This interesting theory has not been confirmed but may at least partially explain the muscle mass gains seen with creatine use.

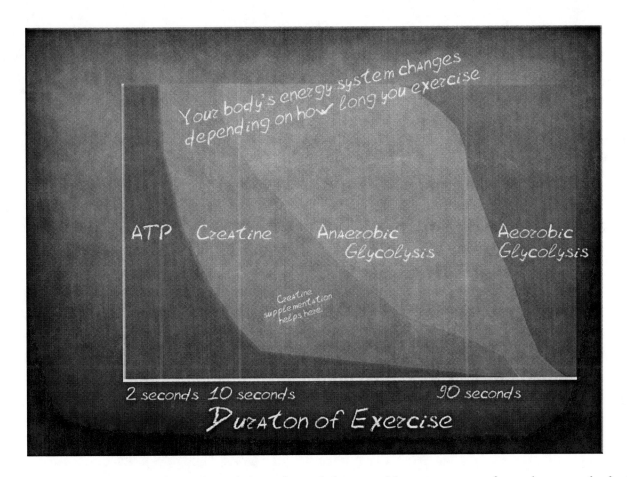

Multiple studies have investigated the safety of short- and long-term use of creatine monohydrate. Over the years, a variety of concerns have been raised about the use of creatine. Some experts have claimed that creatine use will lead to kidney or liver failure or that its use will cause dehydration, muscle cramps, muscle damage, growth retardation in teenagers, and increased incidence of muscle injury in athletes. Most of these reports have appeared in the lay press, on television, and in magazine articles. Some have even called for the banning of creatine because of increased use among high school and college athletes. Careful examination of these accusations have been performed over the years and published in a variety of sports medicine journals. Not a single well-controlled scientific study has ever demonstrated any significant deleterious effects from supplementation with creatine monohydrate. Careful study of athletes undergoing vigorous training in hot and humid conditions has failed to show any evidence of increased muscle cramps or injuries.[183] Similarly, no study has shown evidence of impaired kidney function with creatine supplementation. There are, however, some changes in blood parameters related to kidney function that can occur with creatine use that deserve mention in case you see a physician who is uninformed about this supplement.

Both naturally occurring and supplemental creatine is at least partially converted by the body into *creatinine* (an inert substance that is excreted by the kidneys). Blood creatinine levels are one of the parameters on routine tests to measure kidney function. People with kidney failure will have elevated levels of creatinine in their blood because their kidneys are not filtering it out properly. Supplementation

---

183   Kreider R, Rasmussen C, Ransom J, Almada A. Effects of creatine supplementation during training on the incidence of muscle cramping, injuries, and GI distress. J Str Cond Res. 1998; 12.

with creatine monohydrate can slightly increase the amount of creatinine in the blood (one study showed an average increase of 0.2 micromoles per liter [184]). Intense exercise, which naturally leads to increased muscle breakdown, can also temporarily increase blood creatinine levels. Elevations resulting from these sources are by no means signs of impending kidney failure. An important consideration to keep in mind if you already have some degree of kidney disease, you should speak to your physician before starting creatine use because it could potentially make it more difficult for your physician to monitor your kidney function.

Another concern often raised is that there are no good studies on the safety of long-term creatine use. This is true. However, considering that athletes have been using creatine since the 1970s and its use has skyrocketed in the last ten years, one would think that any complications of long-term use would have manifested themselves by this time.

Perhaps the most common reported side effect from creatine use is gastrointestinal upset. This phenomenon is relatively minor and generally subsides over time but for some can be prohibitive. Complaints of nausea, diarrhea, flatulence, and stomach cramping are typically worse during the loading phase and generally remit during maintenance. Ensuring that your creatine powder is fully dissolved, taking smaller divided doses, or using creatine capsules can help alleviate these problems. There are also micronized and effervescent forms of creatine available; these appear to have greater intestinal absorption and less incidence of stomach upset though they are more expensive than standard creatine powder.

Creatine and Caffeine

Several studies have demonstrated that caffeine can potentially negate the beneficial effects of creatine use.[185] The exact mechanism by which this occurs is not exactly clear. It appears that creatine is still able to enter the muscles in the presence of caffeine but may not be able to be properly used during intense exercise in the presence of caffeine.[186] Studies looking at this phenomenon used approximately five milligrams of caffeine per kilo of bodyweight (350 milligrams in an average 154-pound person) in test subjects. It is not known if lower dosages of caffeine also counteract the beneficial effects of creatine or not. The studies showing this effect have been relatively small and should by no means be considered conclusive. Clearly, further research needs to be done to confirm this finding. However, this is something to consider if you find that you are not getting the results you expect from your creatine.

Types of Creatine: Liquid, Effervescent, and Micronized

Creatine initially was only available as a coarse powder that mixed relatively poorly in liquid, tasted terrible, and caused significant gastrointestinal upset. Since that time, various other creatine preparations have been created to try to offset these problems.

---

184   Kreider R, Ferreira M, Wilson M, Grindstaff P, Plisk S, Reinhardy J, Cantler E, Almada A. Effects of creatine supplementation on body composition, strength and sprint performance. Med Sci Sport Exerc 1998;30:73–82.
185   Vandenberghe K, Gillis N, Vyan Leemputte M, Van Hecke P, Vanstapel F, Hespel P: Caffeine counteracts the ergogenic action of muscle creatine loading. J Appl Physiol 80: 452–457, 1996.
186   Vandenberghe K, Van Hecke P, Van Leemputte M, Vanstapel F, Hespel P: Inhibition of muscle phosphocreatine resynthesis by caffeine after creatine loading. (Abstract). Med Sci Sports Exerc 29: S249, 1997.

Micronized creatine is simply finely ground creatine monohydrate. Particle sizes are about twenty times smaller, and as a result, the powder mixes much more easily. There are claims of increased absorption from the manufacturers, but I found no unbiased research confirming this. Nevertheless, micronized creatine does seem to cause less nausea and bloating. If those side effects are a problem and you don't mind the extra cost, you may want to try micronized creatine.

Effervescent creatine formulations come in fizzing tablets or powders. They provide another mechanism for increasing the solubility and presumably the absorption of creatine into the bloodstream from the small intestine. Effervescent creatine appears to cause less gastrointestinal upset, but there are virtually no unbiased clinical studies comparing effervescent creatine to other forms of creatine. What is clear is that this form is substantially more expensive than standard powdered creatine. If you have the money to spend, effervescent creatine appears to be a good option for those who experience stomach upset with standard and micronized creatine.

Supplemental Ingredients

Many creatine formulations come with additional ingredients that claim to boost its performance-enhancing effects. The following is by no means a comprehensive list but does include some of the most commonly encountered ingredients. As you will notice, few if any have significant support in the scientific literature.

L-arginine

This amino acid is found added into many name-brand creatine products. It is considered a "conditionally essential" amino acid, meaning that under most circumstances, your body is able to synthesize all the l-arginine it needs. However, under periods of extreme stress, such as septic shock, severe burns, and possibly prolonged intense exercise, the body cannot keep up with the demand and deficiency results. L-arginine is often touted as increasing insulin levels with and without the ingestion of carbohydrate. Elevated insulin levels are thought to aid in the absorption of creatine into muscle tissue from the bloodstream. Animal studies, particularly in diabetic rats, have shown that L-arginine can stimulate insulin secretion from the pancreas. It is thought that this is accomplished by raising nitric oxide (NO) levels, which is known to stimulate insulin secretion.[187] While it seems plausible that adding L-arginine to creatine could increase its effectiveness, I could not find a single placebo-controlled study demonstrating this effect. There simply is no good research available at this time. Additionally, elevating insulin levels with L-arginine would generally be counterproductive to those of you on the Endomorphic Diet. As we will see later, there may be other reasons to consider supplementing with L-arginine, but at this time, I can't say that it will have any positive effects in terms of enhancing the effects of creatine.

---

187   Adeghate E, Ponery AS, El-Sharkawy T, Parvez H. L-arginine stimulates insulin secretion from the pancreas of normal and diabetic rats. Amino Acids. 2001;21(2):205–9.

D-Pinitol

This substance is found in the *Bougainvillea spectabilis* plant as well as soybeans and has been shown to exhibit glucose-lowering properties similar to insulin. Indeed, research in diabetic rats has shown that it can improve glucose levels when compared to placebo.[188]

In terms of creatine, there is a single study that appeared to show some benefit in terms of augmenting creatine's retention in muscle tissue. This study, from the University of Arkansas, showed that a relatively low dose of D-Pinitol (five hundred milligrams twice a day with five grams of creatine four times per day) enhanced the retention of creatine in much the same manner as a carbohydrate supplement without the associated calories.[189] Higher doses did not confer any benefit. This study only used twenty healthy male subjects and did not specifically look at whether subjects taking D-Pinitol showed any athletic performance improvements over those taking plain creatine plus placebo. D-Pinitol, at least in rodent studies, appears to exert its glucose-lowering effects independent of insulin. This means that it probably does not simply stimulate insulin secretion but rather acts through other less-understood pathways to lower glucose levels and increase creatine retention. As you may have guessed, this has important implications for those of you on the Endomorphic and Mesomorphic Diets. Other than D-Pinitol, the only other option for enhancing the effects of creatine is mixing it with a high-sugar beverage like sweetened grape juice or one of the commercially available high-glycemic carbohydrate powders. Obviously, those products are off-limits on the Endomorphic Diet and should be greatly restricted on the Mesomorphic Diet. If you choose to use a loading phase when you take creatine, ingesting that much sugar will completely sabotage your fat-burning efforts. Therefore, it seems that a creatine product with D-Pinitol may create a loophole that provides the benefits of carbohydrate intake without the accompanying insulin spike and empty calories. As with most nutritional supplements, however, more research is needed to determine if D-Pinitol will truly be a useful adjunct to creatine supplementation. There is also no long-term safety data in humans, so if you choose to use it, you will be doing so at your own risk.

Alpha Lipoic Acid (ALA)

ALA is naturally synthesized in both plants and animals. It is an important coenzyme involved in energy production and can also function as an antioxidant. There is some research showing that supplementing with ALA can increase the uptake of glucose into muscle cells in humans and animals with type II diabetes.[190] There is a single study showing enhanced creatine uptake in humans who supplement their creatine with ALA.[191] This study had sixteen subjects ingest twenty grams of creatine daily along with one hundred grams of sucrose with and without one thousand milligrams of ALA. One week later, the subjects who ingested the sucrose/creatine/ALA formula had higher muscle phosphocreatine levels than those who

188   Bates SH, Jones RB, Bailey CJ. Insulin-like effect of pinitol. Br J Pharmacol. 2000 Aug;130(8):1944–8.
189   Greenwood M, Kreider RB, Rasmussen C et al. (2001) D-Pinitol augments whole body creatine retention in man. J Exerc Physiolonline 4:41–47.
190   Jacob S, Henriksen EJ, Schiemann AL, et al. Enhancement of glucose disposal in patients with type II diabetes by alpha-lipoic acid. Arzneimittelforschung. 1995;45(8):872–874.
191   Burke DG, Chilibeck PD, Parise G, Tarnopolsky MA, Candow DG. Effect of alpha-lipoic acid combined with creatine monohydrate on human skeletal muscle creatine and phosphagen concentration. Int J Sport Nutr Exerc Metab. 2003 Sep;13(3):294–302.

consumed only creatine and sucrose. The study subjects did not exercise, and no measurements of muscle performance were taken.

Unfortunately, this study did not directly compare ALA plus creatine with sucrose plus creatine. Therefore, it is not known if ALA alone enhances the uptake of creatine or if sugar must be ingested along with it to enhance muscle creatine levels. Therefore, I think it is premature to recommend adding ALA to your creatine supplementation.

ALA may have other benefits that go beyond creatine supplementation but don't have much to do with building muscle or losing fat. It is considered a prescription drug in Germany where it is sometimes used to treat alcohol- and diabetes-induced nerve damage. It appears to have antioxidant properties and to improve blood vessel function in diabetics, though large studies demonstrating clear benefit of supplementation with ALA have not been performed. It remains one of many nutritional compounds with some potential that has yet to be fully explored and confirmed. There appears to be no known side effects of oral ALA even at high doses (1200 milligrams per day for two years). Diabetics may potentially experience low blood sugar and need their medications adjusted accordingly. Its use is not proven safe in pregnant or breast-feeding women.[192]

Di-Potassium Phosphate and Sodium Biphosphate

These ingredients are added to many commercial creatine brands. Creatine typically is sold as creatine monohydrate. This means that a single creatine molecule is bound to a single water molecule. In the bloodstream and in muscle, the water dissociates and a phosphate molecule binds in its place, creating creatine phosphate. Companies that add phosphate to their product would like you to think that the more phosphate you ingest, the more will be bound to creatine thereby increasing phosphocreatine levels. The truth is there is no study proving that ingesting additional phosphate beyond what is found naturally in your diet has any effect on phosphocreatine levels or performance. If you purchase a product with added phosphate, you are likely paying extra money for no reason.

20-Hydroxy Beta Ecdysterone

This compound is found naturally in the herbs Maral Root (Rhaponticum carthamoides) and Cyanotis vaga. It appears to have glucose-lowering properties similar to the prescription medication metformin in rats. This action appears independent of insulin, i.e., insulin secretion was not stimulated by administration of ecdysterone.[193]

I was unable to find a single study showing that ecdysterone enhanced the effects of creatine supplementation in any way. Theoretically, its ability to lower blood sugar could increase the retention of creatine in muscle tissue, but this has not been proven. Therefore, any claim that ecdysterone should be taken with creatine cannot be considered legitimate at this time.

---

192   Hendler SS, Rorvik DR, eds. PDR for Nutritional Supplements. Montvale: Medical Economics Company, Inc; 2001.
193   Chen Q, Xia Y, Qiu Z. Life Sci. Effect of ecdysterone on glucose metabolism in vitro. 2006 Feb 2;78(10):1108–13.

Some studies have shown that ecdysterone may have some anabolic properties in animals.[194] The problem with these studies is most, if not all, were performed in the former Soviet Union in the 1980s and early 1990s and not published in English, nor are they widely available in their original form. Many used animal models. Virtually all information available on ecdysterone comes from one or more supplement companies who happen to sell various formulations of these products. The original studies showing a possible anabolic effect have not been repeated in any reputable Western scientific journal. Similarly, any claims regarding lack of side effects should be considered suspect since none of the Soviet studies examined prolonged use. Eventually, more trustworthy research may reveal that ecdysterone has potential uses for muscle building, but I suspect that the hype will likely far exceed what it can actually deliver.

L-Glutamine

Glutamine is the most abundant amino acid in the human body. It is the primary energy source for the intestinal tract and immune system. Glutamine is not considered an essential amino acid since it can be synthesized from other amino acids in sufficient quantities in healthy subjects. There are situations, however, where someone can become glutamine deficient and would benefit from supplementation. These situations primarily involve very sick surgical patients, burn patients, or those struggling with overwhelming infections. It also appears that athletes involved in prolonged endurance exercise or those who are chronically overtraining may also suffer from glutamine deficiency. In those situations, the demand for glutamine is so great that muscle tissue is broken down at an accelerated rate to keep up with it.[195]

One study looking at the addition of glutamine to supplemental creatine showed benefit above what was found with taking creatine alone. In it, twenty-nine track and field athletes were randomized to receive creatine alone (.3 grams per kilo load for one week and then .03 grams per kilo maintenance for seven weeks) or creatine plus glutamine (four grams per day). At seven weeks, the subjects taking glutamine had a greater increase in lean body mass and greater power production during multiple cycle ergometry bouts.[196] The mechanism by which glutamine exerted this effect is not clear and larger studies would need to be performed to confirm this effect.

No study has shown consistent gains in strength or muscle mass for weight-training athletes with glutamine supplementation in the absence of creatine.[197] There are studies showing potential benefit in terms of immune function in endurance athletes. However, given the relatively inexpensive cost of glutamine and the lack of side effects, it would not be unreasonable to try adding glutamine to your creatine to see if you notice any benefit.

---

194   Syrov VN, Kurmukov AG Farmakol Toksikol. Anabolic activity of phytoecdysone-ecdysterone isolated from Rhaponticum carthamoides 1976 Nov–Dec;39(6):690-3.
195   Glutamine: an essential amino acid for the gut. Nutrition. 1996 Nov–Dec;12(11-12 Suppl):S78–81.
196   Lehmkuhl M, Malone M, Justice B, Trone G, Pistilli E, Vinci D, Haff EE, Kilgore JL, Haff GG. The effects of 8 weeks of creatine monohydrate and glutamine supplementation on body composition and performance measures. : J Strength Cond Res. 2003 Aug;17(3):425–38.
197   Candow DG, Chilibeck PD, Burke DG, Davison KS, Smith-Palmer T. Effect of glutamine supplementation combined with resistance training in young adults. Eur J Appl Physiol. 2001 Dec;86(2):142–9.

Simple Carbohydrates

It has long been known that adding a simple sugar to creatine increases its ability to enter muscle tissue. Increased insulin levels mediate this phenomenon, which causes muscle tissue to absorb glucose, amino acids, and creatine at increased rates. As a result, many creatine preparations come mixed with a simple carbohydrate like dextrose or sucrose. Unfortunately, regular consumption of these high-sugar supplements will sabotage your fat-loss efforts on the Endomorphic and Mesomorphic Diets, and they are strictly off-limits. You may consider them on the Ectomorphic Diet, but even then, consumption of those types of carbohydrates should be limited. Fortunately, consuming protein with your creatine appears to allow you to take in less carbohydrate while still achieving the same benefits of creatine plus a much higher carbohydrate intake.[198]

Non-responders

There are individuals who do not seem to derive much benefit from creatine supplementation. The exact number of these so-called "non-responders" is not known but may be as high as 20 percent. These individuals do not experience significant performance improvement from creatine. It is theorized that they may already have higher than normal creatine levels or have some other condition that prevents additional creatine from exerting its benefits[199]. If after several weeks of creatine supplementation, you don't notice much of a performance boost in the gym, then you may be a non-responder.

198   Steenge, G. R., Simpson, J., and Greenhaff, P. L. Protein- and carbohydrate-induced augmentation of whole body creatine retention in humans. *Journal of Applied Physiology* 2000 Volume 89: pages 1165–1171.

199   Syrotuik DG, Bell GJ. Acute creatine monohydrate supplementation: a descriptive physiological profile of responders vs. nonresponders. J Strength Cond Res. 2004 Aug;18(3):610-7.

In our society, the women who break down barriers are those who ignore limits.

—Arnold Schwarzenegger

DIFFERENCES BETWEEN MEN AND WOMEN

Men and women are obviously different. In the diet and exercise industry, this has led to a plethora of books and articles geared specifically to either male or female readers. Exercise books for women in particular are big business. Scientific researchers have also directed a significant amount of attention to closely examining the differences between male and female athletes of all ages. From neurology to sports science, there has been a great deal of research attempting to quantify these differences and make specific recommendations from them. Unfortunately, this has led to the assumption in the minds of many members of the general public that women and men have fundamental differences that require different approaches to building muscle and losing body fat. The results of these studies may come as a surprise to some. The more we learn, the more it becomes apparent, at least for most areas, the differences between men and women are differences in degree but not in kind. What I mean by this is that men and women at the fundamental cellular level are very similar—almost identical.

On the cellular level, men and women contain identical mechanisms for ATP production and metabolism of nutrients. Muscle tissue in men and women shows the same distribution of fast- and slow-twitch muscle fibers, and both require intense exercise in order to hypertrophy. Even the internal organs, reproductive organs aside, are nearly identical. The differences are largely in degree, meaning that while men and women have nearly identical internal machinery, they do differ in the size, strength, efficiency, and the manner in which that machinery is used.

The most obvious difference between men and women is in muscle size. Though there are clearly exceptions, males tend to carry far more muscle mass and as a result be much stronger than females. This difference is largely a result of the exposure of male muscle tissues to the hormone testosterone. This also explains the increased density of male bone as compared to female bone. Studies show that biopsies taken from male and female athletes are remarkably similar. Male and female muscles have the same general percentage of fast- and slow-twitch muscle fibers. They have the same number of total muscle cells as well as a similar number of motor units. The primary difference is in the size of the muscle cells. Across all muscle fiber types, males tend to have significantly larger muscle cells and therefore are able to generate more powerful contractions. By virtue of their increased muscle fiber size, males are also able to store larger amounts of muscle glycogen for use during exercise. Male and female muscle fibers experience similar degrees of damage when exposed to high-intensity eccentric exercise, though men tend to have a somewhat increased inflammatory response afterward.[200] Both male and female muscle tissue experiences optimal levels of hypertrophy when exposed to heavy, high-intensity resistance training. Males, with the aid of their naturally elevated levels of testosterone, obviously experience far greater amounts of hypertrophy, but females also respond well to this type of training.

Women also carry more body fat than men and do so in a different pattern than males. Under the influence of estrogen, women store additional body fat in the thighs, hips, and buttocks, while men tend to store fat primarily around the abdomen. This is an evolutionary adaption that allows women to store needed calories for potential pregnancy and breast-feeding. Reducing these deposits, as well as overall body fat levels, too drastically (usually less than 11 to 12 percent) will lead to a number of hormonal irregularities in women that contribute to irregular menses and significant bone loss. Therefore, it is not recommended that women drop their body fat levels significantly below this level for any great length of time. Female bodybuilders and fitness athletes typically stop menstruating as they approach a contest but rarely maintain such low body fat levels year-round. Elite distance runners, as well as gymnasts, however, do maintain such low levels for prolonged periods of time and are at very high risk for osteoporosis later in life.

Estrogen has been found to increase the number of alpha-2A-adrenergic receptors in fat tissue. These receptors actually inhibit the breakdown of fat in the subcutaneous tissue.[201] It is likely that the increased prevalence of these receptors in "problem areas," like the buttocks and thighs, contribute to the increased difficulty in burning fat from these areas that some women experience. It is interesting to note that males will also develop this pattern of fat distribution when given female hormones. The discovery of the link between the alpha-2A receptor and the inhibition of fat loss has led to speculation that the supplement yohimbe, which selectively blocks this receptor, may be useful in reducing stubborn fat deposits. There are several studies that suggest this may be a valid assumption. Look for more information about yohimbe as research will undoubtedly develop a clearer understanding of its effects. The take-home point is that elevated estrogen levels make fat loss more difficult for women than men. Additionally, fat tissue promotes the conversion of precursor hormones into estradiol, which compounds the problem in both men and women.

Despite estrogen's effect on fat deposits, there is no significant difference between men and women when it comes to the overall mechanics of fat and carbohydrate metabolism. There are some subtle differences, but they do not lead to drastic differences in overall metabolism. For example, when exercising at high intensity, women tend to burn blood sugar preferentially instead of glycogen to a greater degree than

200   Stupka, N, et al. Gender differences in muscle inflammation after eccentric exercise. J Appl Physiol 89: 2325–2332, 2000.
201   Pedersen, S. et al. Estrogen Controls Lipolysis by Up-Regulating alpha 2A-Adrenergic Receptors Directly in Human Adipose Tissue through the Estrogen Receptor alpha. Implications for the Female Fat Distribution. *The Journal of Clinical Endocrinology Metabolism* 89(4):1869–1878.

men do.[202] This difference makes sense when you consider that men have larger livers and greater amounts of muscle tissue available to store glycogen. Despite this difference, the overall contribution of glucose, whether it comes from serum glucose or glycogen, to total energy expenditure during exercise is the same between men and women. The same can be said for fat metabolism. The oxidation of fatty acids and their contribution to overall energy expenditure, while not identical, is similar in men and women. Therefore, while dieting on The Program, there is no need to alter your macronutrient levels based on gender. Male and female athletes should stick to the same relative proportions of carbohydrates, fats, and proteins.

Hormonal, as well as genetic differences, also contribute to the up to 25 percent larger heart and 25 percent greater lung capacity that men have as compared to women. Women also tend to have lower blood hemoglobin levels, which reduce the amount of oxygen in the blood that can be carried to working muscles. This gives men, in most cases, the ability to exercise longer, run faster, and train harder than their female counterparts. Women do appear to have an advantage in terms of flexibility, however. This is likely a result of their higher progesterone levels as well as lower amount of muscle mass. When I describe these differences, of course, I am speaking in general terms. There are certainly elite female athletes that are far superior to the average male, but when average males and females are compared, as well as when elite male and female athletes are compared, these differences remain.

The take-home point here is that the same stimulus for building muscle is required by both men and women: high-intensity resistance training. Therefore, despite the obvious physical differences, men and women should not engage in different training programs if they have the same goals. If you are a female following The Program, you will be performing the same diet and exercise protocol as the men. The calories you consume and the weights you will be lifting will, in most cases, be less, but you should not alter the fundamental structure of the system as it is described.

---

202   Ruby B, et al. Gender differences in glucose kinetics and substrate oxidation during exercise near the lactate threshold. J Appl Physiol 92: 1125–1132, 2002.

The secret of all victory lies in the organization of the non-obvious.

—Marcus Aurelius

WHAT TO DO BEFORE STARTING THE PROGRAM

Set Goals

One of the essential first steps before starting The Program is deciding exactly what you want to get out of it. What are your goals? When starting an exercise program, most people give relatively vague answers like "I want to get in better shape" or "I want to lose a few pounds." They aren't very specific about how much weight they want to lose or gain, how much stronger they want to get, or how they want to look. I would argue that without explicitly defining your goals, you are starting off on the wrong foot and making it less likely that you will be satisfied with the end results of your training.

If you are very out of shape or have never been on a structured workout program, you may find it hard to convince yourself that you will ever achieve a lean, strong physique. Your previous failures may leave you convinced that you will never have the body that you desire, and your past failures may be exerting an undue negative influence on your thinking. You may feel that you have so far to go that maybe even trying isn't worth the work and sweat you know you will have to put forth. I agree that if you need to lose one hundred pounds or more, the goal of reaching a body fat percentage less than 10 percent might seem fairly daunting. I encourage you, however, to set your sights high. You are following a proven system. You must convince yourself that you will not fail. If you apply the correct knowledge and put forth the effort and discipline required, you will get there!

Your first step is to decide what your long-term goals are. Take an honest assessment of your body and decide exactly what you want to change. This is not the time to be vague. Pick a specific goal body weight, a specific goal body fat percentage, a specific goal strength level in a particular lift, a specific goal measurement…it can be anything you want, but pick some ultimate goal and decide then and there that you will achieve it. Then *write it down*. There is something far more concrete, far more permanent, about a goal when you write it down. Stating explicitly what your goals are and then writing them down will make it far more likely that you will achieve them. I encourage you to post those goals in places where you are bound to see them several times per day. The refrigerator, your desk, your workout journal, in your car, anywhere where you will see them and be constantly reminded and motivated. As stated previously, I want you to choose lofty, long-term goals. This system will work for you and, if followed properly, will deliver the results you are looking for.

Once you have decided on your long-term goals, it's time to start breaking this journey down into achievable steps. You must decide on some short-term goals. In fact, defining and ultimately achieving your short-term goals is even more important than doing the same for your long-term goals. You won't burn fifty pounds of fat, gain forty pounds of muscle mass, and increase your bench press by one hundred pounds in eight months if you don't have a specific day-to-day plan to get you there. (By the way, for most, that would be a very achievable long-term goal when training with The Program.) And when I say day-to-day plan, that is exactly how short term I want your goals to be. For maximum success, you should literally have daily goals that you want to achieve. They don't have to be extraordinary. Something as simple as stating "Today, I am going to add five minutes to my cardio routine" or "Today, when I go out with my friends, I am going to stick to my diet no matter what" or "Today, at the gym, I am going to try for that extra rep at the end of every exercise I do." Achieving little goals like that adds up over time. They build your confidence, your discipline, and your self-esteem, and they boost your motivation.

After setting daily goals, look out a little further and set weekly ones. Again, they don't have to be anything extraordinary; they should be realistic but at the same time challenging. For example, you may decide that "This week, I will lose 1.5 to 2 pounds of body fat" or "This week, I will do one to two more reps on the squat than I did last week" or "This week, I will ensure I get at least eight hours of sleep every night" or "This week, I won't skip a single meal." Write these goals down as well. Don't be too hard on yourself if you slip up and don't achieve one or more of these short-term goals. In all of our lives, things happen that are out of our control and can sabotage our efforts. What you are looking for are trends. You should be meeting most of your short-term goals. If not, step back and make sure that your goals are realistic. If you think you are going to gain ten pounds of muscle in one week, then prepare to be disappointed. Even with massive doses of steroids, that is not going to happen. Take a look at the rest of your lifestyle and see if there are extraneous factors that are standing in your way. If possible, try to modify them so you can proceed onward.

It's important to say a few things regarding choosing realistic goals. Though we are all anatomically and physiologically essentially identical, there are obvious differences in the way each individual responds to high-intensity weight training and to changes in eating habits. Try not to compare yourself to others. Your training partner may be following the same diet and exercise program but be making faster progress than you are. That does not necessarily mean you are doing something wrong. There is tremendous variation in people's ability to build muscle mass and burn body fat. Not everyone has the genetics to burn two pounds of body fat every week and all year long. What you are looking for are trends. Are you consistently getting stronger week-to-week even if only by a few pounds or reps? Are you consistently getting leaner week to week, even if it's by less than a pound per week? If that is happening, you are on the right track. Keep up the good work. The only person you should be comparing yourself to is *you*.

Before Photos

Taking photos of your body before starting The Program is optional, but I highly encourage you to do it. You may be embarrassed to stand in front of a camera with your body exposed, but I believe you will find it to be one of the most useful tasks you will do before starting. First, they give you an honest assessment of where you stand. The camera doesn't lie. You may not have realized it, but yes, your gut really is that big or you really are that skinny. Seeing those photos can give you an additional motivational boost. As you progress in your training, you may find it difficult to see the changes yourself. Those initial photos can serve as a reminder of just how far you have come. Finally, placing those "before" pictures up next to your "after" photos and seeing the huge strides you have made will give you an awesome boost of confidence and the knowledge that all your hard work has paid off.

Blood Work

There are various recommendations put forth by physicians' groups and academies about medical screening prior to beginning an exercise program. For the vast majority of you, no special tests or studies will be needed before beginning this exercise and diet program. Just get out there and get started. Having said that, if you have a history of heart disease of any kind, uncontrolled high blood pressure, diabetes, or any other medical condition that concerns you, I strongly urge you to consult a physician to obtain clearance prior to beginning any sort of exercise program. There are a few simple blood tests that you may want to get prior to starting The Program and again at a later date to chart your progress. These include:

Fasting Blood Sugar—an elevated fasting blood sugar level is an ominous finding. Current standards define a fasting blood sugar level between 100 and 125 as "glucose intolerance" or "pre-diabetic." In reality, if your fasting blood sugar level is in this range, you already have the same risk for heart disease, kidney and nerve damage, and arteriosclerosis as someone with full-blown diabetes (defined as two fasting blood sugar readings greater than 126). Therefore, the label of "pre-diabetes" is really a misnomer. If your fasting blood sugar is over 100, for all practical purposes you have type II diabetes and you better start doing something about it! I consider a fasting blood sugar between 90 and 100 as an early warning sign. You have a significant amount of insulin resistance and are at high risk for progressing to diabetes if you do not lose weight and begin exercising. The good news is that by losing fat and gaining muscle on a vigorous exercise program and carbohydrate-controlled diet, you can dramatically lower your fasting blood sugar and greatly reduce your risk of developing type II diabetes.

Fasting Lipid Panel—Healthy appearing people often have poor cholesterol profiles. The standard fasting lipid panel consists of total cholesterol, triglyceride level, LDL (low-density lipoprotein) level, and an HDL (high-density lipoprotein level). Triglycerides are often elevated in individuals with insulin resistance and are a marker for potential diabetes. They are also elevated by excessive carbohydrate intake.

LDL cholesterol is the bad, artery-clogging cholesterol. High LDL levels are directly related to your risk of heart disease and stroke. HDL cholesterol is the good cholesterol. High levels of HDL are actually protective against heart disease and stroke. There is a significant genetic component to an individual's cholesterol levels, but diet plays an important role as well. As you continue on the diets outlined in The Program, you will see favorable changes in all these values. Your triglycerides and LDL will plummet, and your HDL will increase. Your heart and blood vessels will thank you! The following are the currently recommended values for LDL cholesterol based on NCEP (National Cholesterol Education Program) guidelines. HDL cholesterol should be no lower than forty milligrams per deciliter in both men and women. The higher your HDL level, the lower your risk for heart disease. Keep in mind these are just guidelines and not hard and fast rules. As more information regarding the effects of cholesterol on heart and vascular disease becomes available, you can expect that these recommendations will change.

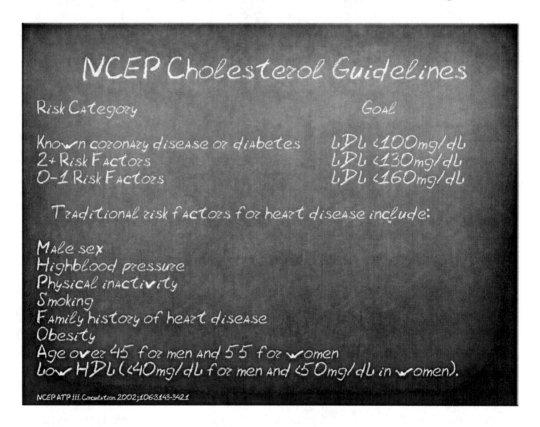

NCEP Cholesterol Guidelines

Risk Category	Goal
Known coronary disease or diabetes	LDL <100mg/dL
2+ Risk Factors	LDL <130mg/dL
0-1 Risk Factors	LDL <160mg/dL

Traditional risk factors for heart disease include:

Male sex
High blood pressure
Physical inactivity
Smoking
Family history of heart disease
Obesity
Age over 45 for men and 55 for women
Low HDL (<40mg/dL for men and <50mg/dL in women).

NCEP ATP iii. Circulation 2002;1063143-3421

- **Liver Function Tests**—abnormal liver function tests can result from dozens of different medical conditions, from infectious hepatitis to various genetic syndromes. In obese individuals, an increasingly common condition causing elevated liver function tests is known as "fatty liver." Individuals with this condition have large amounts of fat surrounding and infiltrating their livers. This leads to impaired liver function and destruction of liver cells. It is a condition directly related to type 2 diabetes, excess insulin production, and poor diet. The good news is that with fat loss and exercise, this condition is also reversible. If your blood tests show that you have abnormal liver function, you and your physician will need to pursue further testing to rule out other serious conditions.

- **Other tests**—A number of other blood tests are available and may be of interest to those on The Program. Given the prevalence of vitamin D deficiency in the northern hemisphere, a baseline 25(OH) D level is not unreasonable for the otherwise healthy athlete. If you have a family history of thyroid disease or feel you are at risk for it, then a baseline TSH level can accurately assess this. If you have undiagnosed thyroid dysfunction (either over- or underactive), then your efforts will not yield optimal results. Testosterone deficiency is also more prevalent than previously suspected. If you have low libido, difficulty achieving or maintaining an erection, or a history of past anabolic steroid use, measuring serum testosterone levels may be helpful. When requesting a testosterone level from your physician, you should request not just a total testosterone level but also a bioavailable testosterone (BVT) as well. Obviously, a low testosterone level will greatly hamper your ability to build muscle mass and should be corrected. If you have a history of any other chronic medical problems, you should consult with your physician to see if any other tests are required prior to starting your diet and exercise program.

- **Blood Pressure**—Getting an accurate evaluation of your blood pressure is important before starting an exercise program. Hypertension is strongly associated with early heart disease, stroke, kidney failure, and a host of other medical problems. Dubbed the "silent killer," hypertension can often manifest itself as early as the teenage years, and because many individuals with hypertension have no symptoms, it often goes unrecognized. Meanwhile, the damage to the body's organs and blood vessels continues with the individual completely unaware that there may be a problem. Fortunately, it is fairly easy for most individuals to get their blood pressure taken. Many grocery stores have free automated machines that take blood pressure and automated and manual blood pressure cuffs for home use are easy to find in most store pharmacies. You may be surprised to find out that what you considered to be "normal" blood pressure is in fact elevated and puts you at higher risk for heart disease in the future.

The Seventh Report of the Joint National Committee on Prevention, Detection, Evaluation, and Treatment of High Blood Pressure (JNC 7) now defines blood pressure as follows:

JNC-7 Blood Pressure Classification		
	Systolic (mmHg)	Diastolic (mmHg)
Normal	<120	<80
Pre-hypertension	120-139	80-89
Stage 1 Hypertension	140-159	90-99
Stage 2 Hypertension	>160	>100

Fortunately, weight loss and exercise do make a difference. Systolic blood pressure will drop anywhere between five and twenty points for every ten kilograms of weight lost.[203] Regular exercise of at least thirty minutes duration can drop systolic blood pressure four to nine points even if no weight is lost.[204]

In order to get an accurate blood pressure reading, you should do the following: Sit quietly in a chair for about five minutes. Try to relax. Your feet should be on the floor and the arm in which the measurement will be taken should be supported at heart level. Make sure the cuff is not too small. Those of you with large, muscular arms will get falsely elevated numbers if you use a cuff that is too small. The air chamber or bladder of the cuff should circle at least 80 percent of your arm. Your doctor may have to use a leg cuff if your arms are too big for a regular cuff. After the first reading, a second should be done in approximately five minutes. Following these steps will ensure you get the most accurate reading possible. If you sit down and check your blood pressure immediately after a hard workout or after rushing around all day, naturally your numbers will be high. Take the time to relax beforehand so you get an accurate reading.

Regardless of your age, if you find that you fall into the stage 1 or stage 2 categories, do yourself a favor and go see your doctor. You may need to be on blood pressure medication at least until you have a chance to drop a few pounds and get serious about your exercise program. High blood pressure *is* a big deal, and if you have it, the sooner you know it and start treating it, the better.

Estimate Your Body Fat Percentage

There are various ways to measure one's body fat percentage, and it's useful to do so for several reasons. It will help you not only track your progress as you lose body fat but also help you calculate an ideal body weight. As stated previously, most men should shoot for a body fat percentage no higher than 15 percent and women no higher than 22 percent. The gold standard for body fat measurement is probably hydrostatic weighing. Unless you have access to a physiology lab, however, this type of measurement is impractical for most. There are other similar (and expensive) highly accurate methods including DEXA scans, MRI, and CT, none of which are widely available to the average person. For the rest of us, two methods are likely to be most useful: skin-fold measurements and bioelectrical impedance (BIA) measurements. Skin-fold caliper measurements, when done correctly, are an accurate way to measure body fat and require only a set of calipers to perform. BIA is built into many commercially available scales and measures the impedance (resistance to flow) of an electrical current throughout the body. Water (the primary constituent of muscle) provides less impedance than fat. Therefore, it is possible to estimate one's body fat percentage based on height, weight, and gender using calculations performed by a microprocessor contained within the scale.

Skin-fold measurements, while generally accurate, should only be performed by someone trained in their use. If possible, have the same person perform your measurements each time and in precisely the same location. This will minimize some of the error potential inherent in this method. Skin-fold caliper

---

203   He J, Whelton PK, Appel LJ, Charleston J, Klag MJ. Long term effects of weight loss and sodium restriction on incidence of hypertension. Hypertension. 2000; 35: 544–9.F.

204   Kelley GA, Kelley KS. Progressive Resistance Exercise and resting blood pressure: A meta-analysis of randomized controlled trials. Hypertension. 2000;35:838–43.M.

kits with instruction books are easily found through various Internet companies and local health food stores. If you use a BIA scale, make sure you are adequately hydrated. Performing a BIA measurement if you are dehydrated will give you a falsely elevated body fat measurement. There are various Internet-based body fat calculators you may use as well. They have varying degrees of accuracy. An example can be found at: http://www.freedieting.com/tools/body_fat_calculator.htm.

Estimate Your Caloric Needs

Whether your goal is to gain muscle, lose fat, or both, it is important when planning your diet to have an idea of just how many calories your body requires. Despite what you may have heard from other diet gurus, calories *do* count. Quite simply, if you consume more calories than you expend, you will gain weight and if you consume less calories than you expend, you will lose weight. As you will learn later though, where those calories come from is just as important as how many of them you are consuming.

The first step is figuring out how many calories your body needs to simply maintain its current weight at rest. This means determining how many calories are needed to carry out the basic life-sustaining activities of your internal organs while you are essentially performing little to no physical exercise. For example, while sleeping. This concept is often referred to as the basal metabolic rate (BMR). Your BMR depends primarily on your height, weight, gender, and certain genetic factors. There are many ways to calculate your BMR. They all will give you a fairly accurate measurement. It doesn't matter too much which one you choose. The following are two popular ways to estimate your BMR.

Schofield Equation

This simple equation is based on your age, gender, and weight in kilograms. The SEE (standard error of estimation) is a built-in "fudge factor." It is the degree to which your calculated BMR may be off (either over- or underestimated). As a general rule, if you are close to the young end of your age range, you should add the SEE to your total since younger people have higher BMRs. If you are toward the upper end of your age range, you should subtract your SEE from your BMR. Similarly, if you already have a lot of muscle, you should add the SEE to your total since you will naturally have a higher metabolic rate. Obese individuals should subtract the SEE from their total.

Men:

10–17 years BMR = 17.7 x W + 657	SEE = 105
18–29 years BMR = 15.1 x W + 692	SEE = 156
30–59 years BMR = 11.5 x W + 873	SEE = 167

Women:

10–17 years BMR = 13.4 x W + 692	SEE = 112
18–29 years BMR = 14.8 x W + 487	SEE = 120
30–59 years BMR = 8.3 x W + 846	SEE = 112

W = Body weight in kilograms

SEE = Standard error of estimation

The Harris-Benedict Equation

This is another formula used to calculate BMR.

Men:

BEE = 66.5 + (13.75 x kg) + (5.003 x height in cm) – (6.775 x age)

Women:

BEE = 655.1 + (9.563 x kg) + (1.850 x height in cm) – (4.676 x age)

The next step is using your BMR to calculate your maintenance calorie level. This is the number of calories needed per day to maintain your body weight at its current level given the amount of exercise you are doing. To do this, simply multiply your BMR by the following activity-level factor:

Sedentary—none or very little exercise = BMR X 1.2

Program workout + no cardio = BMR X 1.4

Program workout + cardio 3/week = BMR X 1.6

Program workout + cardio 5–6 times/week = BMR X 1.7

Higher activity levels (e.g., Program workout + cardio 5–6/week + other sporting activity = up to 2 x BMR)

When you decide which diet plan you will follow, this is the number that you will use as your baseline regardless of whether you are trying to gain or lose weight.

Example:

This is an example of how to calculate your BMR using the above methods on a real subject—a thirty-two-year-old male weighing 220 pounds.

I will use the Schofield Equation.

BMR = 11.5 x 100 kg + 873 = 2023 calories. Since he is near the younger end of the spectrum for this age group, the SEE of 167 calories should be added to the total:

BMR=2023+ 167= **2190 calories**

This athlete is following the program by lifting weights and performing cardio three times per week. Therefore, his BMR should be multiplied by 1.6. This gives the approximate number of calories needed to maintain his current body weight of 220 pounds: 2190 x 1.6 = **3504 calories**

These formulas are fairly accurate for average individuals. However, for those of you who are very muscular, it may underestimate your caloric needs and for those of you who are very obese, it may overestimate the number of calories you require. In these cases, it can be useful to calculate an ideal bodyweight (IBW) and use that value as your actual body weight in the above equations. The most accurate way to do this is by using the body fat percentage you calculated previously. Don't be intimidated by a little math. This is basic grade-school arithmetic. The steps are:

1. Determine your actual weight and body fat percentage (for example 250 pounds at 28 percent body fat).
2. Determine how much of your body weight is actually fat (250 x 0.28 = 70 lbs).
3. Subtract your total fat from your total actual body weight (250 - 70 = 180 lbs).
4. Pick a reasonable goal body fat percentage, for example 12 percent. Your ideal body weight if you had 12 percent body fat is then (180 x 0.12) + 180 = 201.6 lbs.

Choose a Diet

There are three dietary approaches discussed in The Program. The one you choose will depend largely on your personal goals. Each diet is designed to achieve a specific metabolic effect. Simply put, the Ectomorphic Diet is for those looking to gain as much weight in the form of lean muscle as possible when body fat is a secondary factor. The Endomorphic Diet, on the other hand, is geared toward transforming your body into a fat-burning machine. The Mesomorphic Diet can serve both functions as well as be a healthy, sustainable, life-long eating plan. Once you set your goals, choosing the right eating plan for you should be fairly straightforward.

Join a Gym

If you don't belong to a local gym already, you should strongly consider it. Despite the plethora of home gym equipment available today, you will never be able to duplicate the variety of equipment found in a gym (unless you have several thousand dollars to spend). You will also find that as you progress on The Program, you may quickly grow too strong for most home gym equipment. In the event of a training injury, most gyms will have enough equipment variety that you can work around your injury until it heals. I have also found that the variety of both weight and cardio equipment allows you to vary your workouts periodically, which can be very refreshing and a great way to keep yourself from getting bored. The simple act of going to a gym and seeing everyone else around you working out while knowing that your training partner will be there waiting for you can be very motivating as well.

Clean House

Once you decide to start The Program, you have to create an environment that will help you succeed. I promise you there will be days when your willpower will be tested and you will be tempted to stray from your plan. The first and most important thing you can do to alleviate this is to clean house. By that, I mean go through your kitchen, pantry, and anywhere else you store junk food, and throw it all out. Put it in the trash, take it to the curb, and let the garbage man take it away! Out of sight...out of mind. Keeping junk food around while you are following your diet will only serve to tempt you away from achieving your goals. If it isn't in the house, it is far less likely that a moment of weakness will cause you to blow it. If there are others in the house not following your diet, things can be more challenging. I hope they will understand what you are trying to achieve. You may want to ask them to keep their junk food in a separate area where you don't see it as easily. In extreme cases, you could ask them to put it in a locked cabinet or drawer. Regardless of your situation, the bottom line is that you should mold your environment to give you the best chance of succeeding. That means getting rid of all the negative distractions (food or otherwise) in your life.

Set a Start Date

Once you have committed to starting The Program, seal your commitment by picking a start date for your new diet and exercise program. In the time leading up to this point, you should thoroughly read this manual, plan your diet and exercise routine, and perform the necessary grocery shopping. If possible, choose a date that works best in terms of your work and social life. Choose a time when you will be under the least amount of extraneous stress and be well rested. Once you have chosen your date, make the necessary preparations and get started!

Track Your Progress

Some method of record keeping is a must while on The Program. Whether you decide to use a simple notebook or a fancy computer program, keeping accurate records of your progress can be an invaluable tool. With an accurate record of the changes your body is experiencing, you can notice trends and make adjustments as needed, as well as derive a great deal of satisfaction when you see how far you have come. At a minimum, start with a record of some basic anthropometric measurements like your body weight, body fat percentage, and measurements of your waist, chest, arms, and legs. Also of importance are the exercises you will be doing week to week and the amount of weight used and number of repetitions performed. Bring your workout log with you to the gym so you can remember exactly what you did the week before. You will be surprised to see that you will be making steady and significant progress every week.

There are a number of professional workout- and diet-tracking tools available. There are also software programs that perform the same function. If you find one that you like, by all means, use it. Regardless of what method you choose, make sure that you use something. Tracking your progress is a key ingredient in reaching your goals.

"Who ever hears of fat men heading a riot, or herding together in turbulent mobs?
No - no, your lean, hungry men who are continually worrying society, and setting the
whole community by the ears."

-Washington Irving

THE ENDOMORPHIC DIET

For those of you with a great deal of body fat to lose or those looking to lower their body fat levels as much as possible, the Endomorphic Diet is the place to start. This diet is a ketogenic diet. It is designed to alter your metabolism from a carbohydrate-using system to one that burns primarily fats for fuel. Ketogenic diets are not new. They have been used for weight loss and even to control seizures for decades. They have risen and fallen in popularity over the years and attracted a great deal of scientific interest for their ability to treat obesity-related diseases, such as diabetes, hypertension, and high cholesterol. Despite their effectiveness and the generous amount of scientific literature supporting their use, mainstream nutritionists are still hesitant to recommend them and continue to perpetuate a variety of misconceptions about ketogenic diets. Fortunately, the success of previous low-carbohydrate diet plans, like the Atkins Diet and the increasing number of scientific studies showing their safety and efficacy are beginning to change the opinion of many in the health-care industry.

The Endomorphic Diet differs from most commercial low-carb diets in several important ways. You will be maintaining a very low carbohydrate intake throughout the duration of the diet. Most low-carb diets like Atkins and South Beach start off with a short period (usually two weeks or less) of low carbohydrate intake and then transition to gradually increasing carbohydrate intake. As many of you are aware, the greatest amount of weight loss occurs during this early phase, when the body transitions to a fat-burning ketogenic state. Increasing carb intake after this point takes the body out of ketosis and can slow fat loss. You can avoid this problem entirely and maintain the optimum degree of fat burning by keeping carbohydrate intake low for the duration of the diet. Consuming no greater than thirty grams of carbohydrate per day is sufficient for most individuals to maintain at least a low level of ketosis. This figure may vary between individuals. With proper monitoring, you will discover the optimal carbohydrate level for your particular metabolism and be able to adjust your diet accordingly. Additionally, unlike in other ketogenic diets, you will limit the amount of saturated fats you consume to some degree. You will consume most of your fats from healthier monounsaturated and polyunsaturated sources. There is a great deal of research showing that foods rich in these healthier fats have important cardiovascular benefits and are good sources of antioxidants and vitamins.

The Endomorphic Diet is designed to rapidly produce and then maintain a state of diet-induced ketosis. This state is induced by significantly reducing your intake of carbohydrates and replacing them with high-quality proteins and polyunsaturated and monounsaturated fats. This plan is the ideal method for reducing body fat. Without a steady supply of carbohydrate, your body will be forced to activate its own innate fat-burning mechanisms to provide the energy it needs. Carbohydrate restriction will also lower your insulin levels. Insulin is the primary hormone responsible for stimulating fat deposition. This is of central importance for those of you with insulin resistance or full-blown diabetes. With little or no swings in your blood sugar, you will notice that you have steady energy levels throughout the day without the post-meal sugar crash typical of a carbohydrate-rich diet. Additional benefits of the Endomorphic Diet are improved cholesterol levels, decreased hunger, and decreased cravings for sweets.

The Endomorphic Diet is also an anti-catabolic diet. Obviously, one of the worst things that can happen on any weight-loss diet is the loss of lean muscle mass. The amount of muscle tissue you possess is one of the most important factors in determining your metabolic rate. Losing muscle tissue will slow your metabolism and decrease the amount of fat you are able to burn. As compared to conventional diets, ketogenic diets promote the retention of lean muscle tissue to a much greater degree. Studies looking at the effects of ketogenic diets on lean muscle mass have shown increased levels of protein synthesis and preservation of fat-free body mass as compared to conventional high-carbohydrate diets with similar calories.[205] This phenomenon occurs for a number of reasons. Ketones appear to have anti-catabolic and anabolic properties in and of themselves. The most prevalent ketone in the human body, beta-hydroxybutyrate, which is produced in large quantities while one is on a ketogenic diet, has been shown to reduce the loss of nitrogen in the urine (a marker of protein degradation). As discussed in the chapter on protein, leucine is one of the most important amino acids responsible for stimulating protein synthesis. Beta-hydroxybutyrate has been shown to decrease the breakdown of leucine by up to 40 percent as well as stimulate its incorporation into muscle tissue by over 15 percent.[206] The Endomorphic Diet is also high in quality protein and fats. This provides the body with a steady supply of energy substrate in the form of fatty acids and ketone bodies so that there is little need for the body to break down its precious muscle tissue to meet its energy needs.

It's important to note, however, that the Endomorphic Diet's anti-catabolic properties do have limitations. If you skip meals or cut too many calories too quickly from your diet, you will lose muscle tissue. No diet can completely prevent muscle loss, but no diet is better for the non-steroid-using athlete at preserving as much of your muscle tissue as possible.

205   Harper MP, Schenk S, Barkan AL, Horowitz JF: Effects of dietary carbohydrate restriction with high protein intake on protein metabolism and the somatotropic axis. J Clin Endocrinol Metab 2005, 90(9):5175–81.
206   Nair KS, Welle SL, Halliday D, Campell RG: Effect of B-hydroxybutyrate on whole-body leucine kinetics and fractional mixed skeletal muscle protein synthesis in humans. J Clin Invest 1988, 82:198–205.

Hydration

You will likely notice a significant drop in your body weight during the first week or two of the Endomorphic Diet. Some of this weight will be body fat, but a significant portion of it will be water weight. This phenomenon is typical of ketogenic diets. As the amount of stored glycogen in your liver and muscles decreases, the water that binds to it is released and filtered by the kidneys. This is a normal process and not anything to be worried about. However, it is important for several reasons that you increase your water intake during the Endomorphic Diet. You will be exercising intensely and will, therefore, lose water, electrolytes, and minerals through perspiration. These must be replaced. You run the risk of dehydration if you do not compensate for your increased water losses. Water is essential for all bodily functions and should never be restricted on your diet. Aim for at least ten to twelve glasses of water daily. Feel free to mix in your favorite carbohydrate-free drink mix to make achieving this goal easier. Soda, tea, or coffee is not an adequate replacement for water and does not count toward your daily water intake.

Set Yourself up for Success

Before you move on and begin the Endomorphic Diet, you should have gone through the prelaunch checklist detailed in the previous chapter. Make sure you have set yourself up for success by calculating your maintenance calorie requirements, getting rid of the junk food in your home, setting your goals, and formulating your training regimen based on the recommendations in the chapters on exercise. By preparing in this way, you will set yourself up for success and greatly increase your chances of meeting your goals. The Endomorphic Diet, perhaps even more than the other diets, requires precision to work optimally. You can't fly by the seat of your pants, "ball-park" your calorie and carbohydrate intake, and just hope for the best. You won't get the results you are looking for, and you will probably end up frustrated. *When the Endomorphic Diet is done correctly, the results are spectacular.* You will be burning fat twenty-four hours a day while preserving (and likely building) your muscle mass. It is not uncommon to steadily lose two or more pounds of body fat per week (and many lose much more than this) while on the Endomorphic Diet.

How Many Calories Should You Eat?

Once you have determined your maintenance calorie level, it's time to calculate the number of calories you will have to cut to optimally burn body fat at the maximum possible rate. Precision here is important. Though ketogenic diets create a potent anti-catabolic environment that lends itself to preserving your hard-earned muscle tissue, cutting calories too severely will invariably lead to loss of muscle mass in addition to fat tissue regardless of what type of diet you follow. Conversely, consuming too many calories will lead to suboptimal fat loss and potentially fat gain if you overeat.

This begs the question "What is the optimal calorie deficit to maximize fat loss while preserving muscle tissue?" This is a tough question. I'm sure you have heard the conventional recommendations that if you want to lose a pound of fat (which has roughly 3500 calories), you need a five-hundred-calorie per day deficit. This makes sense mathematically but does not take into account hundreds of variables that influence the metabolism of fat and often doesn't necessarily reflect the true deficit you will need to achieve.

Macronutrient ratios, type of exercise, sleep, and a myriad of other variables play a role in the amount of fat loss you can achieve, so I consider this recommendation to be overly simplistic.

There is some scientific literature that can help sort this question out, but clear-cut answers are still lacking. None of the available research was performed on subjects on a high-intensity weight-training regimen, let alone on a ketogenic diet, so the best we can do is try to extrapolate those results into some practical guidelines. One particular study looking at calorically restricted individuals involved in "moderate exercise" estimated that the average person can burn approximately 69.3 (let's just say 70) calories of fat for every kilogram of body fat that they have per day.[207] I won't go into the painful mathematics involved in arriving at this number, it is sufficient to say that the researchers who calculated it did their best to use real-world measurements on human subjects and have arrived at what I consider to be a reasonably accurate figure. This equation explains what most of us have seen in the real world—that the more obese an individual is, the more rapid and dramatic their *initial* weight loss is when they begin their diet. Conversely, this also explains why individuals who are already relatively lean will lose body fat at a slower rate than a morbidly obese individual despite having similar basal metabolic rates, similar caloric deficits, and similar exercise programs.

Consider an average twenty-five-year-old 100-kilogram man (220 lbs) with a body fat percentage of 20 percent. He is carrying 20 kilograms (44 lbs) of fat. Using the above formula, he would be able to burn a *maximum* of 1400 calories from fat per day (70 calories x 20 kg of fat). Extrapolated over seven days and assuming that one pound of fat has 3500 calories, then this individual could lose a *maximum* of 1.28 kilograms or 2.8 pounds of fat every seven days (1400 calories x 7 days = 9800 calories of fat burned per week and 9800 / 3500 = 2.8 lbs).

In the above scenario, our one-hundred-kilogram male, if the above estimate is accurate, could reliably cut *1400* calories from his maintenance caloric intake (estimated to be about *3500 calories* via the Schofield Equation (if he is following The Program workout with cardio three times a week), and his weight loss would be almost exclusively from fat. If his caloric intake was cut beyond 1400 calories, then he could expect that further weight loss would theoretically come from his fat-free mass, i.e., his lean muscle tissue and organs. Therefore, his starting daily calorie intake based on the above equation should not go below (3500-1400 =) *2100* calories. Also note that, according to the above formula, the fatter you are to begin with, the greater your ability to lose fat will be. As you get leaner, it becomes more difficult to lose body fat and your calories must be further restricted. As stated above, this makes real-world sense for most people as we have all heard of morbidly obese individuals dropping huge amounts of weight in the first few weeks of dieting. This rapid weight loss inevitably slows down as the body adapts through multiple mechanisms to the lower caloric input.

It's important to remember that this is the theoretical *maximum* number of calories that could be cut without dipping into your hard-earned stores of muscle mass to supply your needed caloric requirements. Given the difficulty in building lean muscle mass to begin with; it is my opinion that cutting calories this much, to the very edge of where you begin to lose muscle mass, is not a good idea for many dieters.

---

207   Alpert SS. A limit on the energy transfer rate from the human fat store in hypophagia. J Theor Biol. 2005 Mar 7;233(1):1–13.

Remember, this is a mathematical model. It won't fit everyone perfectly, and there will be variations in individual metabolism and activity levels that need to be considered. In the real world, there are a large number of individuals just like the one used in this example for which a 1400 calorie daily deficit is too severe and will result in the loss of lean muscle mass. Therefore, there should be a little "cushion" in that deficit to allow for individual variation. After a few weeks of dieting, if you don't think you are losing as much fat as you would like, then you can reduce that cushion as much as necessary. At the beginning, however, I think it would be wise not to cut calories quite so drastically to provide an extra margin of safety against muscle loss. How much of a margin should you factor in? There is no scientific data available at this time to give any guidance on this issue, but my personal opinion, based on real-world subjects, is that cutting about 75 percent of your calculated maximum caloric deficit appears to be a reasonable place to start. That would mean in the above example that instead of starting out with a 1400-calorie deficit, our theoretical hundred-kilogram male would have an initial caloric deficit of *1050* calories (1400 x 0.75 = 1050). He would then create a diet with *2450* calories (3500 - 1050) and go from there. If after about two weeks of dieting, he is not satisfied with the amount of fat loss he is experiencing, then he could consider decreasing his calories by 10 to 20 percent and see what happens. Similarly, if his weights in the gym are plummeting, and he feels like he is losing too much muscle mass, then he could increase his calories by 10 to 20 percent and reevaluate his results.

From this point onward, he would stay at his current caloric deficit for as long as he is satisfied with his degree of fat loss. After all, if it ain't broke, don't fix it. Inevitably, however, there will come a time when his fat loss will slow down and he will reach a plateau. The body will adapt to its current calorie level through changes in a host of hormonal and metabolic pathways by becoming more efficient at utilizing those calories. Additionally, as you reach a significantly lower body weight, the simple cost of maintaining that weight will decrease, i.e., your basal metabolic rate will slow. At this point, an additional caloric deficit needs to be created for fat loss to continue.

This is where things can get a little tricky if you try to use the above equation to calculate what your new calorie deficit should be. If you simply plug in your new numbers and use the seventy-calories-per-kilogram rule, you will find that, according to the equation, you should *increase* your calories instead of cut them to continue losing fat, which is clearly counterintuitive.

Let's continue with the above example to demonstrate this point. Let's say our theoretical hundred-kilogram (220 lbs) individual has been dieting for four weeks. He has cut approximately 1050 calories from his daily maintenance regimen and lost a total of four kilograms (8.8 lbs) of fat. He now weighs ninety-six kilograms (211.2 lbs). He previously carried twenty kilograms (44 lbs) of fat but now has only sixteen kilograms (35.2 lbs) of fat giving him a body fat percentage of approximately 15 percent. At this new weight and body fat percentage, he is now capable of burning *1134 calories* of fat per day. His new maintenance calorie requirement using the Schofield Equation is now approximately *3426 calories*. As mentioned earlier, the leaner you are, the less fat you are capable of burning per week. Therefore, it makes sense that after four weeks and a loss of almost nine pounds of body fat, the maximum amount of fat you can lose per week will decrease. Using our seventy-calorie-per-kilograms-of-fat equation, his new maximum caloric deficit is *1120* calories (a 20 percent drop from 1400), and the maximum amount of fat he could now burn per week is a still very respectable 2.2 pounds per week. However, we are going to keep our 25 percent calorie buffer, which would mean a cut of *840* calories (1120 x 0.75), which must now be subtracted from his new maintenance level. This would leave him with a diet that provided *2586* calories, a 136-calorie increase!

For obvious reasons, *adding* calories is not the right answer when you have reached a fat-loss plateau on your diet. You must create a further calorie deficit to compensate for the normal metabolic slowdown that occurs anytime you restrict calories below maintenance level for an extended period of time. Therefore, I'd recommend the seventy-calorie-per-kilogram rule only as a starting point for your diet. After you have been dieting for an extended period of time and your weight loss ceases, using it again will not yield an accurate estimate of what your caloric needs will be. Again, this is because it doesn't take into account the normal metabolic slowdown that occurs during prolonged calorie restriction.

To continue losing weight, you have to create an additional calorie deficit. The question is how much of a deficit should you make? How many additional calories should you cut? For the time being, there is no hard scientific data using weight-training athletes on a ketogenic or moderate-carbohydrate diet to help us make this determination. Real-world practical experience would suggest that cutting calories by an additional 10 percent is a reasonable place to start. Remember, maintaining your hard-earned muscle mass is of crucial importance. You don't want to cut your calories too low and begin sacrificing muscle tissue. Not only will you look and feel worse, but this will make it even more difficult to burn body fat. If after two weeks with a 10 percent deficit you aren't losing as much fat as you would like, then consider cutting an additional 10 percent. Unless you have particularly bad fat-burning genes, I wouldn't recommend cutting more than 10 percent at a time from your total calories. For most individuals, 10 percent seems to work well and be a modest enough decrease so as not to put one's muscle mass at risk. Whether this deficit comes from further cutting calories from your diet or from an increase in exercise is up to you. I personally think it easier to simply add some additional time on the treadmill or exercise bike to make the difference, but for those of you who feel like you may be bordering on overtraining, you may want to reduce your portion sizes sufficiently to create the same deficit.

In our above example, our athlete started out on a 2450-calorie-per-day diet. He did well for eight weeks at which point his fat loss began to slow and he reached a plateau, no longer losing fat for two weeks. He would then need to either drop his daily caloric intake by 10 percent (245 calories) or perform an additional 245 calories of exercise per day.

It's important to state again that losing body fat, like trying to gain muscle mass, is a dynamic and ever-changing process. There are significant genetic differences among individuals in regards to the ability to build muscle tissue and burn body fat, as well as differences in the degree to which individual metabolisms respond to a calorie deficit. This is important to remember because following any of the diets in The Program requires surveillance and occasional adjustments on your part. It is impossible to throw out a specific formula that can be applied perfectly to every human being on earth. What has been presented here is not a diet that you can simply start and then leave on autopilot. No diet that actually works in the long term can do that. Use the guidelines presented above to start yourself on the right path but make adjustments in your total calories and exercise level based on the results you are achieving. If you start losing strength and energy in the gym and feel like you are losing muscle mass on your initial caloric estimate then, by all means, increase your calories by 10 to 20 percent as recommended above and see what happens. Similarly, if your fat loss is lower than you wish, use the 10 percent rule mentioned above to further restrict your calories or increase your physical activity level. Fortunately, for most people, the starting recommendations given above are pretty close to optimal and will result in sustained, steady fat loss for months at a time.

Translating these guidelines into a practical day-to-day diet you can follow may seem a little daunting at this point. Don't worry; it's not as difficult as you might think. After you have calculated the number of calories you will be consuming over six meals, create the target number of grams for each macronutrient (carbohydrate, protein, and fat) and roughly how many calories of each you will consume per day. Remember that carbohydrate and protein both have four calories per gram, while fats have nine calories per gram. You can then create a chart like that shown here to better visualize what your daily intake will be. Keep in mind that you don't have to be perfect here. Your diet doesn't have to have *exactly* the amount of calories or grams of fat, protein, and carbohydrate that you have calculated for yourself. These are target figures. Your diet should, however, come as close as possible to these numbers as you can make them.

Let's continue with the example used above of our hypothetical 220-pound male athlete with 20 percent body fat who starts his diet with approximately 2450 calories and see what a real-world diet would look like for him. First, here is how his daily macronutrients would look:

Carbohydrate: 30 grams (120 calories)
Protein: 200 grams (800 calories)
Fat*: 170 grams (1530 calories)

*No more than 1/3rd of total fat calories (~500 calories/57 grams) should come from saturated fat. The remainder is split between monounsaturated and polyunsaturated fats.

Carbohydrates are limited to a maximum of thirty grams per day. Protein intake is at two grams per kilogram of bodyweight, and the remainder of his calories comes from fats.

This leaves us with a diet that has its calories split as follows: 60 percent fat, 30 percent protein, and 10 percent carbohydrate. When you create your diet, these are the ratios you should aim for.

In an ideal scenario, his macronutrient intake could be broken down roughly evenly across six meals as shown below. This sort of precision isn't really possible when you are eating real foods, but, as stated above, looking at things in this way can help you plan your meals and ensure that you aren't overloading one meal with too much protein or fat at the expense of another. Not all meals have to have exactly the same macronutrient breakdown, obviously, but you should make an attempt to spread out your calories through the day.

The following is an example of what a real-world diet that comes very close to achieving the numbers calculated for total calories and macronutrient grams for our hypothetical 220-pound athlete would look like. This is not intended as the best diet for everyone. Rather, it simply serves as one example of a nearly infinite combination of foods that could be combined to meet the goals mentioned above. The foods you choose to meet your particular goals may be very different from those shown here, and that's fine. Use your calorie counter book to choose the foods you prefer. As long as you are meeting the diet's requirements, feel free to include any food that you like. Staying on the Endomorphic Diet for a prolonged period of time is challenging. You can make it easier by picking foods you enjoy and including as much variety as possible. I would recommend that when you create your first diet, you take the time to create two or three others, all of which meet the same requirements but have different food choices. You can then rotate these different diets so you don't tire of eating the same thing every day. Having some variety in your diet is important, not just for ensuring you get the nutrients you require but to help keep you sane.

Sample Diet

Meal 1: 5-whole-egg omelet made with 2 teaspoons olive oil (may add small amount of cheese, spinach, or other veggies for a negligible amount of carbohydrate and calories):

> Calories: 545
> Carbs: 2 grams
> Fiber: 0 grams
> Fat: 39 grams fat (6 poly, 21 mono, 11 saturated)
> Protein: 30 grams

Meal 2: one cup of flaxseed hot cereal

> Calories: 300
> Carbs: 4 grams
> Fiber: 24 grams
> Fat: 12 grams—all polyunsaturated
> Protein: 24 grams

Meal 3: 1 Buffalo burger patty (or oily fish) with 1 cup asparagus + spinach salad (with feta cheese, bacon bits, 3 tablespoons of olive oil, and vinegar salad dressing.)

> Calories: 540
> Carbs: 6 grams
> Fiber: 6 grams
> Protein: 57 grams
> Fat: 33 grams (9 saturated, 28 monounsaturated)

Meal 4 (pre-workout): Whey protein isolate shake (1 scoop) +1 cup of 2% milk

> Calories: 227
> Carbs: 12 grams
> Fiber: 0 grams
> Protein: 25 grams
> Fat: 6 grams (3 grams saturated, 3 monounsaturated)

Meal 5 (post-workout): Whey protein isolate shake 1 scoop + 2 tablespoons flax oil w/ lignans

Calories: 320

Carbohydrates: 0 grams

Fiber: 0 grams

Protein: 25 grams

Fat: 23 grams (16 grams polyunsaturated, 4 grams monounsaturated)

Meal 6: Pure egg-protein powder (1/2 cup):

Calories: 150 calories

Carbohydrate: 2 grams

Fiber: 0 grams

Protein: 32 grams

Garden salad (1 cup lettuce, 1 tomato, 1/4 cucumber) + 1 Tablespoons of olive oil + vinegar dressing

Calories: 126

Carbohydrate: 5 grams

Fiber: 3 grams

Protein: 0 grams

Fat: 14 grams (monounsaturated)

Cheat Day

Following the Endomorphic Diet can be more difficult for some than others. Those of you used to consuming regular meals and snacks consisting of junk-food items like fast food and sweets can find the transition to a healthier diet trying. Fortunately, the steady blood sugar and energy levels, as well as the excellent fat loss you will experience, keep cravings for these items to a minimum for most. However, you should periodically reward yourself for your hard work and discipline by giving yourself one day per week when you can loosen up and eat whatever you feel like. Not only will this give you something to look forward to each week, but it will satisfy those occasional cravings you may get. Most dieters choose to have their "cheat day" on the weekend so they can go out with friends and eat freely at restaurants without having to forgo what everyone else is eating. On your "cheat day," you may eat any particular food item you wish. The day starts on waking with breakfast and should end no later than ten o'clock that night. Though you may structure your meals however you wish, attempt to consume six meals with at least some quality protein included in each. Your "Cheat Day" should not degenerate into "Binge Day." Just because you can eat the foods of your choice does not mean that you should wake up and go clean out the local bakery on a ten-thousand-calorie sugar binge. After eating a healthy diet, you will find that your body is no longer accustomed to eating unhealthy sugar-loaded items, and you will likely feel quite ill. Use a certain degree of moderation on your cheat days, and you will enjoy them much more.

Useful Adjuncts

Flax , Hemp and Chia

As discussed in the chapter on polyunsaturated fats, both flax and chia seeds are an excellent source of ALA (alpha-linolenic acid) as well as fiber. Hemp is also a rich source of both omega-3 and omega-6 fats as well as protein. Consuming large amounts of healthy fats is one of the corner stones of the Endomorphic Diet and important in the Mesomorphic and Ectomorphic Diets as well. While it is easy to consume large amounts of saturated fats on a ketogenic diet, consuming adequate amounts of polyunsaturated fats can be difficult for some, especially while trying to maintain a low overall carbohydrate level. Consuming flax, hemp and chia, whether in ground or oil form, can make this much easier.

Whole flax- and chia seeds are easily added to most foods. Flaxseeds should be milled, however, because they are otherwise very difficult to digest. Milled flaxseeds can be used for baking and can even be used as a replacement for butter or margarine. Virtually all of the carbohydrate found in flax, hemp and chia are in the form of insoluble fiber, making them an excellent addition on a low-carbohydrate diet. There are a large variety of commercially available products on the market today from granola mixes to instant hot cereals, making their addition into your diet that much easier. Hemp, chia and flaxseeds are high in fiber and can be purchased as flour for use in baking. All three are loaded with polyunsaturated fats and readily available in most health food stores. Chia oil in particular works well in soups, sauces, or as an ingredient in salad dressings. It makes an excellent addition to most protein shakes as well. Flax and hemp seeds have a nutty flavor that most people find quite pleasant, and chia's mild flavor also makes it a delicious addition to your protein shakes. For vegetarian athletes, hemp protein provides one of the few complete protein sources that is readily available as a powder.

Keto Sticks

It is useful, though not mandatory, to obtain some commercially available keto-sticks. These specially treated strips are designed for use by diabetics. They change color when exposed to ketones in the urine. They can be very useful for monitoring your metabolic state while on the Endomorphic Diet. Typically, you will notice ketones in your urine within forty-eight hours of beginning the Endomorphic Diet. Later, you can use them to ensure that you are maintaining ketosis throughout the diet. Remember, the daily thirty-gram carbohydrate limit is a general recommendation that fits most people well. However, there are those who will not be able to maintain ketosis at this level and will need to go slightly lower. Similarly, some of you may be able to get away with slightly higher carb intake and still maintain ketosis. The easiest way to determine this is to use keto sticks on a regular basis. The goal during the Endomorphic Diet is to maintain at least trace ketone levels in the urine. This is usually manifested by a light-pink color change on most keto strips. There are several factors besides carbohydrate intake that will influence the results you see on your strips, however. Greater water intake can potentially dilute the ketone levels in your urine and therefore show a falsely lower degree of ketosis on your strips. This is why I advise always maintaining at least trace levels. It is likely that you are underestimating your degree of ketosis if you are consuming the recommended amounts of water. The best time to check your ketone levels is first thing in the morning. After an overnight fast, you should be in at least moderate ketosis. If not, you may need to adjust your carbohydrate diet downward somewhat. If you find that you are consistently in heavy ketosis, it is likely that you are not consuming enough water. By the end of the day, most dieters are in moderate to trace ketosis. If you find that you are consistently getting no color change in your strips at day's end you are either drinking a tremendous amount of fluid or taking in too many carbohydrates. Take a closer look at your diet, especially serving sizes, and ensure that you are not breaking your carbohydrate limit.

Low-Carb Recipe Books

You have probably noticed that there are no sample recipes and no mini-cookbook included in The Program. This was not an accidental omission. The truth is that the market is literally flooded with a multitude of low-carbohydrate cookbooks, meal planners, and guides. Rather than simply rehash those in this text, I've decided to recommend a few resources you can find yourself. Unless you have an incredible amount of discipline or were born without taste buds, you are going to have to create some variety in your diet while on the Endomorphic Diet. It's easy to fall into the trap of just eating the same thing day in and day out. Doing this will not only make you miserable but will inevitably lead to burnout. That's why you should strongly consider making at least three different diets, all of which have the proper calories and ratios of macronutrients, and rotate them throughout the week. Having several good low-carbohydrate recipe books on hand can be very helpful when doing this. There are a few good resources that you may find helpful online as well.

Recommended Supplements

There are no supplements that are mandatory for you to take while on the Endomorphic Diet. However, you may wish to include the following items to ensure you are consuming a complete range of nutrients and to make meeting your dietary requirements easier.

Multivitamin and mineral supplement are generally recommended to ensure you are consuming adequate levels of antioxidants and minerals. For those of you without a great deal of time or a personal chef, finding a palatable low-carbohydrate whey protein powder or bar can make meeting your daily protein and calorie needs much easier while you are on the go. An egg- or casein-based protein powder can also be useful as a quick source of "slow" protein before bed. Creatine monohydrate has been shown to be beneficial in terms of improving muscle strength. Its use may help you maintain your strength levels while you lose weight. A fish oil supplement is also strongly recommended unless you consume fish as daily part of your diet. Consider supplementing with vitamin D especially if you live in a cooler climate or get minimal sun exposure.

How Long Should You Stay on the Endomorphic Diet?

The answer to this question is "It's up to you!" The Program is designed to be an individualized system that helps you meet your specific goals. In general, you stay on the Endomorphic Diet until you reach your body fat goals. There are numerous studies showing that there are no long-term problems associated with ketogenic diets going out at least 12 months.[208] Sticking to this, or any other diet, for that long can be difficult, especially if you are traveling or undergoing some other major life stressor. If you find that, despite the great results you are getting, that circumstances dictate you stop the diet, you should transition to the Mesomorphic Diet. This will help you maintain the results you have achieved to date and is a much easier eating plan to follow. You can then resume the Endomorphic Diet when you feel the time is right.

Common Pitfalls

Hidden Carbs

A common pitfall for those trying to cut back on carbohydrate intake is forgetting to look for and count some of the "hidden carbs" found in many foods. With the renewed popularity of these diets, a number of food manufacturers are bringing low-carb products to the market. This has made it much easier to increase the variety of foods and flavors in your diet. Unfortunately, some of these so-called low-carb foods are mislabeled or falsely advertised as having less carbohydrate than they actually contain.

Current FDA regulations allow foods with less than one gram of carbohydrate per serving but more than 0.5 grams per serving to be labeled as having "less than 1" or "1." You can see clearly that an easy way to make a high-carbohydrate food or additive appear to be low carb is to simply reduce the serving size so that it contains less than 1 gram of carbohydrate. Additionally, foods with less than 0.5 grams of carbohydrate can be labeled as having zero carbohydrate per serving. Ordinarily, this wouldn't pose much of a problem, but when you are consuming very limited amounts of carbohydrate on the Endomorphic variant, every little bit can add up. For example, say you are at a restaurant or bar and want to add some sweetness to your ice tea. In the course of the evening, you use six packets of artificial sweetener. Almost all sweeteners contain a high-glycemic carbohydrate base (either dextrose or maltodextrose) to give them some bulk and added flavor. The amount in each packet is usually the equivalent of 0.4 to 0.9 grams of carbohydrate. Depending on the brand you used, you have just consumed 2.4 to 5.4 grams of carbohydrate when according to the packet label you consumed zero! My advice would be to count each packet of artificial sweetener as 1.0 grams of carbohydrate and take that into account when counting your daily intake.

Sometimes, additional carbohydrates are not even listed on food labels. If you look at enough food labels you will notice that occasionally the numbers just don't add up. Fat contains nine calories per gram, and carbohydrates and protein both have four calories per gram.

In a properly labeled food item, the following formula should hold true:

(carb grams x 4) + (protein grams x 4) + (fat grams x 9) = Total Calories

The total calories listed on the label should correspond to the sum of the calories from fat, protein, and carbohydrate. What you will sometimes see is that the total calories listed on the label are actually

---

208   Dashti, H.M. Mathew, C.M., Hussein, T. et al., "Long Term Effects of a ketogenic Diet in Obese Patients", Clinical Cardiology, 2004, 9(3), 200–205.

higher than what you would get by adding the individual calories from its fat, protein, and carbohydrate components. What gives? Is there some fourth form of calories previously unknown to science? No. These extra calories come from carbohydrate sources that are not counted by the manufacturer but can still impact your insulin levels and potentially derail your diet if you don't account for them. They include sugar alcohols, glycerin, cornstarch, and milk solids among other ingredients. When looking for hidden carbs, keep a particular eye out for the following ingredients. They are often found in so-called low- or zero-carbohydrate foods/beverages but are actually very high carbohydrate items. Be sure you account for these extra calories and carbohydrates in your diet. Remember, the more precise you are with your diet, the better your results will be.

Cheating

It goes without saying that if you cheat regularly on your diet, you won't achieve your goals. Sneaking the occasional candy, cookie, or chocolate while on the Endomorphic Diet doesn't seem like it would sabotage your diet, but it will. While in ketosis, your metabolism is geared to burn fat as its primary fuel source. This fat-burning metabolic state is absolutely dependent on maintaining a low insulin state. Remember, in the setting of elevated insulin levels, dietary fat will be shunted into fat cells instead of being burned as fuel, cholesterol levels will rise, and insulin resistance will be promoted. Therefore, it is absolutely essential that you don't screw up your finely tuned fat-burning metabolism by exceeding your daily carbohydrate limit. You are allowed a full "cheat day" once a week to indulge your cravings for sweets and junk food. For the rest of the week, you must stay within your carbohydrate limits. If you don't, the Endomorphic Diet will certainly backfire on you and you will likely end up gaining fat instead of losing it.

Consuming Too Many Calories

This would seem like a no-brainer, but it is probably the most common reason (along with cheating) that individuals get suboptimal results on their diet. High-fat foods are calorically dense, and it can be easy to consume more calories than you intend, especially if you are used to eating larger portions of less calorically dense foods. Fortunately, the longer digestion times and satiety induced from a higher-fat meal can offset this, but excessive calorie consumption can still be a problem. The reason you go through the trouble of calculating your optimal caloric deficit and why you have a caloric reference guide on the Endomorphic Diet is so that you can create a diet that allows you to burn as much fat as possible. If you don't take the time to measure your portions or just chose them arbitrarily, you won't get optimal results. Despite the fact that ketogenic diets are relatively forgiving when it comes to excess calorie intake, they still don't violate the basic laws of human physiology. If you take in more calories than you burn, you will gain weight.

Too Much Protein

One of the most common pitfalls encountered by athletes attempting to follow a ketogenic diet like the Endomorphic Diet is consumption of excessive protein at the cost of dietary fats. Most dieters don't have a problem restricting their carbohydrate intake since it's fairly simple to identify prohibited items. Many dieters, however, become fixated on the protein component of their diet and make extra effort to include lean sources of protein like chicken, fish, and lean red meats to the exclusion of nearly all else. Additionally, many higher-fat food items, even those rich in healthier mono- and polyunsaturated fats, are high in protein as well.

Previously, it was noted that there is a safe upper limit to the amount of protein a person's liver can safely process. However, even intake well under this limit can cause problems with achieving ketosis on your diet if you exceed the recommended ratios of protein, carbohydrate, and fat. On a low-carbohydrate diet, the body cannot maintain a stable blood sugar level by relying on dietary carbohydrate alone. It must convert some of its dietary protein into glucose via the process of gluconeogenesis. This process, though not terribly efficient, can impact blood glucose levels negatively if large amounts of protein are ingested. Certain amino acids are particularly favored by the body for the production of glucose. These so-called glucogenic amino acids are easily converted to glucose by the liver and can directly impact blood glucose levels. Only two amino acids are so-called ketogenic amino acids: leucine and lysine. As discussed in the chapter on protein, leucine is one of the key amino acids responsible for increasing protein synthesis after a meal. A few other amino acids, namely threonine, isoleucine, phenylalanine, tryptophan, and tyrosine, can be either ketogenic or glucogenic depending on the needs of the body. Animal studies looking at diets where protein is the predominant macronutrient (generally greater than 50 percent of total calories) have shown that both fasting blood sugar and insulin levels of participants are elevated when compared to those of people with lower protein intakes.[209] High protein intakes also stimulate both glucagon and insulin secretion and can lead to elevated levels of both hormones.[210] As discussed previously, elevated glucagon levels cause blood sugar to rise, which in turn results in elevated insulin secretion as a compensatory mechanism. Additionally, high protein intake in and of itself can stimulate the secretion of insulin, independent of blood sugar levels. Dietary fat, however, does not influence insulin secretion. If dietary protein is kept around 30 percent of total calories, then this property can be minimized and numerous studies have shown a favorable decrease in insulin levels in those following ketogenic diets in which less than 30 percent of total calories are derived from protein. Remember, insulin is the body's storage hormone. It promotes the shunting of calories from all sources into fat cells and inhibits fat loss from fat cells, both of which will make losing body fat much more difficult.

If you find that you are having difficulty achieving or maintaining ketosis while on the Endomorphic Diet, examine your diet a bit closer and make sure your macronutrient ratios are in line. Your total protein intake should not be much higher than 30 percent of your total calories. For the rare individual with poor genetics, it may be necessary to decrease your protein intake closer to the 20 percent range to achieve ketosis and replace the calories missed with calories from fat. Another option is to change the source of your protein calories to favor foods that are higher in the ketogenic amino acids leucine and lysine. As shown above, egg whites and soy protein isolate are high in both of these amino acids.

---

209   Usami, et al. Effects of High Protein Diet on Insulin and Glucagon Secretion in Normal Rats. J. Nutr. 112: 681–685, 1982.
210   Eisenstein, AB. Increased glucagon secretion in protein-fed rats: lack of relationship to plasma amino acids. Am J Physiol. 1979 Jan; 236 (1): E20–7.

Skipping Meals

This is another no-brainer. Skipping meals is a surefire way to sabotage your fat-loss goals on any diet. By skipping meals, you will likely be cutting far more calories than you intended and the result will be that you sacrifice more of your hard-earned muscle tissue to compensate. As you lose muscle tissue, your metabolic rate will slow and it will make further fat loss even more difficult. Additionally, by skipping meals, you will be more likely to be hungry, irritable, and resort to quick, easily obtainable junk foods to satisfy your appetite. By spacing your meals out properly, you ensure a steady supply of high-quality protein to maintain a positive nitrogen balance and avoid overeating. It can be a challenge to ensure you meet the demands of the Endomorphic Diet when you have a busy schedule. With a little bit of forethought and planning, however, you can prepare your meals in advance and anticipate times when you will be at risk for missing meals.

Medications that Can Interfere with Ketosis

There are a few prescription medications that can interfere with ketosis. This obviously won't be an issue for the majority of dieters, but if you do take prescription medication on a regular basis, you may wish to read on.

Acetazolamide is a diuretic medication used for a wide range of conditions. Most chronic users have a condition like pseudotumor cerebri that causes elevated pressure in the fluid surrounding the brain or a similar condition. Patients on acetazolamide should not undertake a ketogenic diet because of the risk of severe metabolic acidosis.[211]

Phenobarbital is an older medication that is still used commonly to treat seizures. Ketogenic diets can cause phenobarbital to accumulate in the brain, leading to significant sedation. While starting a ketogenic diet while taking phenobarbital isn't absolutely contraindicated, it is not something that should be undertaken without the strict supervision of a physician. It is very likely that the dose of phenobarbital will need to be lowered and blood levels checked closely.[212]

Valproate is another seizure medication that is in wide use for a variety of conditions from bipolar disorder to migraine headaches. Valproate has a number of metabolic side effects and can interfere with ketone production and cause a carnitine deficiency. The combination of valproate and a ketogenic diet can cause nausea, vomiting, lethargy, liver injury, and in severe cases, coma.[213]

---

211   Dodson WE, Prensky AL, DeVivo DC, Goldring S, Dodge PR. Management of seizure disorders: selected aspects. Part II. J Pediatr 1976;89:695.
212   Freeman JM, Kelly MT, Freeman JB, eds. Initiating the ketogenic diet. In: The epilepsy diet treatment: an introduction to the ketogenic diet, 2nd ed. New York: Demos Vermande, 1996:65–164.
213   Gerber N, Dickinson RG, Harland RC, et al. Reye-like syndrome associated with valproic acid therapy. J Pediatr 1979;95:142–4.

If you are taking any diuretic medications like furosemide (Lasix) or hydrochlorothiazide (HCTZ) you should check with your doctor before starting a ketogenic diet. Ketogenic diets cause a natural diuresis, and the addition of diuretic medications can leave you prone to dehydration.

Finally, a large number of over-the-counter medications have added sugar as a way to make them more palatable. This is particularly true for cough and cold remedies. Read drug labels closely and look for added sugar in your medications before taking them. A useful reference for medications that can influence your diet can be found at www.ketomeds.com.

The Endomorphic Diet in a Nutshell

Total Calories: as calculated below

Carbohydrates:

Begin with a total of 30 grams total per day. Less than 10% of total calories should come from carbohydrate. Keep carbohydrates low for breakfast. Composition of carbohydrates should come, as much as possible, from high fiber, leafy green vegetables.

Optimal time for bulk of carbohydrate intake is prior to the daily workout.

Protein:

- Total protein intake should be 2.0 grams per kilogram of body weight divided roughly equally between 6 daily meals.
- Approximately 30% of total calories will come from protein.
- Fast proteins should be consumed immediately before and immediately after the daily workout. Slow proteins should be consumed before bed.
- Goal is for a minimum of 20 grams of leucine and 100 grams of BCAAs per day divided between 6 meals.
- Protein should not exceed 40% of total calories

Fats:

- Approximately 60% of daily calories come from fat
- Saturated fat no more than 1/3 of daily fat calories
- Goal is near equal omega-6 to omega-3 fat intake
- Omega-3 fatty acid supplementation with a goal of 2–3 grams of DHA+EPA total per day from fish oil or flax

"Cheat Day"

Once a week, you may break from the diet and eat however you like. Attempt to consume the same amount of quality protein you would normally consume, but you may eat any carbohydrate or fat foods that you wish. Do not consume carbohydrates after 10:00 p.m.

The Endomorphic Diet Checklist

1. Estimate your body fat percentage and kilograms of body fat carried:

Use the method of your choice—skin callipers, hydrostatic weighing, bioelectrical impedance (BIA), et cetera. and calculate how many kilograms of body fat you are carrying:

> *Weight in kg x body fat % expressed as a decimal=* kg of body fat
> (ex: 100 kg individual with 15% body fat has 100 x 0.15 = 15 kg of body fat)

2. Estimate your maintenance calorie level:

As detailed previously, use either the Schofield Equation or Harris-Benedict Equation to estimate what your basal metabolic rate is and then adjust for your current activity level.

3. Estimate your maximal caloric deficit:

Your maximum allowable calorie deficit is 70 calories per kilogram of body fat per day. As an added safety margin, this number is increased by 25 percent to give you the initial number of calories you should subtract from your maintenance calorie level.

> *Kg of body fat x 70 x 0.75 =* maximum caloric deficit
> (Ex: an individual with 15 kg of body fat could burn 15 x 70 = 1,050 calories of fat per day x 0.75 = 788 calories subtracted from his/her maintenance calorie level)

4. Calculate your starting calories:

> *Maintenance Calorie Level - Maximal Caloric Deficit =* Starting Calories

5. Divide your calories roughly evenly over six meals.

"Many's the man/ who thought himself wise/ but what he needed/ he did not know..."

—Richard Wagner, The Ring of the Nibelung

THE MESOMORPHIC DIET

The Mesomorphic Diet is the eating plan that most adherents to The Program will eventually end up on even if they start with the Ectomorphic or Endomorphic Diets. The Mesomorphic Diet is an eating plan that can be followed for life. It is far less restrictive than the Endomorphic Diet yet more limited in carbohydrates than the Ectomorphic Diet.

The Mesomorphic Diet serves several purposes. It is an ideal long-term eating plan to maintain the gains you have made while on the other diets and maintain optimal health throughout your life. It can also serve as a temporary break from the requirements of the other diets, which, particularly in the case of the Endomorphic Diet, can be quite demanding. Finally, the Mesomorphic Diet can be manipulated to provide ongoing gains in muscle mass or continued fat loss depending on your particular needs.

The Mesomorphic Diet could be considered a low-carbohydrate diet, but a more accurate term is a "correct-carbohydrate diet." Over one-third of your total calories will be coming from carbohydrates on this diet, but the source of those carbohydrates is of paramount importance. High-glycemic carbohydrates like processed sugars and breads, pastas, juice drinks, and other items are strictly limited. In their place, however, you can consume a broad range of delicious and healthy carbohydrate sources like vegetables, fresh fruits, bean, legumes, nuts, et cetera.

On the Endomorphic Diet, carbohydrates are limited to thirty grams or less, so the source of those carbohydrates is not of paramount importance. On the Ectomorphic Diet, carbohydrates from all sources are allowed. On the Mesomorphic Diet, however, the type of carbohydrate you ingest is far more impor-tant than the total amount. By consuming "correct" carbohydrates, you can achieve many of the same goals of the Endomorphic and Ectomorphic Diets: you can keep insulin levels under control so as to limit the amount of body fat you gain while also providing enough carbohydrate so that your protein intake is spared for the production of additional muscle mass. Finally, the wide range of food choices, despite the restriction on high-glycemic items, makes sticking to the Mesomorphic Diet much easier and makes it a healthier diet for long-term use.

Starting the Mesomorphic Diet

In preparation for starting the Mesomorphic Diet, you will perform several of the same tasks required of the other diets. You will need to estimate your body fat percentage and the number of kilograms of body fat you currently carry. Then you will determine your basal metabolic rate using one of the equations provided previously. From there, you need to decide what your goals are. If you have achieved a certain level of muscularity and definition and wish to maintain it, then construct your diet in such a way that you are consuming calories at your maintenance level. If you would like to shed a few more pounds but for whatever reason don't want to try the Endomorphic Diet, then estimate what your maximum allowable caloric deficit is by multiplying the number of kilograms of body fat you currently possess by seventy calories. Cut this number by 25 percent, and that will leave you with the number of calories you can safely cut from your maintenance level. Using that number, then decide how you will construct your diet. From there, you should evaluate your results about every two weeks. If you are losing body fat at the desired rate, then continue without changing your diet. If your fat loss slows or halts, follow the recommendations laid out in the Endomorphic Diet and create an additional 10 percent caloric deficit by increasing your physical activity, cutting back on calories, or both. Then re-evaluate your results in another two weeks.

If your goal is to gain weight, but you don't wish to try the Ectomorphic Diet, then simply calculate your daily maintenance calories and add an additional five hundred +calories per day to that total. There is very little good data available on how many additional calories are required to optimally build muscle tissue, so the five-hundred-calorie recommendation is somewhat arbitrary. In real-world training situations, it appears to be a sufficient caloric surplus to ensure the growth of new muscle tissue without significant spillover into the growth of fat cells. Is it the optimal number of calories to maximal muscle growth? I'll be the first to say I don't know, and you should be wary of people who say they do but can't show you the scientific study proving their answer. What I can say is that adding more calories than this runs the risk of adding fat weight instead of pure muscle. So, with a five-hundred-calorie surplus, you are probably making a bit of a trade-off. You may not be gaining muscle at the fastest possible rate, but at the same time, you aren't gaining additional body fat. Given the broad genetic variation in individual muscle fiber types, testosterone levels, and numerous other metabolic factors, it seems likely that no single recommendation in terms of optimal caloric surplus will suffice for all people. What can be said with confidence is that you must first give your body a reason to grow additional muscle tissue. That's where a properly performed high-intensity weight-training regimen like the one presented in The Program comes in. Without the proper stimulus in the form of high-intensity exercise, you can consume all the calories you want but won't gain an ounce of muscle tissue. Additionally, you must provide the body with a caloric surplus, a surplus that contains the necessary building blocks for muscle tissue, which is protein.

On all the diets presented in The Program, you will be consuming 2.0 grams of protein per kilogram of bodyweight, which will provide those building blocks. There is no proven benefit to consuming more than this amount so any additional calories you consume should come primarily from fat and carbohydrate sources. Additional carbohydrate has a protein-sparing effect, meaning that less of your consumed protein will be used for creating energy and will instead be utilized for the building of new muscle tissue, which is precisely what you are looking for. Too much carbohydrate, however, will raise insulin levels and could potentially lead to additional fat deposition. The recommendation to consume and additional five hundred calories per day will give you a theoretical 3500-calorie surplus after seven days. One pound of muscle contains approximately 1800 calories if completely devoid of water. Muscle tissue is over 70 percent water, however, so in the real world, a single pound of muscle tissue contains about 500 to 600 calories depending on your hydration state and the amount of stored glycogen.

Therefore, on the Mesomorphic Diet, if your goal is to gain muscle mass while minimizing the amount of body fat you accrue, you should aim for a five-hundred-calorie daily surplus.

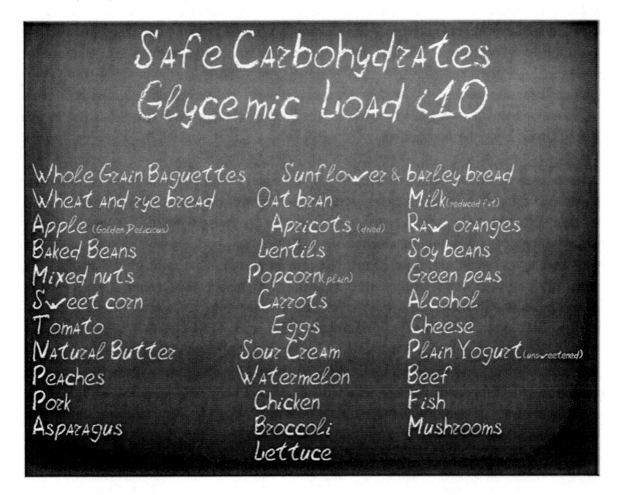

The macronutrient breakdown of the Mesomorphic Diet is rather simple. On all Program diets, you will be consuming two grams of high-quality protein per kilogram of body weight. What varies between the diets is the ratio of carbohydrates to fat and total calories ingested. On the Mesomorphic Diet, carbohydrate calories are split equally with fat calories and will compose approximately 35 percent of your total calories in most cases. They will be divided roughly equally over six daily meals. These calories should come almost exclusively from high-fiber, low-glycemic sources. Specifically, foods with a glucose load (GL) of ten or less are simply the best choice. These include raw vegetables, legumes, nuts, meats, eggs, et cetera. Only a small fraction, 5 percent or less, should come from high-glycemic carbohydrates (i.e., those with a GL over 20). In the table, you will see a sample list of carbohydrates classified as "Safe," "Restricted," and "Forbidden." This is by no means a comprehensive list of the foods you should be eating; it is presented just as an example of the sorts of foods falling into those categories. It's crucial that you obtain a reference book listing the glycemic loads of common foods so that you can provide some variety to your diet and not inadvertently consume foods that you should be avoiding.

"Safe" carbohydrates will form the backbone of your diet. "Restricted" items (those with a GL greater than eleven) can be consumed every now and then in small quantities but should generally be avoided. Finally, "Forbidden" items have no redeeming qualities and are actually harmful to your body. They should never be part of your diet save for your one cheat meal. These include regular soda, which is nothing more than an unnatural toxic concoction of sugar and chemicals. In truth, diet sodas are only slightly better in that they don't have the massive amounts of sugar that regular sodas do, but they are still very unhealthy and should generally be avoided. Trans fats, as discussed in the chapter on fats, are pure poison and should be completely avoided on all Program diets. Finally, use your GL reference to avoid foods with very high-glycemic loads (greater than forty). Their caloric density and ability to very rapidly elevate blood sugar and insulin levels will surely sabotage your fat-loss efforts. In virtually all cases, you can find a lower-glycemic variation or alternative for those particular foods that tastes just as good but won't wreak havoc with your metabolism.

Calories from fat, as mentioned above, are roughly equal to carbohydrate calories. However, since fat contains nine calories per gram to carbohydrates' four calories per gram, your total grams of fat will be lower than your total from carbohydrates. Fat calories on the Mesomorphic Diet should come almost exclusively from mono- and polyunsaturated sources. It's not realistic for you in most cases to cut out all saturated fats, but you should make the effort to limit them greatly. Obviously, trans-fats of any kind, in any amount, are totally off-limits. Good sources of healthy fats include nuts, legumes, flax, oily fish, olive oil, and vegetable oils.

Sample Diet

To illustrate what a real-world Mesomorphic Diet would look like, we will use the same example used previously of a 220-pound (100 kg) male with 20 percent body fat who is following The Program Workout. The first step he must take is to estimate how much body fat he is carrying. In this case, the equation looks like this:

100 kg x 0.20 = 20 kg of body fat

Next, he will estimate his maintenance calorie level while following The Program's exercise routine. This can be done using the Schofield Equation or Harris-Benedict Equation. In this case, we will use the Schofield Equation, but feel free to use either one.

BMR = 15.1 x weight in kg + 692 x activity factor (1.6)

15.1 x 100 kg + 692 = 2202 x 1.6 = 3523 calories (let's just say 3500)

If our sample athlete is looking to maintain his current weight, he would build his diet with approximately 3500 calories spread out over six meals. If his goal is to lose body fat, then a little more math is required to determine just how many calories he should cut from this maintenance level. The maximum amount of body fat he can burn is seventy calories of fat per kilogram per day, which in this case leaves us with a maximum of 1400 calories of fat burned per day. For reasons explained more thoroughly in the chapter detailing the Endomorphic Diet, this is not the number of calories you should cut from your maintenance. Rather, using about 75 percent of this value is more optimal as it will prevent you from potentially losing muscle mass while cutting your calories. Therefore, if he would like to adapt the Mesomorphic Diet for fat loss, his daily caloric intake should be approximately:

75% of 1400 = 1400 x 0.75 = 1050 calories.

3500 - 1050 = 2450 calories

He would then go about dividing these calories more or less evenly over six meals.

If our athlete decided he wanted to use the Mesomorphic Diet to put on some additional muscle mass, then he would simply add five hundred calories to his maintenance level for a total of approximately four thousand calories per day divided over six meals. As mentioned earlier, these additional calories should come from low-glycemic carbohydrates and healthy fats and not from consuming additional protein. If he is following the diet correctly, he is already consuming the optimal amount of protein and adding more does not confer additional benefit.

The Mesomorphic Diet requires that macronutrients be divided up so that protein, fat, and carbohydrates compose *roughly* 30 percent, 35 percent, and 35 percent of total calories respectively. It is *not* imperative that you achieve these ratios exactly in your own diet. You should first calculate your total protein intake (two grams per kilogram of body weight) and then fill in the remainder of your calories with an even split between healthy fats and carbohydrates. In the majority of cases, this will get you the above ratio, but don't fret if you are getting a little bit more carbohydrate and fat. You will still get great results.

For our 220-pound athlete who is trying to consume maintenance calories, his macronutrient breakdown would look something like this:

Protein: (2g/kg) 800 calories
Carbohydrate: (0.35 x 3500) 1233 calories
Fat: (0.35 x 3500) 1233 calories

Notice that the total here only comes to 3266 calories…not 3500. Don't fret! Simply divide the difference (234 calories) and split the added calories evenly between carbohydrates and fats.

This gives him a diet that looks like this:
Protein: 800 calories
Carbohydrate: 1350 calories
Fat: 1350 calories

For those of you who like to nail down the detail, this gives a diet with 38.5 percent of its calories coming from fat and carbohydrate and 22.8 percent of its calories from protein.

Here is what this diet would look like when charted out in terms of macronutrient grams and calories:

Carbohydrate: 338 grams (1350 calories)
Protein: 200 grams (800 calories)
Fat: 150 grams (1350 calories)

The sample diet given here differs somewhat in its distribution of macronutrients but still aims for a close to even ratio of protein, carbohydrates, and fats for each meal. Obviously, you can spread things out differently if you prefer, but you should attempt to keep each meal roughly similar if at all possible. This will help prevent wide swings in insulin levels thereby keeping you from getting hungry or having lapses in energy throughout the day as well as preventing you from stuffing yourself at one sitting and having little to nothing at another.

The following is a sample daily meal plan for our 220-pound male who is eating at a maintenance level of approximately 3500 calories per day while on the Mesomorphic Diet. This is just an example of a single day on the Mesomorphic Diet using foods that I like, but you obviously can create your own diet using the foods you prefer. You will notice that I have included meal-replacement shakes for two of the six daily meals. I keep a very busy schedule and find that having a meal-replacement powder on hand ensures that I don't skip meals. It is not mandatory that you use them, so feel free to include real food meals if you are able. Indeed, whole foods are preferable as they are better sources of vitamins, antioxidants, and other important nutrients. However, the reality for most people leading busy lives and trying to balance work, family, and time at the gym is that including a meal-replacement powder for one or more meals makes getting adequate quality protein much easier. I don't endorse any particular brand of meal-replacement product. My recommendation would be to find one that has a quality protein derived from whey protein isolate and is relatively low in sugar. A list of recipes that are compatible with the Mesomorphic Diet has been deliberately left out of this book. There are hundreds of available cookbooks and websites that you can reference to find sample meals you can include on your diet, so listing many of them here would be redundant. The Mesomorphic Diet offers you substantial flexibility in terms of choosing a wide variety of foods so it is fairly easy to create several different daily meal plans that fulfil the basic requirements of the diet. Indeed, you should create at least three different daily diets and rotate them periodically so you don't grow tired of eating the same thing day in and day out.

Meal 1:   Three-egg whole omelette with mushrooms
                Two slices of whole-wheat toast with Benecol spread
                One turkey sausage patty
                One-half cantaloupe
                655 calories
                31 grams of fat
                64 grams of carbohydrate
                30 grams of protein

Meal 2: Meal-replacement shake with two tablespoons of flaxseed oil and two cups of non-fat milk
776 calories
40 grams of fat
46 grams of carbohydrate
58 grams of protein

Meal 3: Grilled chicken and veggie salad
550 calories
30 grams of fat
40 grams of carbohydrate
30 grams of protein

Meal 4: Meal-replacement shake plus 1 tablespoon of flaxseed oil
436 calories
20 grams of fat
22 grams of carbohydrate
42 grams of protein

Meal 5: Whey protein isolate shake plus toasted rye bread with grilled veggies and melted Swiss cheese sandwich.
350 calories
6 grams of fat
43 grams of carbohydrate
31 grams of protein

Meal 6: 6 oz spinach salad with 2 cups of grilled mixed veggies and grilled asparagus shoots. Egg protein shake at bedtime.
764 calories
28 grams of fat
94 grams of carbohydrate
34 grams of protein

Recommended Supplements

There are no supplements that are mandatory for you to take while on the Mesomorphic Diet. However, you may wish to include the following items to ensure you are consuming a complete range of nutrients and to make meeting your dietary requirements easier.

A multi-vitamin and mineral supplement is generally recommended to ensure you are consuming adequate levels of antioxidants and minerals. For those of you without a great deal of time or a personal chef, finding a palatable meal-replacement powder or bar can make meeting your daily protein and calorie needs much easier while you are on the go. An egg or casein-based protein powder can also be useful as a quick source of "slow" protein before bed. Creatine monohydrate has been shown to be beneficial in terms of improving muscle strength. Its use may help you maintain your strength levels while you lose weight. A fish oil supplement is also strongly recommended unless you consume fish as daily part of your diet. I personally like adding flaxseed oil to my protein shakes for added polyunsaturated fat calories and for a little flavoring. You may have noticed in the sample diet that I include the margarine substitute Benecol in place of butter as a toast spread. Benecol, Take Control, and other similar products are spreads made with plant sterols that have been shown to lower cholesterol. They are rich in polyunsaturated fats primarily from rapeseed and therefore make an excellent addition to all Program diets.

Common Pitfalls

The Mesomorphic Diet is a much easier diet to follow and is an eating plan you can perform for life. There is quite a bit more leeway in terms of carbohydrate and calorie intake. However, there are still a few ways you can screw things up. These common pitfalls are the same ones you can encounter on the Endomorphic Diet. The most obvious one is cheating on your diet outside of your allowed "cheat meal." Eating junk food gives you calories you don't need, and these calories usually come from the worst possible sources—high-glycemic carbohydrates and saturated and trans-fats.

Along the same lines, consuming too many calories when you are trying to maintain or lose weight will sabotage your diet as well. This can be easy to do, even when you are trying to follow the diet as closely as you can. Be aware of portion sizes and consider using a scale or measuring cups to make sure you are eating the number of calories you think you are. Skipping meals is also a setup for failure. It will make you hungry, irritable, and more likely to binge on foods you shouldn't be eating.

Cheat Meal

The cheat meal is something most Mesomorphic dieters look forward to each week. While on the diet, you are allowed *one* meal per week where you can eat and drink whatever you want—beer, pizza, onion rings…whatever you like. This lets you loosen up your diet a bit, go out to a restaurant or party with friends, and not feel like you constantly have to miss out. Keep in mind though that this is one meal only—and you can't stretch that meal out into a three-hour binge session. Enjoy your cheat meal every week and then get right back on the wagon again.

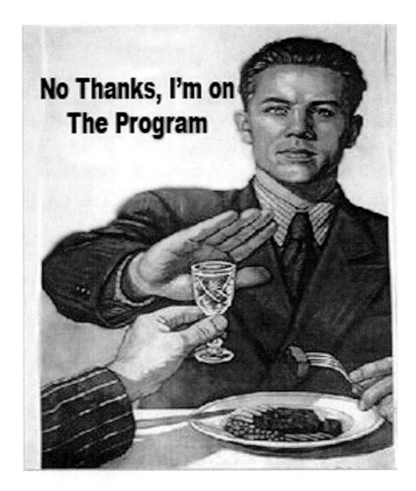

The Mesomorphic Diet in a Nutshell

Total Calories: as calculated above

Carbohydrates:
- Approximately 35% of your total calories
- Less than 25% of total carbohydrate items from the "restricted" list
- Composition of carbohydrates should come, as much as possible, from high fiber, leafy green vegetables, fresh fruits, nuts, legumes, and whole grains.

Protein:
- Total protein intake should be 2.0 grams per kilogram of body weight divided roughly equally between 6 daily meals
- Approximately 30% or less of total calories will come from protein
- Fast proteins should be consumed immediately before and immediately after the daily workout
- Slow proteins should be consumed before bed
- Goal is for a minimum of 20 grams of leucine and 100 grams of BCAAs per day divided between 6 meals
- Protein should not exceed 40% of total calories

Fats:
- Approximately 35% of daily calories come from fat
- Saturated fat no more than 10% of daily fat calories
- Goal is near equal omega-6 to omega-3 fat intake
- Omega-3 fatty acid supplementation with a goal of 2–3 grams of DHA+EPA total per day from fish oil or flax
- Zero trans fats

Cheat Meal: Once a week, you may break from the diet and eat one meal containing whatever you like.

The Mesomorphic Diet Checklist

1. Estimate your body fat percentage and kilograms of body fat carried:

Use the method of your choice—skin calipers, hydrostatic weighing, bioelectrical impedance (BIA), et cetera, and calculate how many kilograms of body fat you are carrying:

Weight in kg x body fat % expressed as a decimal= kg of body fat

(ex: 100 kg individual with 15% body fat has 100 x 0.15 = 15 kg of body fat)

2. Estimate your maintenance calorie level:
As detailed previously, use either the Schofield Equation or Harris-Benedict Equation to estimate what your basal metabolic rate is and then adjust for your current activity level. If your goal is to maintain your current body fat and muscle mass, then this will be your daily caloric intake.

If your goal is to lose weight...

3. Estimate your maximal caloric deficit:

Your maximum allowable calorie deficit is seventy calories per kilogram of body fat per day. As an added safety margin, this number is increased by 25 percent to give you the initial number of calories you should subtract from your maintenance calorie level.

Kg of body fat x 70 x 0.75 = maximum caloric deficit

(ex: an individual with 15 kg of body fat could burn 15 x 70 = 1,050 calories of fat per day)

Subtract this deficit from your maintenance caloric level calculated above.

If your goal is to gain weight...

4. Add approximately five hundred calories to your maintenance calorie level and monitor your progress. If you aren't gaining enough weight, add an additional 250 calories every two weeks until you are gaining weight at the rate you are happy with. If you are gaining too much fat, then cut back your calories by 250 and reevaluate your results in two weeks.

5. Divide your calories roughly evenly over six meals.

"You can always tell an old soldier by the inside of his holsters and cartridge boxes. The young ones carry pistols and cartridges: the old ones, food."

-George Bernard Shaw

THE ECTOMORPHIC DIET

The Ectomorphic Diet is the eating plan designed for the true hard-gainer. Its goal is to provide the ideal environment for building as much muscle tissue as your particular genetic profile will allow. The training program described previously will create the stimulus your body needs to set its muscle-building machinery into motion, and this diet will provide, in abundance, the nutrients your body needs to build every last possible ounce of muscle tissue that it can.

The goals of athletes on the Ectomorphic Diet differ from those on the other diets described in this book. Therefore, this diet differs in several important ways as well. Ectomorphic dieters are those with one goal in mind: building as much muscle tissue as possible. Fat loss is not an issue or at best a secondary issue. Carbohydrates, because of their effect on insulin secretion, form the cornerstone of each meal along with high-quality protein and healthy fats. The source of these carbohydrates, while critical in the other diets, is of less importance on the Ectomorphic Diet. In fact, you will be using the ability of high-glycemic carbohydrates to spike insulin levels at key times to drive your body to build muscle tissue at an acceler-ated rate and maintain a near round-the-clock positive nitrogen balance. You will be able to eat a wide range of carbohydrates including fruits, breads, pastas, vegetables, and even the occasional candy bar if you like! This elevated carbohydrate intake will allow you to make the most of carbohydrate's protein-sparing ability. This means that, even though you will be consuming the same amount of protein as in the other diets, you will be using as much of it as possible purely for building and maintaining muscle tissue rather than having it diverted for use as energy. Fat intake will be the lowest of all the diets in this book but will still be an important part of your diet. You will still need to consume a large portion of your fat intake from healthy mono- and polyunsaturated sources while keeping your saturated fat intake relatively low.

This combination of high carbohydrate and moderate protein and fat intake in excess of mainte-nance requirements, with both their timing and composition adjusted to take advantage of certain key physiologic windows, provides the ultimate anabolic environment for muscle building. It goes with-out saying, therefore, that the Ectomorphic Diet is not a weight loss diet. In fact, the diet is designed specifically for those who are naturally quite thin and want to gain as much weight as possible in the form of lean muscle mass. However, for the non-steroid-using athlete, this will invariably mean the gain of some degree of fat tissue. This, in virtually all cases, is an unavoidable side effect of creating an environment conducive to round-the-clock muscle building. The optimal caloric surplus for building muscle tissue without spillover into adipose tissue varies between individuals. Therefore, to guarantee you are getting every possible building block your body needs, you will almost certainly have some degree of caloric spillover. Those excess calories, as you would expect, will be stored as body fat. For skinny ectomorphs, this is hardly a concern, however. They need to build as much muscle mass as possible as quickly as their genetics will allow. Their metabolisms generally make the burning of any accumulated body fat at a later date a relatively easy process. It is not uncommon for many individuals to cycle back and forth between the Ectomorphic and Endomorphic or even the Mesomorphic Diets. They may spend three to four months gaining as much muscle as possible and then transition to one of the other diets with a slight caloric deficit for a few months to remove any fat they may have accumulated before going back to the Ectomorphic Diet.

Starting the Ectomorphic Diet

The initial steps of the Ectomorphic Diet are similar to those described in the Endomorphic and Mesomorphic Diets. As part of your initial overall assessment of your current state of fitness, you should estimate your body fat percentage and the total amount of fat you are currently carrying. While body fat is not your primary concern on this diet, it is still important to get an idea of where you are starting in terms of your body fat percentage. You can then make adjustments in your total calories if you are gaining too much body fat as you progress.

The next step is the calculation of your maintenance caloric level. You can use either the Schofield Equation or Harris-Benedict Equation. Depending on whether or not you decide to include regular aerobics in your training program, your maintenance calories will vary slightly. Once you have determined the number of calories you require to maintain your current body weight, add one thousand calories to that total and divide your calories over seven total meals in twenty-four hours. To reiterate, the precise amount of caloric surplus required to provide all the necessary building blocks for building muscle tissue at the maximum possible rate without spillover into body fat will vary between individuals. There is no solid scientific data that allows a precise measurement like this to be made and applied to all individuals. However, as mentioned previously, one pound of muscle contains approximately 1800 calories if completely dehydrated. Since at least 70 percent of muscle tissue's weight is from water, that number drops to about 500 to 600 calories per pound of muscle. Now, this does *not* necessarily mean that all you need to do to gain a pound of muscle is consume an additional 500, 600, or even 1800 calories above maintenance requirements. There is a metabolic cost to building muscle tissue. The conversion of calories to muscle tissue is not an efficient process and does not occur in a 1:1 fashion. Therefore, the precise amount of caloric surplus needed to build a pound of muscle for a given individual is unknown. For the purposes of this diet, you will be starting with a 1000-calorie-per-day surplus divided over a total of seven meals. This, obviously, will give you a 7000-calorie surplus by the end of the week. Let's assume, for the sake of argument, that muscle tissue has 600 calories per pound but the conversion of surplus calories into muscle tissue is three to one, meaning that 1800 additional calories would need to be consumed to create one pound of muscle tissue. The remaining calories are used in various metabolic pathways along the way but are not directly transformed into muscle tissue. In this case, a 7000 weekly caloric surplus would provide enough calories for the building of approximately 3.9 pounds of muscle per week. The real confounder is your particular conversion ratio for surplus calories to muscle tissue. Is it three to one, five to one, or ten to one? Your guess is as good as mine. This is why the 1000-calorie surplus is used. Even for conservative estimates of this figure, it should be more than enough to provide the extra calories you need. For many, 1000 extra calories per day will be too much. For others, it may be just right. As with all the diets in The Program, you should evaluate your results every two weeks or so and make adjustments. If you feel like you are gaining too much fat, then eliminate 250 calories from your daily total. Do this every two weeks until you are at a level that works best for you. Similarly, if you aren't gaining enough weight on a 1000-calorie-per-day surplus (something that will likely only apply to a small number of dieters), add 250 or more calories and revaluate your results.

Finally, you will need to disperse those calories roughly evenly over seven meals in twenty-four hours using the following guidelines. Carbohydrates should make up roughly 60 percent of your total calories. For three of your meals—the post-workout meal, the late-night meal, and the early morning meal, these carbohydrates should consist of high-glycemic carbohydrates from the source of your choice. The easiest way to do this is by consuming a weight-gainer protein powder or meal replacement containing fifty to one hundred grams of maltodextrin, dextrose, or some other high-glycemic carbohydrate source, but if you prefer fruit juice or some other source, then feel free. It's crucial that all your meals contain protein, however. Do not consume any meal that does not contain both protein and carbohydrates. For your other meals, you should attempt to consume healthier, lower glycemic items like whole-wheat breads and pastas, fruits, vegetables, et cetera.

Now you are likely raising an eyebrow at the mention of not only consuming seven meals per day, but eating late at night and then waking up in the early morning to eat as well. I can't say I blame you. However, if these two windows of opportunity (one after 11:00 p.m. and the other three hours before breakfast) are available why not take advantage of them? I fully realize the inconvenience of having to do this. However, there are some ways to make it a bit easier. Before bed each night, set up a serving of a protein-containing, high-glycemic carbohydrate beverage at the bedside. You can then set your alarm to wake you up, roll over, down your meal, and then go right back to sleep.

Now, do you *have* to do this? No, you don't *have* to do anything, but doing this has two advantages. First, you spike insulin levels and put your body's protein synthesis into overdrive during a time when you would ordinarily be breaking down muscle tissue for fuel. You also spread out some of the calories you have to consume over seven meals instead of five or six. Eating a thousand calories over maintenance levels can be a lot of food for some people; many have difficulty keeping up and resort to force-feeding themselves throughout the day. If you drink some of those calories at night, then you don't have to eat quite so much food during the day. Many of you have lifestyle, family, or work commitments that will prevent you from getting up in the middle of the night to eat. In those cases, you will have to consume your calories during the day. I would advise, however, that you make every effort to at least consume a large dose of slow protein right before bed to help keep you in positive nitrogen balance for as long as possible and minimize the duration during which you are breaking down muscle tissue for fuel in the early morning.

Protein intake will be similar to that on the other diets. Shoot for two grams per kilogram of body-weight of high-quality protein. Every meal should contain protein. Breakfast and the pre- and post-work-out meals should contain at least some fast-acting proteins. The meal just before bed should contain an ample amount of "slow" protein like egg, casein, or soy. As with the other diets, you should aim for at least twenty grams of leucine and one hundred grams of branched chain amino acids per day, something that won't be difficult with the inclusion of a quality whey protein supplement. Your real food protein sources should be made up primarily of lean cuts of beef, chicken, and fish. These types of foods will provide you with the protein you need but also keep your total fat intake under control.

Fat intake will be moderate and make up around 20 to 25 percent of your total calories. Most of these calories should come from healthy monounsaturated and polyunsaturated sources like olive oil, nuts, flax, and fish, but some saturated fat intake is allowed and inevitable. Supplementation with fish oil capsules is, as always, recommended. No trans-fats should be consumed on any of the diets in The Program...ever.

"But wait...what about my cheat meal?" you may be asking. Sorry, my friend, no such thing. Well, sort of. While you don't have a specific scheduled cheat meal or cheat day, the nature of this diet does allow you quite a bit of leeway to include some items that would ordinarily be off-limits on the other eating plans. During your high-glycemic meals, you are allowed to consume some sugary snacks and treats as long as they help you fulfill your dietary requirements in terms of macronutrients and calories and don't prevent you from eating healthier food items. What you are not allowed do is fill up on junk food to the point where you exclude the healthy carbohydrates, fats, and protein that you should be eating. If you want to have a candy bar every now and then, that's fine as long as you factor it in to your daily requirements. If you stuff yourself with a box of Double Stuff Oreo cookies and are too full or nauseated to eat the fruits, veggies, and protein you are supposed to be eating, then that's not okay.

A Word on Aerobics

On the Endomorphic Diet, performing regular cardiovascular exercise is recommended to help speed your fat loss and maintain ketosis. Similarly, while on the Mesomorphic Diet some cardiovascular training is recommended to help you maintain a low body fat percentage and overall fitness. On the Ectomorphic Diet, however, cardiovascular exercise should be greatly reduced if not eliminated entirely. Performing additional aerobic exercise not only taxes your recovery ability (something that may already be somewhat limited for the natural ectomorph), but it potentially diverts calories away from the building of muscle tissue. If you feel like you must perform some aerobic exercise, then try to limit it to no more than thirty minutes per session two days a week.

A Sample Diet

To give you an idea of what a sample Ectomorphic Diet would look like, let's take the hypothetical case of a six-foot-tall, twenty-five-year-old male, weighing 150 pounds with an ectomorphic body, who is looking to pack on some quality muscle mass.

His first step in preparation for this diet is to measure his body fat percentage. Being an ectomorph, he is quite lean and discovers that via bioelectrical impedance that his body fat percentage is 10 percent. This means he is carrying about fifteen pounds of total body fat.

Next, he would calculate his basal metabolic rate (BMR). In this case, we will use the Harris-Benedict Equation:

BMR = 66 + (13.7 x weight in kg) + (5 x Height in cm) - (6.8 x age in years)

BMR = 66 + (13.7 x 68.2 kg) + (5 x 180 cm) - (6.8 x 25)

BMR= ~1730 calories per day

Next, he will multiply his BMR by his exercise-level correction factor. In his case, he will be performing The Program workout without performing regular aerobic training.

1730 x 1.4 = ~2422 calories per day to maintain his current body weight

Now, he will start his diet with an additional daily surplus of 1000 calories giving him a goal of 3422 calories consumed per day.

His calories are then divided up in the following manner:

Protein: (2g/kg) = ~136 grams per day (544 calories)

Carbohydrates: Roughly 60% of total = 513 grams (2052 calories)

Fats provide the remaining calories:

Fats: ~91 grams per day (819 calories)

To summarize, this is how his macronutrient breakdown would look:

Carbohydrate: 513 grams (2052 calories)
Protein: 136 grams (544 calories)
Fat: 91 grams (819 calories)

What follows is just one way this particular athlete could approximate the above requirements over the course of seven meals. This is by no means necessarily the best way; it serves only as an example of one way you can set up your diet. There are a near-infinite number of food combinations you can choose to create your own diet. As long as you are meeting the calorie and macronutrient requirements of the diet, you can include whatever foods you prefer most. As with the other diets, you should make several different daily diets and rotate them periodically, so you don't get tired of eating the same thing day in and day out. Having some variety will make sticking to your diet much easier.

Meal 1 (breakfast): One cup of oatmeal (may add sugar and/or butter for flavor)

One slice of whole-wheat toast with Benecol spread

One cup of 2% milk. Three whole eggs—scrambled.

Cantaloupe ½ medium size

693 calories

33 grams of fat

72 grams of carbohydrate

27 grams of protein

Meal 2: 8 oz of low-fat fruit yogurt + ½ cup of natural granola

447 calories

7.5 grams of fat

79 grams of carbohydrate

16 grams of protein

Meal 3: Spinach pasta with crème sauce + fruit salad

455 calories

15 grams of fat

75 grams of carbohydrate

5 grams of protein

Meal 4 (pre-workout): Meal-replacement shake plus 2 tablespoons of flaxseed oil

550 calories

30 grams of fat

50 grams of carbohydrate

20 grams of protein

Meal 5 (post-workout): Weight-gainer protein shake (1 cup)

518 calories

2 grams of fat

100 grams of carbohydrate

25 grams of protein

Meal 6 (late-night dinner): Grilled vegetable and rice burrito with 1 tablespoon sour cream + slow protein shake (egg, soy, or casein)

419 calories

7 grams of fat

64 grams of carbohydrate

25 grams of protein

Meal 7 (early morning meal): (3 hours before meal #1) Weight-gainer protein shake (1 cup)

    518 calories

    2 grams of fat

    100 grams of carbohydrate

    25 grams of protein

Recommended Supplements

There are no supplements that are mandatory for you to take while on the Ectomorphic Diet. However, you may wish to include the following items to ensure you are consuming a complete range of nutrients and to make meeting your dietary requirements easier.

Multi-vitamin and mineral supplements are generally recommended to ensure you are consuming adequate levels of antioxidants and minerals. For those of you without a great deal of time or a personal chef, finding a palatable meal-replacement powder or bar can make meeting your daily protein and calorie needs much easier while you are on the go.

In particular, a high-calorie weight-gainer powder can be a big help, especially for your early-morning meal. Look for one with a fairly high carbohydrate content combined with a quality whey protein. An egg- or casein-based protein powder can also be useful as a quick source of "slow" protein before bed. Creatine monohydrate has been shown to be beneficial in terms of improving muscle strength and is highly recommended on this particular diet. The high insulin levels you will experience on the Ectomorphic Diet will allow you to drive creatine into your muscle cells, thereby maximizing its benefit. A fish oil supplement is also strongly recommended unless you consume fish as daily part of your diet. I personally like adding flaxseed oil to my protein shakes for added polyunsaturated fat calories and for a little flavoring. You may have noticed in the sample diet that I include the margarine substitute Benecol in place of butter as a toast spread. Benecol, Take Control, and other similar products are spreads made with plant sterols that have been shown to lower cholesterol. They are rich in polyunsaturated fats primarily from rapeseed and therefore make an excellent addition to all Program diets. Please thoroughly review the chapter on supplements before including these or any other products into your diet.

Common Pitfalls

The Ectomorphic Diet is a fairly straightforward dietary regimen. The cornerstone of the diet is built on regular consumption of both complex and simple carbohydrates as well as quality protein. Therefore, you shouldn't have too much difficulty in terms of cravings for sugars or desserts because you will be able to incorporate them (to a limited extent) into your diet. However, there are still a few ways you can screw things up. The Ectomorphic Diet requires you to consume a lot of calories. There is just no way around that. Some people have difficulty finding the time to eat so many calories and often find that they are force-feeding themselves. As a result, they may skip meals or eat fewer calories than they need. This can be mitigated to some extent by consuming higher-calorie meal-replacement shakes or weight-gainers because they are somewhat less filling than whole foods, but it can still be difficult. It is also difficult for some to eat late at night or very early in the morning when the natural insulin spikes we discussed earlier occur. While not mandatory, consuming some of your daily calories during this time can speed your weight gain and make your daytime eating schedule a little easier.

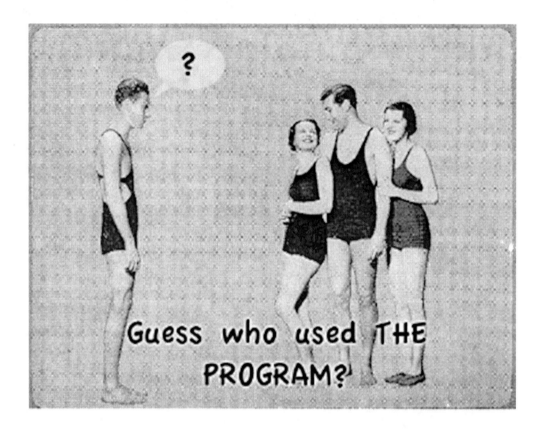

The Ectomorphic Diet in a Nutshell

Total Calories: Maintenance level + 1000 calories per day over 7 meals.

Carbohydrates:
- Approximately 60% of your total calories. Consume at least 50–100 grams of high-glycemic carbohydrate during three critical windows:
  1. After 11:00 p.m.
  2. Approximately 3 hours before breakfast
  3. Immediately after the day's workout
- The remainder of the day's carbohydrate should be a mixture of moderate- and low-glycemic carbohydrates from fruits, vegetables, and grains.

Protein:
- Total protein intake should be approximately 2.0 grams per kilogram of body weight divided roughly equally between 6 daily meals and a seventh early morning meal
- Approximately 20% or less of total calories will come from protein
- Fast proteins should be consumed immediately before and immediately after the daily workout and with the early morning meal
- Slow proteins (egg, soy, or casein) should be consumed before bedtime
- Goal is for a minimum of 20 grams of leucine and 100 grams of BCAAs per day divided between 7 meals

Fats:
- Remainder of total calories will come from fat, resulting in approximately 25% of daily calories from fat
- Limit saturated fat to no more than 10% of daily fat calories
- Goal is near equal omega-6 to omega-3 fat intake
- Omega-3 fatty acid supplementation with a goal of 2–3 grams of DHA+EPA total per day from fish oil or flax
- Zero trans fats

Cheat Meal: Sorry, no such thing!

The Ectomorphic Diet Checklist

1. **Estimate your body fat percentage and kilograms of body fat carried:**
Use the method of your choice—skin callipers, hydrostatic weighing, bioelectrical impedance (BIA), et cetera, and calculate how many kilograms of body fat you are carrying:

Weight in kg x body fat % expressed as a decimal= kg of body fat

(ex: 100 kg individual with 15% body fat has 100 x 0.15 = 15 kg of body fat)

2. **Estimate your maintenance calorie level:**

As detailed previously, use either the Schofield Equation or Harris-Benedict Equation to estimate what your basal metabolic rate is and then adjust for your current activity level.

3. **Add approximately 1000 calories to your maintenance calorie level, and monitor your progress.**
If you aren't gaining enough weight, add an additional 250 calories every two weeks until you are gaining weight at the rate you are happy with. If you are gaining too much fat, then cut back your calories by 250 and re-evaluate your results in two weeks.

4. **Divide your calories roughly evenly over seven meals.**

Out of life's school of war: What does not destroy me, makes me stronger.

—Friedrich Nietzsche

TRAINING

Weight training and cardiovascular training are integral parts of achieving your goal of a leaner, more muscular body. The dietary guidelines in The Program will help you lose fat and build lean muscle mass. However, diet alone is insufficient. You must provide the body with a stimulus to build new muscle tissue. That stimulus comes in the form of resistance training with weights. Building lean muscle mass with weight training not only will enhance your appearance and strength, but will allow you to burn more body fat. Muscle tissue is highly active metabolically. The greater your muscle mass, the greater your resting basal metabolic rate and the more calories you will burn—even when you are not exercising.

The weight-training regimen outlined in The Program has several goals. The first and foremost are to build lean muscle mass and increase strength. These two aspects of weight training go hand in hand but are often misunderstood. As you progress in your workouts, you will be primarily training for strength. This means you will be continually trying to lift heavier weights and/or perform more repetitions than you did previously. Muscle magazines, other bodybuilding or power-lifting literature, and even some trainers make a distinction between training for strength and training for muscle size. The truth is that they are one and the same. The concept of strength itself has led to some of this confusion. People often think of strength in terms of the maximum weight an individual can lift for a single repetition. This is best described by the term "absolute strength." A power lifter is an example of an athlete who trains primarily for this type of strength. However, there is also the ability to generate strength over longer periods of time and over multiple repetitions. Let's look at two athletes of identical bodyweight and compare their bench press weights to show this relationship more clearly.

Athlete A is able to perform a maximum bench press of 300 pounds. Athlete B is able to perform a maximum bench press of 275 pounds. Most individuals would say that clearly Athlete A is the stronger bench presser. Next, each athlete is told to bench press 200 pounds as many times as possible. Athlete A is able to perform eight repetitions. Athlete B is able to perform ten repetitions.

In simple mathematical terms, Athlete A lifted (8 x 200 =) 1600 pounds during his set, and Athlete B lifted (10 x 200=) 2000 pounds during his. Now, who is the stronger athlete? It's not quite so cut-and-dry anymore. I bring up this point not to confuse you but to help you understand that there is more than one way to look at the concept of strength.

Let's explore some of the factors that play important roles in strength. Why is it that the two athletes above, despite having identical body weights, have such different abilities? To understand this, we must understand how your brain controls your muscles and how your muscles work.

The basic unit of movement is referred to as the motor unit. A motor unit is a nerve cell located in the brain and all the individual muscle fibers that it controls. When that nerve cell fires a signal, all the muscle fibers it controls contract with maximum force. It is an all-or-none phenomenon. Some motor units consist of a nerve and thousands of muscle fibers. These are often found in the larger muscles of the body—the quadriceps, the pectorals, gluteals, et cetera. These muscles need to generate powerful contractions to help us jump, run, push, and so on. Other motor units consist of a nerve and only a few muscle fibers. These motor units help control very fine and precise movements. They can be found controlling the muscles of the hands, eyes, and fingers for example.

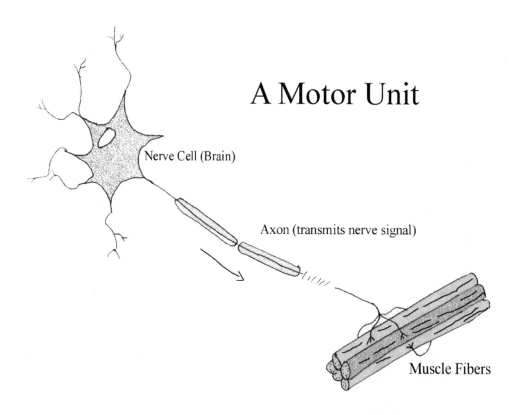

A Motor Unit

Nerve Cell (Brain)

Axon (transmits nerve signal)

Muscle Fibers

One of the primary determinants of one's ability to generate muscular strength, both for single and multiple repetitions is the ability to recruit motor units. The more motor units your brain can recruit to perform, for example, a squat, the greater force you will be able to generate and the more weight you can lift. This is the primary mechanism involved in the early strength gains you will experience using The Program. You will notice that in the first few weeks of training you will make astounding increases in your weights and repetitions, especially if you are new to weight training. Much of this gain is not due to increased muscle mass (though some certainly is). It is a direct result of your central nervous system becoming more efficient and learning to bring more motor units to bear to help you perform your lifts. After several weeks, your brain will have become very efficient at recruiting motor units and further strength gains come largely from increases in muscle size.

The next critical factor in determining an individual's strength is muscle fiber type. There are various types of muscle fibers, each with its own strengths and weaknesses. This is a 100 percent genetically mediated trait. The proportions of the different muscle fiber types in your body are inherited from your parents, and, despite some recent research showing that it may be possible for fibers to change from one type to another under laboratory conditions, for all practical purposes, you are stuck with what your parents gave you.

Humans have varying proportions of three different muscle fiber types. Type I (slow twitch) fibers are relatively small and do not generate a great deal of force but have tremendous endurance. They have large amounts of stored triglycerides for sustained energy production but relatively low levels of glycogen and creatine phosphate, which are used for quick, explosive movements. These fibers are used primarily for aerobic activities, walking, maintaining posture, et cetera. Marathon runners and distance swimmers are examples of athletes with high percentages of type I fibers. These athletes have tremendous endurance but have difficulty developing large, powerful muscles.

Fast-twitch fibers (type II) have the ability to generate much faster, higher force contractions than slow twitch fibers. These fibers tend to be much thicker and store larger amounts of glycogen and creatine phosphate. As a result, they are able to generate very strong contractions but cannot sustain them for long periods of time. Fast-twitch fibers come in two varieties—fast twitch A and fast twitch B. The A fibers hold the middle ground between slow twitch fibers and the B-type fast-twitch fibers. They are able to generate a fair amount of force and maintain it for some time. They store large amounts of glycogen, creatine, and a fair amount of triglycerides. As a result, they are primarily involved in prolonged anaerobic activities like the four-hundred-meter dash. They have a fairly good ability to hypertrophy in response to weight training. Type B fast-twitch fibers are the polar opposite of slow-twitch fibers. They are very large and can generate a tremendous amount of force very quickly. They store very large amounts of glycogen and creatine but very little triglyceride. The high power output of these fibers comes at a cost, however. They fatigue very quickly and are unable to maintain their great strength for very long. These fibers are used primarily for short bursts of speed and strength, like a one-hundred-meter dash, dunking a basketball, and near maximal weightlifting.

The only certain way to determine what percentages of these fiber types you possess is to perform a muscle biopsy and examine the tissue under the microscope. Since most people are not that eager to undergo this procedure, there are some indirect methods that can be utilized to estimate your personal fiber composition. One method that is used commonly is as follows:

Estimating Muscle Fiber Type

1. Determine your 1 rep maximum for a given lift.

2. Perform as many reps as possible with %80 of that weight

<7 reps: More than %50 fast twitch fibers

7-12 reps: Equal parts fast and slow twitch fibers
>12 reps: Slow twitch fibers predominate

For practical purposes, the proportion of your muscle fiber types does not matter when training using The Program. The type of training you will be performing will not change. Despite the differing characteristics of each fiber type, they all respond to high-intensity weight training. Those of you with high percentages of fast-twitch fibers will respond more quickly in terms of size and strength gains, but no matter what the makeup of your muscles, you can still expect steady progress.

Another factor affecting muscle strength is cross-sectional diameter. Essentially, the larger a muscle fiber—the more sarcomeres it contains—the greater force it will be able to generate during a contraction. Therefore, a muscle fiber cannot get larger (hypertrophy) without also getting stronger. The goal of the workouts in The Program is ultimately to give you larger muscles. Therefore, it follows logically that the focus of one's training should be on developing strength. This is precisely what you will be doing week to week on The Program.

Finally, there are anatomic considerations that must be taken into account when looking at strength. Factors such as limb length play important roles. Obviously a shorter, more compact individual has to move a given weight a shorter distance to complete a repetition when compared to a much taller individual. This may explain in part why champion power lifters tend to have shorter limbs and be fairly compact when compared to NBA athletes for example. Variation in tendon lengths and insertions also play important mechanical roles in determining one's strength. As with muscle-fiber type, these anatomic factors are largely hereditary. You won't be able to change them through training.

As mentioned earlier, the focus of the weight training on The Program will be on increasing one's strength. The focus will not be on absolute strength but rather strength over multiple repetitions. In the first few weeks of training, your central nervous system will adapt to the new exercises you are performing and your strength will increase quickly. Beyond that point, the bulk of your strength increases will come from muscle hypertrophy. Therefore, your training must focus on stimulating the maximum number of fibers possible (motor units) and then providing the necessary recovery time to allow those fibers not only to recover but also to grow beyond their previous size.

Repetitions

The goal of each set is to stimulate the maximum number of muscle fibers possible. When performing a set of a given number of repetitions, it is important to realize that only a fraction of the available muscle fibers are being used to perform each repetition. You start the set with all your muscle fibers rested and ready to contract. As you perform the first repetition, your brain recruits the appropriate number of motor units needed to lift the weight. As you go on and perform a second and third repetition, those initial motor units fatigue and fresh ones are recruited to take their place. This allows you to continue your set. Generally, the smaller slow-twitch fibers are used first. If the intensity of the exercise remains relatively low, then these fibers may be all that is needed. If the intensity is high, the weaker, slow-twitch fibers will be insufficient and the larger type II fast-twitch fibers will be used. The A-type fast twitch fibers are recruited first followed by the B-type.

Electromyogram (EMG) studies have shown that lifting very heavy weights—so heavy that one can only perform less than five repetitions—relies heavily on the large fast-twitch fibers and very little on the smaller, slower-twitch fibers. The smaller fibers simply cannot generate enough force to move such heavy weight. The athlete reaches momentary muscular failure as soon as he has exhausted his larger fibers. The training programs of most power lifters emphasize the engagement of fast-twitch fibers, because they have the greatest influence on single-repetition strength. These athletes will have very large fast-twitch fibers, but their slow-twitch fibers may actually atrophy somewhat. Similarly, athletes who perform endurance exercise or light-weight, high-repetition weight lifting will selectively hypertrophy their slow twitch fibers while their fast twitch fibers atrophy.

The training system in The Program differs somewhat. Your goal will be not only to exhaust both the large fast-twitch fibers but also the slow-twitch fibers. This raises the question of optimal rep range. You should perform sets with heavy enough weight to fully fatigue the large fast-twitch fibers but light enough that the slow-twitch fibers are also stimulated. The goal of the training in The Program is overall muscle hypertrophy. Research has shown that the optimal repetition range for achieving this goal is somewhere between eight and twelve.[214] The advantage of this range is that you can still use very heavy weights while keeping the forces placed on your joints, ligaments, and tendons relatively low, thus reducing your risk of injury.

---

214 Fleck SJ and Kraemer WJ (1996) Periodization Breakthrough! Advanced Research Press, New York.

When you begin, you will pick weights that you estimate you can perform eight to twelve repetitions with to failure. Don't worry if you are initially way off and perform only five or six reps or over fifteen. Make a note of it in your workout log, and next time, you will be able to adjust the weights accordingly. As you grow stronger and can perform greater than twelve reps with a given weight, add more weight to bring the reps back down to between eight and twelve.

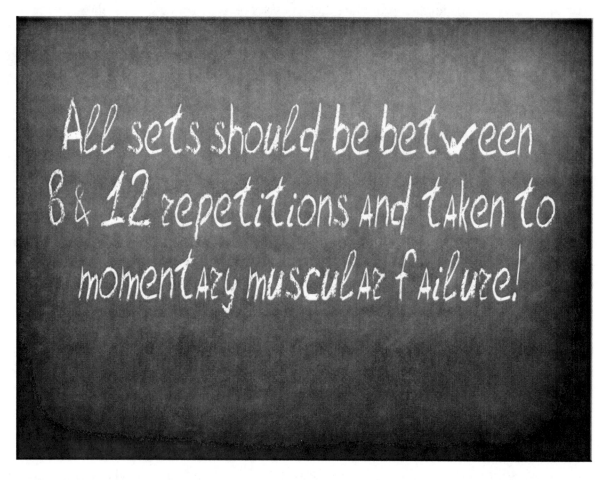

Each rep should be performed in a controlled and systematic manner. Don't fall into the trap that many athletes do and assume that if you move the weight more quickly it somehow makes the set more effective. Explosive lifting has a role in sports like Olympic weight lifting and a few other sports-specific training styles, but the high injury potential and lower return in terms of hypertrophy make it inadvisable for most trainees. Lift the weight in a slow, deliberate, and controlled manner and lower it in the same fashion. There isn't convincing literature proving definitively exactly how long you should spend lifting and lowering a weight for optimal results. Therefore, I advise a speed where you feel comfortable that you aren't cheating the weight up or putting yourself at higher risk for injury. For most individuals, this is about two to four seconds for both the lifting and lowering portions.

Intensity

The concept of intensity is of central importance in weight training. There are many definitions in use. The one I prefer was put forward by Mike Mentzer years ago and is defined as "the percentage of momentary muscular effort exerted during a set." The layman's translation would be "how hard you are working during your set." As you can imagine, trying to quantify intensity is quite difficult. Mr. Mentzer went on to teach that in fact, the only intensity levels you can be certain that you are achieving during a set are zero intensity (before you pick up the weight) and 100 percent intensity (when you reach your all-out failure point and another repetition is impossible). Some authors have attempted to quantify intensity in terms of an athlete's one-repetition max in a given lift, such as the squat. This makes it a little easier to quantify intensity levels between zero and one hundred. Using this definition, working at 50 percent intensity would involve a weight that is half of your one-repetition maximum. This definition is an integral part of periodized training programs. I prefer Mr. Mentzer's definition because it is far more practical in the day-to-day performance of your workouts. Using The Program requires that you give it your all and achieve 100 percent intensity with each set.

The concept of intensity is central to the understanding of athletic performance. Human physiology dictates that very intense exercise, such as sprinting, can only be performed for a short time. It is far too taxing to be maintained for any long period. On the other hand, lower-intensity activities, like jogging, can, in some individuals, be continued for hours and hours. This is because intensity determines which of the two primary energy systems the body uses to perform a given task—aerobic or anaerobic.

Anaerobic metabolism is defined by its ability to be performed without oxygen. Very short, ultra-high-intensity activities, such as a one-hundred-meter sprint or a maximum-weight squat or bench press rely primarily on the anaerobic system. The anaerobic system uses available stores of creatine phosphate and glucose to rapidly provide the working muscles with ATP for energy. These stores are very limited, however, and rapidly depleted by high-intensity activity. As we already learned, the fast-twitch, glycolytic muscle fibers use this energy system almost exclusively. Weight training of the type specified in The Program uses this energy system.

Lower-intensity activities can be maintained for much longer periods of time because they largely rely on the aerobic system. Aerobic metabolism, as you may have guessed, uses oxygen to generate the ATP from glucose and fats. This system is slower but provides a steady fuel supply to working muscles. Slow-twitch muscle fibers have much greater capacity for aerobic metabolism than their fast-twitch neighbours. Marathon runners and other long-distance endurance athletes rely heavily on the aerobic system for performance. It should be noted that as the intensity level gradually increases, there is a point where the working muscles will switch to anaerobic metabolism. A good example of this is the ten-thousand-meter runner who, in the final one hundred meters of his or her race, attempts an all-out sprint to the finish. He or she has been using primarily aerobic metabolism throughout the race but to generate the last burst of speed needed to win, increases the intensity of his or her running and kicks in the anaerobic system for that speed.

The concept of exercise intensity is critically important when your goal is larger, stronger muscles. Intensity of exercise is the key stimulus to muscle hypertrophy. Muscle fibers of all types (but especially fast twitch) will increase in size, and therefore strength, only if they are subjected to a sufficiently intense stimulus. In this case, multiple intense bouts of resistance exercise are needed. By necessity, these high-intensity activities can only be maintained for a short period of time but are the key factor in stimulating muscle growth. Longer bouts of lower-intensity exercise may stimulate very small amounts of muscle hypertrophy, but nowhere near the degree that high-intensity exercise will. A perfect real-world example can be found in track and field athletes. One-hundred and two-hundred-meter sprinters tend to have very large, well-developed thighs, glutes, and hamstrings. Their training is centered on performing very high-intensity, short-duration sprints. It is this stimulus that has developed their physiques. On the other extreme are ten-thousand-meter runners. These athletes tend to have very thin, light muscular development. Their training focuses on long bouts of much lower intensity running. They have tremendously developed cardiovascular systems but not much in the way of muscle strength or size when compared to their sprinter teammates. The important lesson here is that within the constraints of your genetic makeup, form follows function. This means that if you train like a sprinter, your body will begin to take the shape of a sprinter's. If you train like a ten-thousand-meter runner, your body will change to fit those needs as well. Since one of the goals of The Program is building larger, shapely muscles, you must give your body a reason to move in that direction. This means that all of your muscles must be exposed to very high intensity, short-duration weight training. Every set you perform after your warm-up must be carried to muscular failure. For those unfamiliar with this concept, it simply means that you must continue performing repetitions until you can no longer complete a full-range repetition in good form. This is critically important. Because you will only be performing one to two sets per body part, you must make those sets count. You must stimulate as many muscle fibers as possible. If you do not—if you stop short of failure—you will not be providing your muscles with the necessary stimulus for growth, and in the end, you will be disappointed with your results. For example, if you could perform a set of bench presses with three hundred pounds for ten repetitions to failure, but stopped at only six repetitions, you would leave a significant percentage of your muscle fibers unused and without a reason to grow. You would stimulate some growth, but you can be certain that any progress you made would cease very quickly and you would never progress beyond that point. Just "going through the motions" or stopping your set just because it's getting a little uncomfortable is not an option on The Program. You must train to failure to get maximal results.

Rest

The good news about high-intensity training is that because it is so taxing, it can only be performed for a very limited time before your muscles are depleted of the necessary biochemical factors needed for exercise. In fact, there is a direct inverse relationship between the intensity of your training and its duration. The harder you train, the shorter your training session and the longer the recovery period between workouts. I say this is good news because, in addition to helping you achieve the body you have always wanted, training this way will save you tremendous amounts of time. You will never need to spend hours in the gym, training day after day, with little or nothing to show for it. In fact, once you have learned the exercises and chosen the appropriate weights for each, you will rarely need to spend more than thirty minutes performing your workouts. This will free up lots of time for you to pursue hobbies, spend time with your family and friends, read, study, and enjoy the good things in life that many "gym rats" are missing out on. Not only will you have the time to enjoy these things; you will be developing the body you have always wanted. It doesn't get any better than that!

The starting phase of The Program is a three-workout system. If you are in your late teens or twenties, this could take the form of a Monday-Wednesday-Friday system with weekends off, but you may alter your schedule to suit your needs. The only stipulation is that you give yourself at least one day of full rest between workouts. For older individuals, it is recommended that you start with two full rest days between weight-training sessions. You may perform cardio sessions on days you are not weight training if you wish. On weight-training days, try to perform your cardio sessions first thing in the morning or immediately after your weight-training workout. Performing it immediately before lifting will tire your muscles somewhat, and you won't be able to generate as much intensity for your workout. Keep in mind that as you progress and grow stronger, the stresses you place on your muscles will also increase and you will need to insert additional rest days to avoid overtraining. On your off days, try your best to relax and not perform any intense exercise. These days are critically important for your body to replenish your muscles and rebuild them after your workouts. They are also when much of your new muscle mass will be developing. Follow your diet carefully and make sure you provide your body with lots of high-quality protein foods. This will keep your progress steady and help you avoid overtraining.

Over-training

Over-training is perhaps the most common mistake weight-training athletes make. They assume their lack of progress in their training is due to inadequate volume of exercise. So, without much thought, they add more sets to their training and more days per week in the gym. You can't really blame them. In our society, we are rarely taught that you can have "too much of a good thing." We instead hear phrases like "Give more, and you will get more"; "Work harder and longer, and you will make more money"; "Study more, and you will get better grades"; et cetera. Some of these things are true when looked at within their own context. With regard to high-intensity weight training, however, beyond a very precise limit, you can definitely have too much of a good thing.

High-intensity weight training, where each set is taken to the point of muscular failure, is extremely taxing to the physiology. If you were able to examine individual muscle fibers using an electron microscope, you would find that after intense exercise, many of the fibers are torn, shredded, and in disarray. After such a workout, the first thing that happens is the body attempts to replenish muscle glycogen, creatine, and a myriad of other cofactors that were depleted in order perform your workout. At the same time, the repair process begins. It is only after the muscles' energy stores are replaced and the damage from the workout repaired that the final phase of growth and adaptation can occur. It is obvious what would happen if you performed another workout before the growth and adaptation phase had time to complete — you would fail to build new muscle mass and you would be in a continuous state of "catching up" from your last workout. You must provide an adequate rest period between your workouts, or you will be continually frustrated.

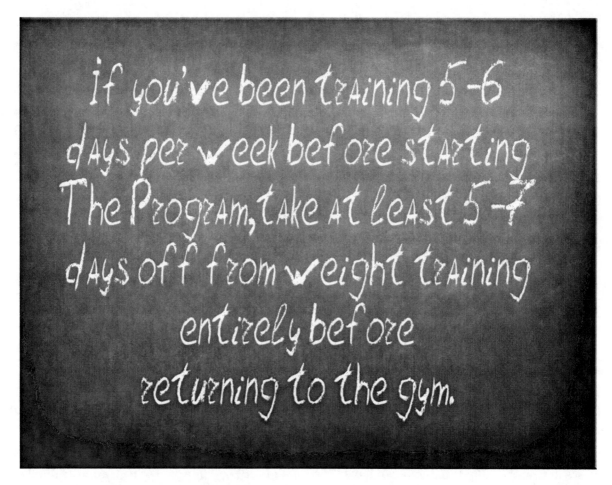

If you've been training 5-6 days per week before starting The Program, take at least 5-7 days off from weight training entirely before returning to the gym.

How long a rest period should you have between workouts? As with many things, the answer to that question is: "It depends." However, it is longer than many athletes realize. The ability to recover and adapt to short bursts of high-intensity exercise varies among individuals. Genetically gifted athletes and younger athletes will obviously recover much more quickly than older and less-gifted athletes. Adequate nutrition and the proper timing of your pre- and post-workout protein also make a difference in recovery time as well. Studies looking at recovery from high-intensity exercise have shown varying results depending on the particular protocols used. What appears clear is that the more intense the exercise stimulus, the longer muscle recovery and adaption take. Exercise routines that emphasize heavy eccentric movements in particular cause the greatest amount of muscle damage and require longer rest periods for adequate recovery to take place. Following intense resistance exercise with eccentric loads, resting metabolic rate and evidence of muscle damage manifested by elevated levels of creatinine kinase in the blood remain high for over forty-eight hours.[215] The inflammatory changes in muscle after high-intensity exercise can last over a week.[216] For most healthy athletes in their twenties starting their training regimen, forty-eight hours of recovery time between workouts will be an adequate amount of time to recover and build new muscle tissue in the body parts just exercised. If you are in your thirties or older, you may need to give yourself two to four full days of rest between workouts to ensure adequate recovery. Remember, you need enough time not only to repair the tissue damage resulting from your workout but also to build new muscle tissue

215   Dolezal, BA, et al. (2000). Muscle damage and resting metabolic rate after acute exercise with an eccentric overload. Medicine and Science in Sports and Exercise, 32, 1202–1207.

216   Friden J, Sjostrom M; Ekblom B. Myofibrillar damage following intense eccentric exercise in man. Int J Sports Med. 1983; 4(3):170–6.

as well. I can recall in my early twenties when I could squat to failure with over five hundred pounds on Monday, go to an intense three-hour rugby practice Tuesday, perform deadlifts to failure with over five hundred pounds on Wednesday, go to rugby practice again on Thursday, perform a heavy chest and arm workout on Friday, and then play in a rugby game Saturday with no difficulty at all. I was a little sore between workouts, but I was still making steady progress in all my lifts. If I tried to perform that sort of training regimen now, I would end up bedridden for a week. Now I may go fourteen days or more between heavy squat workouts depending on my other activities to ensure full recovery. As I approach forty years old, my workout regimen averages three days of recovery between workouts. I know other trainees my age who are less gifted in terms of recovery ability who only train once every five or six days and continue to make good progress. Regardless of your age, you will need to give yourself enough recovery time between workouts if you want to make optimal progress.

For athletes accustomed to training every day, cutting back to an every-other-day or less frequent training regimen can be difficult. Many trainees are fooled by the muscle magazines into following the steroid-fuelled, completely non-scientific, workout routines endorsed by professional bodybuilders. As a result, the very thought of performing only two to three workouts total per week with each body part being exercised no more than once a week can seem preposterous. However, after just a few Program workouts, you will see that the less frequent training regimen presented here not only won't result in all your hard-earned muscle atrophying away but will cause you to put on more muscle and become stronger than you ever have on the high-volume workouts you see in bodybuilding magazines. There is ample evidence in the sports medicine literature demonstrating that extended periods of active rest (light cardiovascular exercise, stretching, et cetera) between workouts do not result in loss of strength or muscle tissue. Even after fourteen days of rest, weight-training athletes do not manifest a loss of strength in standard power exercises like squats and bench press.[217] Anecdotally, I have frequently taken layoffs of a week or more due to military deployments and travel and invariably come back just as strong if not stronger than when I left. As you progress in your weight training, you will find the optimal recovery time for your particular physiology. As you progress over the years and become extremely strong with this type of training, you will find that your training frequency will decline by necessity. Don't be surprised if eventually you are training only once every fourth or fifth day and still making excellent progress.

If you are currently on a four-to-six-day-per-week training regimen and are about to start The Program, I'd recommend taking five to seven days off from weight training entirely. During this time period, you can perform cardiovascular training, sports, or body weight exercises like push-ups and sit-ups if you like, but do not engage in any weight training. This layoff will give your body time to recover from the chronic overtraining you have been experiencing on your previous training regimen. It will also help heal up any minor training injuries you may have.

---

217   Hortobagyi, T, et al. The effects of detraining on power athletes. Med Sci Sports Exerc., Vol 25, No. 8, pp. 929–935, 1993.

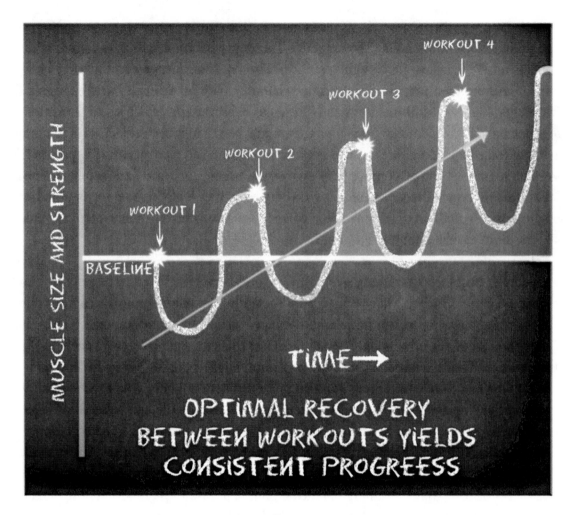

Sets

There is also considerable confusion and controversy among athletes about how many sets should be performed per body part. Indeed, the issue is still debated even among exercise scientists. Most athletes perform some arbitrary number, usually three to five per exercise, based on "feeling," without ever taking the time to examine if that really is the optimal way to train their muscles. Most muscle magazines advise somewhere between five and twenty sets per body part. The important thing to remember is that many if not all these recommendations have little to no scientific evidence to back them up. Most muscle magazines simply copy the routines of various professional bodybuilders and then present them as gospel. The truth is that unless you are on loads of steroids, following the same program as one of these "champs" will lead to certain failure. Lacking the steroid-enhanced recovery ability they possess, you would quickly overtrain. The massive steroid doses professional bodybuilders ingest makes just about any training program effective. As a health-conscious, natural athlete you have to be smarter and much more precise in your training.

The lifting program presented in The Program is not some arbitrary fabrication. It is based on solid scientific research and "real-world" experience in the gym. Its goal is to provide you with the most productive and simultaneously time-saving system possible. While using The Program, you will never perform more than two sets per body part. In the vast majority of cases, one will be all that is needed. It is this idea, which such low volume of exercise is required to stimulate optimal strength and size, which is the most difficult for most trainees to grasp. They have been conditioned to believe that they must spend hours in the gym, performing set after set, to make any progress. Nothing could be further from the truth. Remember, your goal is to enter the gym and perform exactly what you need to in order to stimulate your muscles to grow and then get out of there and let the recovery and growth processes begin. Why waste your time performing more sets than are required? I'm sure you can find better things to do with your time.

For those of you who are having difficulty believing that only one set of an exercise is required, let me review two important scientific studies that clearly demonstrate this point. The first study randomly assigned healthy, untrained men and women to three groups. Group 1 performed one set to failure of leg extensions and leg curls. Group 2 performed three sets of the same exercises, and Group 3 was a control group that performed no exercise.[218] They performed these exercises three times a week for fourteen weeks and did no other exercise. All workout sessions were supervised to ensure that each group was conforming to the test protocol. At the end of the study, there was no statistical difference between Group 1 and 2 in terms of strength gain and muscle size. The only important difference is that Group 2's workouts took at least three times longer to perform. This study looked at individuals with no weight-training experience. Another study looked at individuals with an average of 6.2 years of training experience.[219] They were randomly assigned to either a one-set or three-set group. They performed nine exercises in a circuit three times per week to volitional fatigue. Again, all training sessions were monitored closely, and when the participants could perform greater than twelve repetitions, they were required to increase their weights by 5 to 10 percent. After thirteen weeks, there was no difference in the two groups in terms of strength gained and increase in lean body mass. Again, the only difference was that the three-set group spent at least 300 percent more time in the gym to achieve the same results.

These two studies are just two examples of the validity of one-set training. There are over fifty studies showing similar results.[220] Not all of these studies are perfect (there is really no such thing as a perfect study), but they demonstrate that it is not necessary to spend your time performing set after set to get great results in the gym. One set is sufficient for our purposes. It's important to note that there are no studies I am aware of to date that clearly demonstrate that only one set is superior to three sets in terms of muscle hypertrophy. However, when considering the amount of time you will save in the gym, the superiority of one-set training becomes evident. In fairness to the proponents of multi-set training, there are a few isolated studies suggesting higher-volume, periodized programs may be superior to single-set training in certain circumstances, such as with elite athletes. However, the vast majority of research in this area shows no difference between the two methods. So why spend more time in the gym than you need to? Get in the gym, work hard, and then get out and enjoy the rest of your day.

For many of you, making the transition to the low-volume training in The Program will be mentally difficult. This training philosophy runs counter to everything the general public and many so-called experts

---

218   Starkey DB, Pollock ML, Ishida Y, Welsch MA, Brechue WF, Graves JE and Feigenbaum MS (1996) Effect of resistance training volume on strength and muscle thickness. Medicine and Science in Sports and Exercise 28:1311–1320.
219   Hass CJ, Garzarella L, Dehoyos D and Pollock ML (2000) Single vs multiple sets in long term recreational weightlifters. Medicine and Science in Sports and Exercise 32: 235–242.
220   Carpinelli R N and Otto R M (1998) Strength training: Single versus multiple sets. Sports Medicine 26:73–84.

espouse regarding weight training. I have encountered many trainees who, despite showing them clear scientific evidence, laid out in a simple and straightforward manner, simply cannot make the transition. They adhere dogmatically to the "more sets are better" philosophy. They continue to believe that one set just can't be enough. Unfortunately, these are often the same individuals who make little to no progress in the gym despite training up to six days a week. When you begin The Program, I encourage you to throw away your preconceived notions about weight training. Approach this endeavor with the same rigorous skepticism and enthusiasm that scientists and engineers display when tackling projects in their fields. As in any scientific endeavor, there is no room for arbitrary, dogmatic or imprecise action. Don't do things a certain way simply because that's the way everyone else is doing them. Remember, your goal in the gym is to do the precise amount of exercise needed to maximally stimulate your muscles to get stronger and bigger and not a single set more. As mentioned above, the vast preponderance of scientific evidence shows that a single set will achieve this goal.

Proponents of higher-volume workouts state that more than one set is required, but they are often vague when pressured to give an exact number. The usual answer is three to five. This isn't very precise. Is it three, four, or five? Or does it depend? If so, what does it depend on—the body part? The day of the week? The position of the planets? You will hear different answers from many people. Yet not a single one of them will be able to show you a well-designed scientific study to support their viewpoint. Their assertions are completely arbitrary and have been passed on and taken for gospel since bodybuilding became popularized in the 1950s. Fortunately, beginning in the 1970s with men like Arthur Jones and Mike Mentzer, the high-volume, multi-set approach began to be challenged. Since that time, more and more evidence in favor of high-intensity, single-set training has been generated in sports science labs around the country, and this philosophy is catching on in gyms and fitness centers as well.

The Training Log

Keeping a training log is an important part of The Program. Not only will it help provide you with a framework around which to perform your workouts; it will also serve as an excellent motivational tool. You may set up your training log any way you wish. The following is an example. Your log should have a list of the exercises you are to perform as well as the weight you lifted and the number of repetitions you achieved on your last workout. For your first workout, your starting weight will merely be your best guess at what weight you can perform eight to twelve times. For example, on one particular day, you will be performing leg presses. You consult your log and note that during your last leg-press workout you performed ten repetitions with five hundred pounds. You are still within the desired eight to twelve rep range, so the weight will not change. However, you know that today, your goal will be to perform at least eleven repetitions with five hundred pounds. In order to make constant, steady progress, you must be aware of your prior workouts. Knowing that last week you performed ten repetitions helps you focus on your goal of exceeding your prior performance. Without a log, you will have to rely on your own memory, which, given the infrequent nature of the workouts you will be performing, can be difficult. You should leave yourself some space in your training log to make any relevant notes. If you had a poor workout and didn't achieve your weight or rep goals, was there a reason for it? Did you not sleep well the night before, engage in some other exercise, or eat poorly prior to your workout? Similarly, if you had a particularly outstanding workout, what were the factors that may have contributed to that? This is important information to jot down. It will help you identify any trends in your workouts or lifestyle impacting your training. The most satisfying aspect of keeping a training log, however, is looking over it after you have been training on The Program for eight to twelve weeks. You will derive a tremendous sense of accomplishment when you see just how much strength you have gained in such a short amount of time.

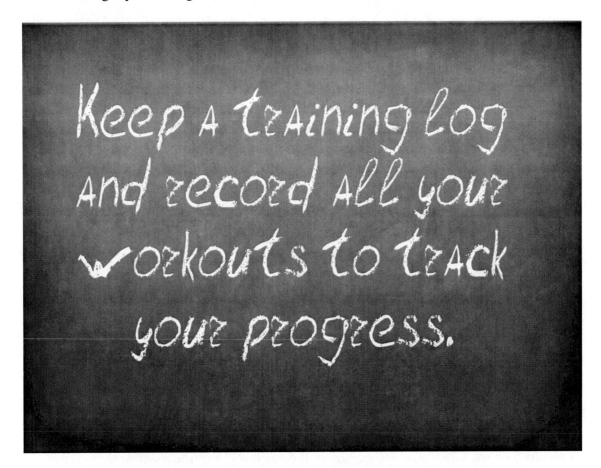

The following is an example of a training log that you may choose to use in your training. Each vertical column represents a workout. Blank copies are included at the end of the book for your use if needed.

For simplicity, only the workouts on day 1 are shown. As you can see, the trainee here started with the ability to squat 225 pounds for eight repetitions to failure and calf press 300 pounds eight times. He continued with these weights until he could perform twelve or more repetitions with that weight. At that point, the weight was increased to bring the repetition range back down to between eight and twelve. Over just seven workouts, the trainee substantially increased his strength in both lifts. For many of you, especially those who have seen little to no progress in your training efforts to date, these kinds of regular strength gains may seem exaggerated or unrealistic. I assure you they are not. When properly implementing The Program, you will grow stronger every workout. After a couple of months, take a look back at your training log and see just how far you have come.

	1	2	3	4	5	6	7	8
Day 1								
Thighs SQUATS	225 X8	225X11	225X13	245X10	245X12	265X9	265X12	275 X10
Calves SEATED CALF RAISE	300 X8	300X12	325X8	325X10	325X12	350X8	350X11	350X13
Day 2								
Front Deltoid								
Side Deltoid								
Biceps								
Triceps								
Abs								
Day 3								
Chest (Press)								
Chest (Fly)								
Deadlift or								
Narrow-grip Back								
Wide-grip back								

Training Partners

One of the best ways to get the most out of The Program is to find a friend who will do it with you. Having a reliable training partner is one of the best ways to maximize your progress and maintain your motivation. The workouts you will be doing, though brief, require considerable mental effort and energy. Inevitably, there will be days when you just don't have a lot of that to spare. Having a workout partner there to push you and encourage you during your workout can mean the difference between a mediocre workout and an outstanding one. Similarly, when you feel like you might cheat on your diet, a good training partner can keep you focused and away from the foods you know you shouldn't be eating. As you progress in your training, many of you will want to use more advanced intensity techniques. Having a training partner there to spot you and help load the weights for you makes it easier to get the most out of these techniques. A workout partner also provides an added safety net. Your partner (one hopes) won't let you get stuck while lifting a weight, will make sure you use proper form, and will warn you if you are doing something that may lead to an injury. Obviously, a training partner is not required to succeed on The Program. Many individuals prefer working out alone and are able to find the necessary motivation and intensity within themselves. This is perfectly fine. If you choose to rely primarily on machines for your workouts, you won't require a spotter for safety since you won't have to worry about dropping the weight or becoming stuck under a bar. Nevertheless, many of you will find that a good training partner will not only enhance your enjoyment of The Program but improve your results as well.

A poor training partner, however, can be far worse than no training partner at all. Make sure you choose someone who shares your commitment to both the diet and training aspects of The Program. A great workout partner who constantly tries to offer you pizza and Coke will sabotage your efforts and ultimately lead you to fail in your quest to improve your body. A partner who takes shortcuts or is unwilling to work hard in the gym will do the same thing.

Aerobics

If you have a good deal of body fat to lose or simply want to lower your body fat to its lowest possible level, you will need to incorporate regular aerobic exercise into your training routine. Those of you on the Endomorphic Diet should schedule at least thirty minutes of cardiovascular training daily. If you have a great deal of fat to lose, you may consider gradually increasing your aerobic work to forty-five to sixty minutes. The ideal time to perform aerobic exercise is first thing in the morning on an empty stomach. When you wake, your body has very little in the way of stored glycogen, having used most of it while you slept. As a result, you will more quickly turn to your fat stores for energy if you exercise first thing in the morning. This isn't always feasible for some people, so the next best time is immediately after your weight-training workout. After lifting, you have also burned some of your stored muscle glycogen and will similarly turn to your fat stores for fuel during your cardiovascular training. Do not perform your cardiovascular training before your weight training since this will inevitably cause your weight training to suffer.

Choose a low-impact activity that raises your heart rate to approximately 75 to 80 percent of your predicted heart rate maximum and try to maintain it for about thirty to forty-five minutes. You can calculate your maximum heart rate using the formula [220-age] for a rough estimate. Depending on your initial condition, you may not be able to start out at thirty minutes and that is okay. Start with shorter increments like ten or fifteen minutes. Add an additional five minutes every week until you are able to reach the goal of thirty minutes. It's up to you what activity you choose for your aerobic work. Some people prefer stair-climbing machines, treadmills, or elliptical trainers. Others prefer a structured aerobics class or getting outside for a brisk walk. The activity doesn't matter as much as just getting out there and doing it. For you mesomorphs and ectomorphs, try to limit your cardiovascular training to your workout days. This will allow for more complete recovery between your sessions and give you a mental break from training on your days off.

Some form of aerobic training is mandatory for maximum fat loss on the Endomorphic Diet. This will accelerate fat loss to the highest degree and help you achieve your fat loss goals more quickly. Cardiovascular training on the Mesomorphic variant is considered optional. I encourage you to do it to maintain your heart health and keep your body fat low. However, if you are satisfied with your current body fat level and are focusing on gaining maximum amounts of muscle, you may forgo aerobic training for the time being. Those of you on the Ectomorphic variant presumably already have very low body fat levels. Your training is going to center around gaining muscle mass. In this case, you should generally avoid or greatly limit your aerobic activities, as they will only tax your body's limited recovery ability and potentially compromise your muscle growth. When you have met your muscle-building goals and transition to the Mesomorphic variant, you may then consider adding aerobic exercise into your routine.

Warming Up

Before you begin your workouts, it is important in most cases to prepare your muscles by warming up and stretching. There isn't a tremendous amount of scientific literature on the best ways to go about doing this. However, there has been some research that I will summarize for you, and I will provide some basic principles that you can follow.

Stretching before working out is generally recommended. There are obviously many different ways to stretch. You will see some athletes performing rapid, short-duration stretches (so called "ballistic" stretching). Others stretch more slowly and hold the stretch for various lengths of time (static stretching). In general, ballistic-type stretching is not recommended. This sort of stretching does not give the muscle adequate time to fully lengthen and appears to be inferior to static stretching in achieving an improvement in muscle range of motion. So how long should you hold a stretch? Fortunately, there has been some research looking into this question. It appears, that holding a stretch for approximately thirty seconds increases range of motion to a greater degree than fifteen seconds does. Holding the stretch for sixty seconds does not seem to give any additional benefit.[221] Therefore, a thirty-second static stretch seems like a reasonable place to start. How many times should you stretch before working out? In the long term, it appears that a single thirty-second stretch was as effective as three thirty-second stretches in improving range of motion over six weeks.[222] In the short term (just before working out), it is unclear just how many times one should stretch for optimal benefit.

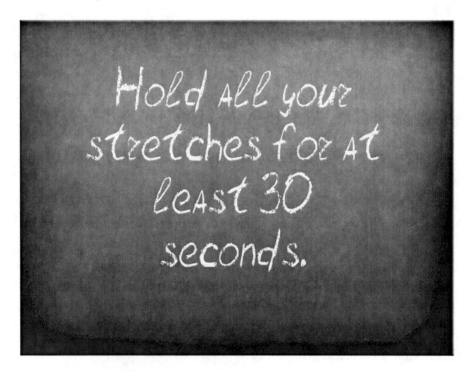

---

221   Bundy WD, Irion JM: The effect of time on static stretch on the flexibility of the hamstring muscles. Phys Ther 1994:74(9):845–852.
222   Bandy WD; Irion JM, Briggler M: The effect of time and frequency of static stretching on flexibility of the hamstring muscles. Phys Ther 1997;77(10):1090–1096.

It is also often recommended that individuals perform some sort of warm-up activity in addition to stretching. Indeed, it appears that performing an active warm-up followed by stretching does seem to increase range of motion beyond just stretching alone.[223] The activity you choose may vary. Some prefer a brisk walk on the treadmill or a few minutes on a stair-climber machine. I tend to recommend performing an activity that closely mimics or is identical to the lifts you are planning to perform that day. For example, on squat day, I may briskly walk to the gym and perform a few repetitions of deep knee bends followed by quadriceps, hamstring, and low back stretching. I then begin with a very light weight on the squat bar. I gradually increase the weight over two to three sets before performing my final all-out set to muscular failure. In between warm-up sets, I will perform the same stretches. Obviously, when performing exercises that work large muscle groups and when using heavy weight, you may want to perform a more extensive and gradual warm-up than when working small muscle groups like biceps or calves. For those muscle groups, a single warm-up set with light weight is usually sufficient.

The following are some basic recommendations that you can follow when deciding how to best warm up before exercising:

1. Perform the minimum amount of warm-up and stretching needed prior to exercise. Do not expend unnecessary energy performing a prolonged and complicated warm-up. This will only serve to fatigue you and detract from your workout.

2. For most muscle groups, a single thirty-second static stretch is sufficient.

3. Stretch until you feel a certain degree of tension on the muscle. Hold this until the muscle lengthens and the tension relaxes. Then stretch beyond this point until you feel the original amount of tension recur. Continue this for the thirty-second duration of your stretch.

4. Consider daily stretching. A daily stretching program performed over weeks has been shown to increase both muscle strength and running speed.[224] The effect is fairly modest: about 2 to 5 percent. However, if you are a competitive athlete, this small margin may mean the difference between winning and losing. If you are not a competitive athlete and are participating in The Program primarily to get in shape, then daily stretching is optional.

223   Wiktorsson-Moller M, Oberg BA, Ekstrand J, et al: Effects of warming up, massage, and stretching on range of motion and muscle strength in the lower extremity. Am J Sports Med 1983;11(4):249–252.
224   Shrier I: Does stretching improve performance? A systematic and critical review of the literature. Clin J Sports Med 2004;14(5):267–273.

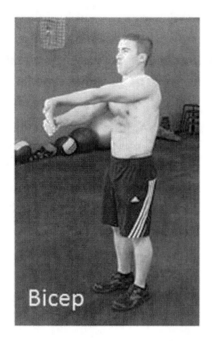

Bicep

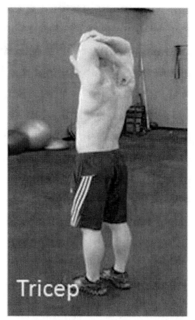

Tricep

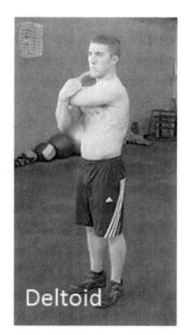

Deltoid

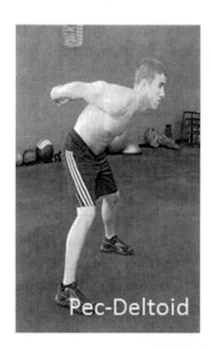

Pec-Deltoid

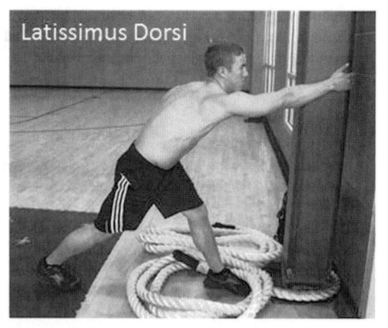

Latissimus Dorsi

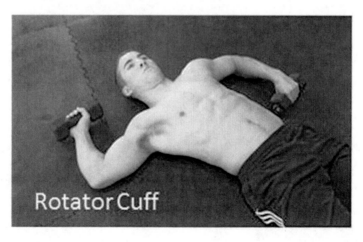

Rotator Cuff

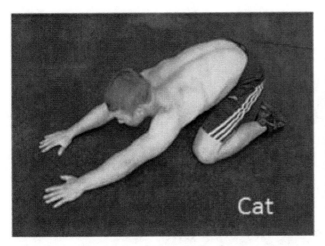

Cat

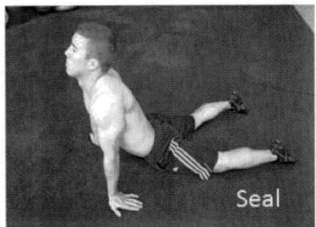

Seal

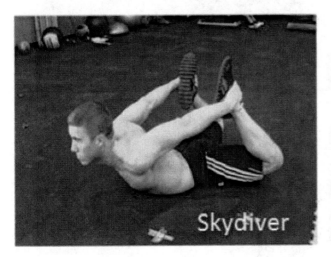

Skydiver

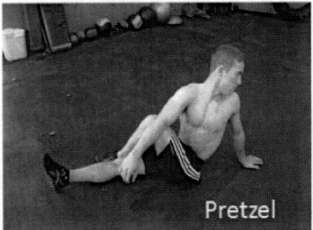

Pretzel

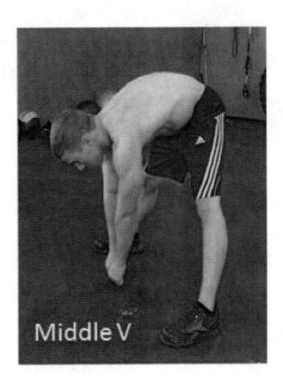

Middle V

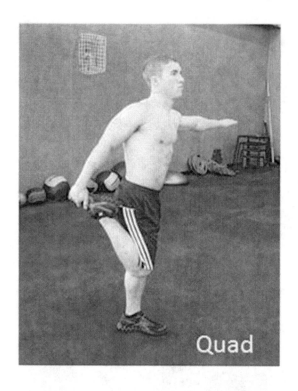

Quad

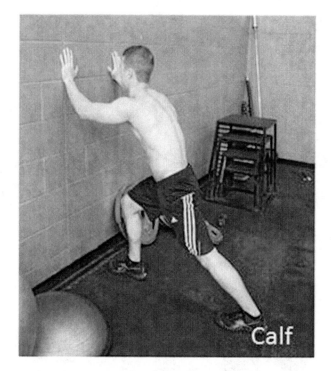

Calf

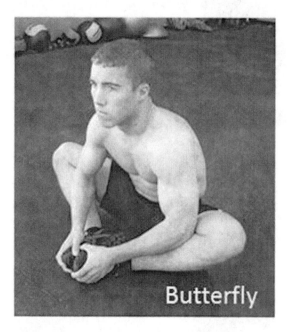

Butterfly

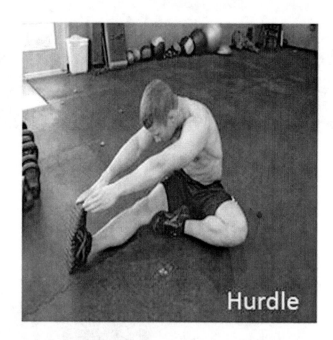

Hurdle

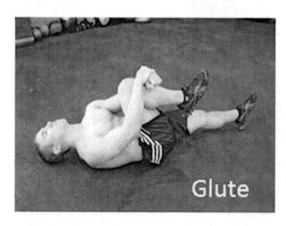

Glute

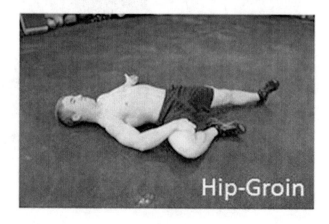

Hip-Groin

Machines Versus Free Weights

There has always been considerable debate in bodybuilding over the use of weight-training machines. Bodybuilders since even before the 1950s have built outstanding physiques with free weights alone. In the 1970s, with the emergence of Arthur Jones and Nautilus, machines became more and more popular. In recent years, the number of companies producing weight-training machines has continued to increase. Many proponents of high-intensity training claim that training with machines is actually superior considering the high-quality equipment available in most gyms. When I began training as a teenager, I trained exclusively with free weights. The machines available at the gym I trained in were awkward, and I never felt that I was able to stimulate my muscles to the same degree as I did with free weights. As a result, I developed a bias toward free weights that I maintained for years. Recently, having had the opportunity to train using some of the newer Hammer Strength, Cybex, and Med-Rx equipment, I have changed my opinion. The truth is that both free weights and machines have advantages that you should exploit if you wish to develop your physique fully.

Free weights are available in every gym. They are relatively cheap compared to machines. With a power rack, an Olympic bar, and a few plates, you can perform a highly effective whole-body workout in your garage if need be. Free weights are also able to move in all planes of motion. As a result, when you lift a free weight, you not only have to contract the primary muscle(s) you are training, but you must activate numerous smaller stabilizing muscles to keep the weight under control. Machines typically move through a controlled range of motion thereby decreasing the need for these smaller stabilizers. As a result, the potential for developing muscle imbalances exists. This may not have a big impact if you are primarily training for bodybuilding purposes, but if you are engaged in explosive sports, the possibility of injury should be considered. The downside to the increased range of motion offered by free weights, of course, is an increase in the probability of injury if the exercise is not performed with good form. Free weights can be dropped and can drift in unsafe directions. While straining to reach muscular failure, it is easy to travel outside of a safe arc of motion and suffer a strain, muscle tear, or worse. In almost all cases, high-intensity training with free weights mandates a competent spotter who can help keep you safe during your lift.

The new generations of weight-training machines are valuable tools in your arsenal of training equipment. They are carefully designed to work with the natural biomechanics of the human body and effectively isolate specific muscle groups. As mentioned above, machines provide an additional safety factor that free weights cannot. With most, it is impossible to move the weight outside of a safe movement arc. Even if you reach complete muscle failure and the weight comes crashing down, it usually returns safely to its starting position. This is particularly advantageous if you train alone and have a hard time finding a good spotter. Machines are also valuable when you have an injury. You will inevitably develop minor aches and pains while weight training. If you ignore these warning signs, you may develop a more chronic condition like tendonitis. When this happens, you need to lay off the offending exercise for a while to let your body heal. Fortunately, because machines are better at isolating specific muscle groups, you can often find a machine that will allow you to continue your workouts without aggravating your injury. Unfortunately, with machines, one size does not fit all. They are designed to accommodate most sizes and shapes, but you may find that if you are particularly tall or short, you simply cannot fit comfortably in a particular machine. This problem rarely exists with free weight exercises. Another important consideration is that only a limited amount of weight can be loaded onto a machine. This may not be an issue for you now, but as you grow stronger on The Program, don't be surprised if you outgrow the ability to use certain machines simply because you have become too strong.

You will notice that most of the primary exercises listed in the Exercise Database are free weight exercises. Despite the progress that machines have made, it is still to your advantage to start with a workout built primarily around free weight exercises. Certainly, if you have an injury, train alone, or simply prefer machines, you may substitute them as needed. There is only one free weight exercise that, unless you have an injury, should never be removed from your workout. That exercise is squats. No machine yet built can provide the high-intensity, deep muscle-stimulating properties of a set of heavy squats performed to failure. A set of squats to failure is like running a mini-marathon. This type of very intense training stimulus not only stimulates your legs to grow tremendously but also raises testosterone levels in men and leads to whole-body muscle growth. Substitute other exercises for other body parts if you must, but think twice before removing squats. Along with deadlifts, they will be your most result-producing exercise.

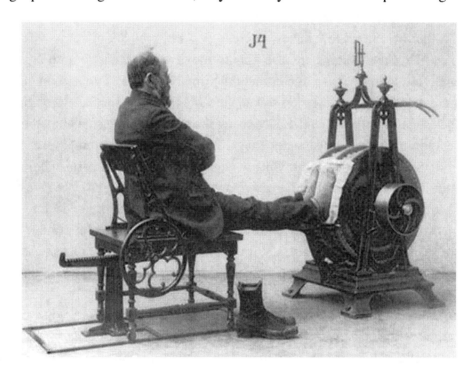

The Beginner's Workout

Many of you starting The Program will have no weight-training experience. The two-week beginner's workout was designed for you. Its goal is to familiarize you with the core exercises you will be performing later on. During this two-week period, you will have the time to learn proper exercise form and adjust to regular exercise. Training to absolute failure is not required during this time, though you may if you wish. You will also get an idea of approximately how strong you are and how much weight you will be using when you graduate to the core workout. Your workouts will take a little longer during this phase since you will be learning new movements and performing a few more sets than you will later. You will be able to choose which exercises you perform from the exercise database provided below. In general, try to stick to the exercises listed first in the database, as they are the ones generally considered to be the most productive. If you have an injury or some other good reason to change an exercise, you may choose a replacement from the exercise database. After two weeks, you should be ready to transition to the core workout. If you have prior weight-training experience and feel confident that you know how to perform all the exercises listed, then you may move directly to the core workout.

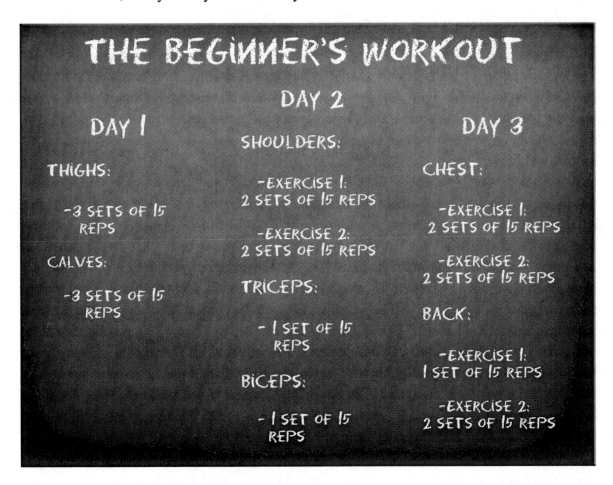

THE BEGINNER'S WORKOUT

DAY 2

DAY 1

SHOULDERS:

THIGHS:
- -EXERCISE 1:
  2 SETS OF 15 REPS

-3 SETS OF 15
REPS
- -EXERCISE 2:
  2 SETS OF 15 REPS

CALVES:

-3 SETS OF 15
REPS
TRICEPS:

- 1 SET OF 15
REPS

BICEPS:

- 1 SET OF 15
REPS

DAY 3

CHEST:

- -EXERCISE 1:
  2 SETS OF 15 REPS

- -EXERCISE 2:
  2 SETS OF 15 REPS

BACK:

- -EXERCISE 1:
  1 SET OF 15 REPS

- -EXERCISE 2:
  2 SETS OF 15 REPS

The Core Workout

The Core Workout forms the foundation of the workout you will be performing while using The Program. All the major muscle groups are exercised over three workouts. This system fits well into a Monday-Wednesday-Friday routine, which is convenient for most people and leaves the weekends free to pursue other activities. As stated previously, however, do not feel constrained to limit yourself to this schedule. You may schedule your workouts as you see fit, as long as there is a minimum of one day of rest between workouts. Keep in mind that this type of split, with only a single day between workouts may, depending on your recovery ability, constitute over training. As you get stronger, the stresses you apply to the musculoskeletal system will increase and additional rest days will be needed. Most individuals will eventually end up on a one-on/two-to-three-off program or an even less frequent workout system. If you are over age thirty I recommend starting with a one on-two off split. That is if you work out Monday, you would then take Tuesday and Wednesday off before training again. Keep accurate training records, and if you notice that your progress is slowing down or stalled for more than a couple weeks, consider adding an additional rest day between exercise sessions.

The Core Workout is designed to allow you a certain amount of flexibility in choosing which exercises you perform. For each body part, you will select an appropriate exercise from the Exercise Database. The exercises are ranked in order of their overall effectiveness in stimulating the specific muscle group involved. Unless you have an injury that prevents you from performing the primary exercises for each muscle group, you should make every effort to incorporate them into your workouts. Certainly, if you feel like you are becoming mentally stale with a particular exercise and want to introduce some variety into your routine, feel free.

The body parts in the Core Workout are scheduled in such a way as to allow you to focus maximum attention to the particular muscle group you are training. Day 1 is thighs and calves. The most common response I get when trainees see this workout on paper is "One set for legs? That's it?" I usually chuckle because I know anyone who says this has never had the experience of performing an all-out, slow, and controlled set of squats or leg presses to complete muscular failure. Believe me, one set is more than enough. In fact, in most cases, you will be so exhausted from that one set that you will be physically unable to perform a second set, even if you wanted to (almost nobody does). Thigh workouts are the most physically taxing of all the workouts you will perform. You will need all your mental and physical energy to get the most out of this workout. That is why the only other body part that is worked that day is calves. After training, those two body parts should be physically drained. If you performed additional exercises for other muscle groups, it is doubtful you would be able to generate the needed intensity to maximally stimulate their growth.

For those of you who really want to ramp up the intensity of your thigh workouts, you may combine two exercises into a single set called a superset. A more detailed explanation of supersets is provided in the advanced high-intensity techniques chapter. Squats and leg presses or leg extensions followed immediately by squats are just two examples of exercises that can be combined into one super-high-intensity set that will make your thigh workout all the more intense and productive.

Day 2 involves working the arms. Overall, it is a much easier workout than days 1 or 3 since smaller body parts are involved. After a brief warm-up, you start with two shoulder exercises. The shoulder is a complex joint and able to move within a wide range of angles. Therefore, two exercises are needed to stimulate the entire deltoid. The first exercise is performed to stimulate the front deltoids. In reality, most front deltoid exercises that involve pressing movements work the entire deltoid, but the frontal portion of the muscle carries the bulk of the load. The side and rear deltoids are then finished off with a single set that primarily targets those regions. This system encourages even and symmetric development throughout the entire muscle group. Biceps are worked next. The arm biceps are perhaps the most overtrained body parts in all of bodybuilding. Everyone wants to have well-developed arms, and they assume that set after set of all kinds of biceps curls are needed to get there. The truth is that the biceps are a relatively small muscle group. Its primary function is to flex the arm and supinate the wrist. That's it. Uninformed trainees often perform ten or more sets for their biceps one day and then go on to perform ten to twenty sets for their backs on another. What they fail to realize is that the biceps also take a beating during their back workouts. In reality, they are performing up to thirty sets a week for their biceps! And they wonder why they aren't growing like they want them too. A single set to failure is all that is needed to stimulate optimal growth in your biceps. Remember, you will be working them again indirectly during your next back workout. The same principle applies to the triceps muscle group. You will be indirectly stimulating them during your chest workout with any pressing movement you perform. Therefore, only a single set is needed. Day 2 is concluded with a set of abdominal exercises. Again, only a single set is required. Abdominals are another muscle group that receives a great degree of indirect stimulation from other exercises. Exercises like squats, deadlifts, and triceps pushdowns require intense contraction of the abdominals to maintain trunk stability. It is difficult to find abdominal exercises that will provide enough resistance to perform only eight to twelve repetitions. Therefore, a higher number of reps are allowed to ensure that you maximally fatigue the muscle group.

Day 3 is another challenging workout. After warming up the chest, you will perform a single pressing movement. After a brief rest, you will go on to perform a flying movement that will stretch the chest. Combining these two different types of chest exercises ensures optimal strength and muscular development. After another brief rest, you will perform the deadlift exercise of your choice. This particular type of exercise is very taxing but also extremely rewarding in terms of muscle growth and strength development. Make sure you take the time to learn proper form, as there is some potential for injury if these exercises are not performed properly. For those of you unable to perform a deadlift type exercise due to injury, you may substitute a narrow-grip rowing movement for the back from the list below. Day three is concluded with the performance of a single set of a wide-grip movement for the upper back and latissimus muscles.

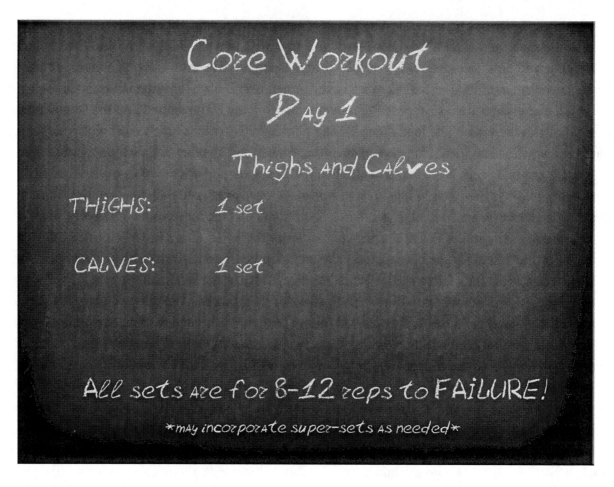

Core Workout
Day 1

Thighs and Calves

THIGHS: 1 set

CALVES: 1 set

All sets are for 8-12 reps to FAILURE!
may incorporate super-sets as needed

The exercise arrangement in the Core Workout is not set in stone. However, they are arranged in such a way to optimize recovery of individual muscle groups while allowing you to focus on generating as much effort and intensity as possible. If you have a compelling reason to rearrange the order of these exercises, you may do so as long as you do not violate the basic principles outlined at the beginning of the chapter. All your workouts should be very intense, infrequent, and short in duration. Resist the temptation to perform additional sets. The system laid out in The Program is tried and tested and designed to give your body exactly what it needs to build new muscle as quickly as possible. Follow this system as closely as possible, and you will be rewarded with gains in strength and lean muscle beyond what you have ever experienced with any other program.

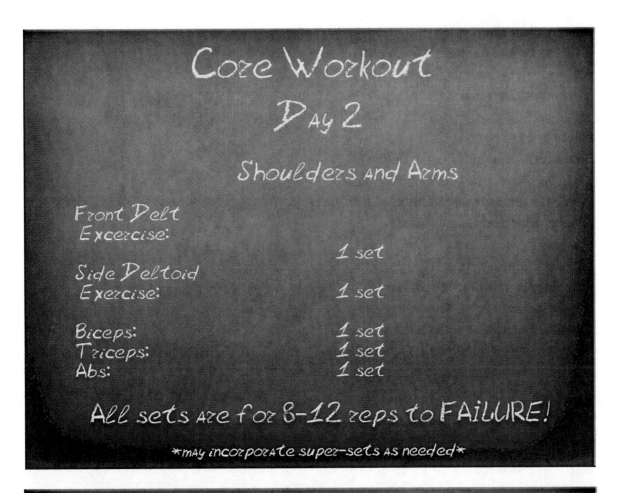

Core Workout
Day 2

Shoulders and Arms

Front Delt Excercise:	1 set
Side Deltoid Exercise:	1 set
Biceps:	1 set
Triceps:	1 set
Abs:	1 set

All sets are for 8-12 reps to FAILURE!

may incorporate super-sets as needed

Core Workout
Day 3
Chest and Back

CHEST:	
Pressing Exercise:	1 set
Fly Exercise:	1 set
BACK:	
Dead lift Exercise:	1 set
Wide grip Exercise:	1 set

or narrow-grip row if injury prevents doing deadlifts!

All sets are for 8-12 reps to FAILURE!

may incorporate super-sets as needed

Day 1: Thighs and Calves
- Thighs: 1 set to failure
- Calves: 1 set to failure
- Abdominal Exercise: 1 set to failure

Day 2: Shoulders and Arms
- Front Delt Exercise: 1 set to failure
- Side Delt Exercise: 1 set to failure
- Biceps Exercise: 1 set to failure
- Triceps Exercise: 1 set to failure

Day 3: Chest and Back
- Pressing Exercise: 1 set to failure
- Fly Exercise: 1 set to failure
- Deadlift Exercise: 1 set to failure
- Wide-Grip Row Exercise: 1 set to failure

Exercise Database

Most of the recommended exercises are pictured below, however, anyone with access to the internet will be able to find multiple variations of each in picture or video formats. The most important factor is to make sure your choice engages the target muscle groups.

Thighs

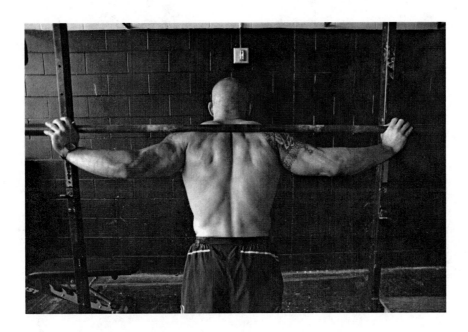

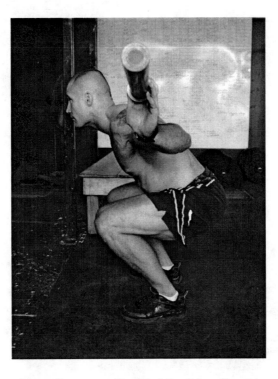

Free Squat or Smith Machine Squat

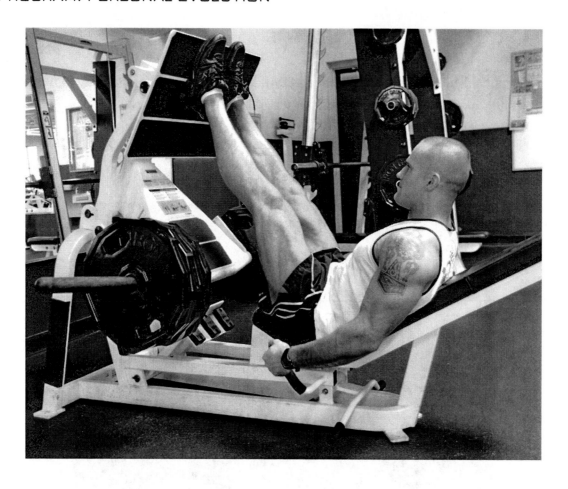

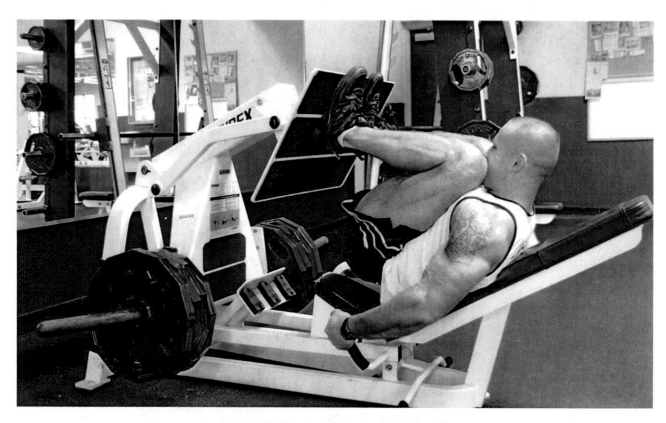

Leg Press or Hack Squat

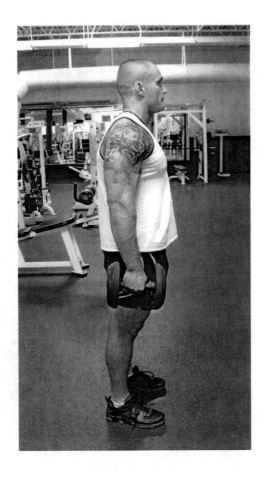

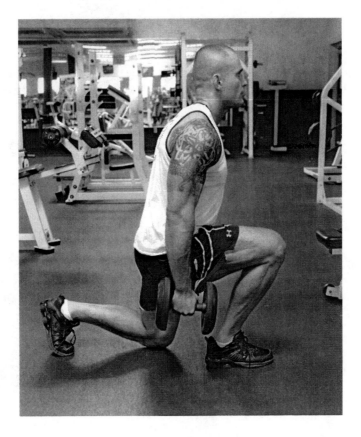

Lunges

Calves

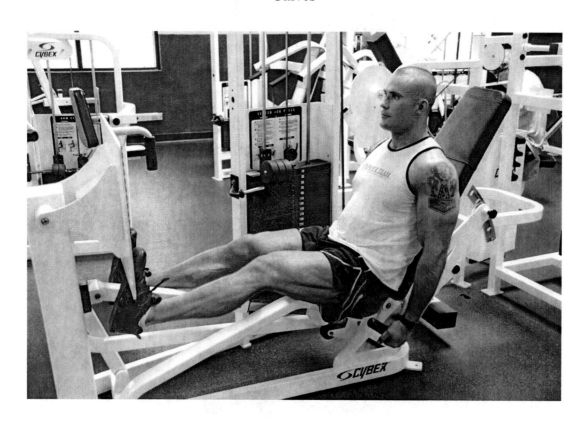

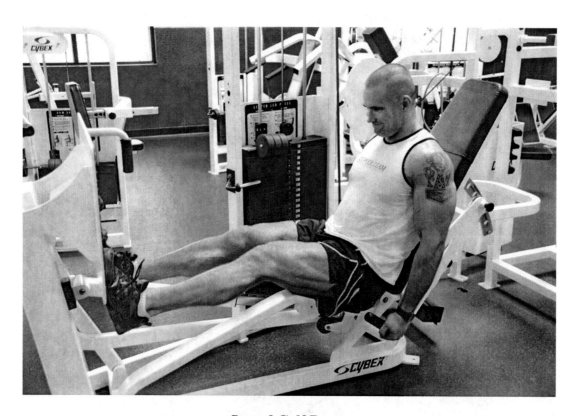

Seated Calf Press

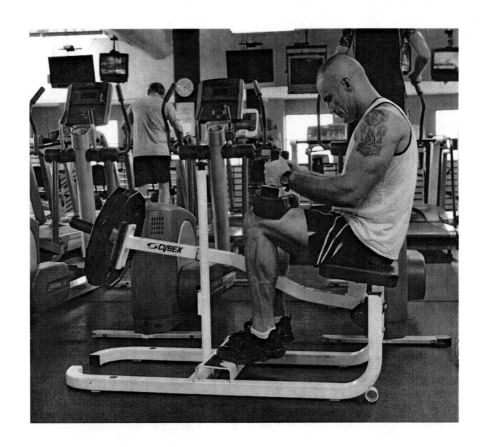

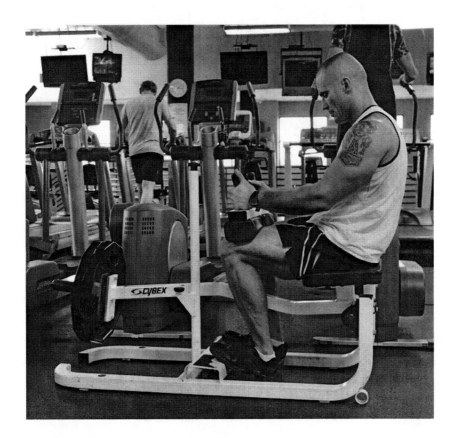

Seated Calf Raise

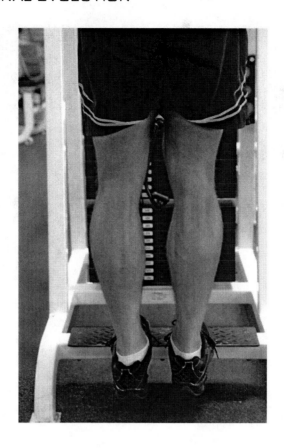

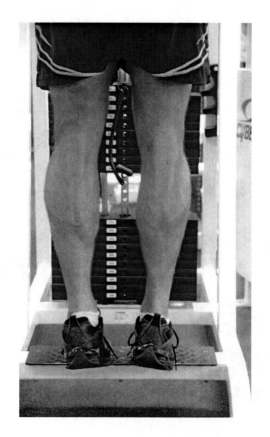

Standing or Donkey Calf Raise

Shoulders (Front Deltoid)

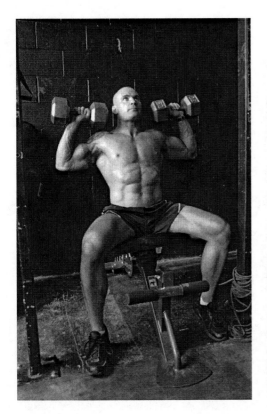 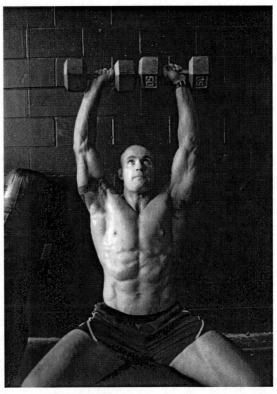

Dumbbell Shoulder Press

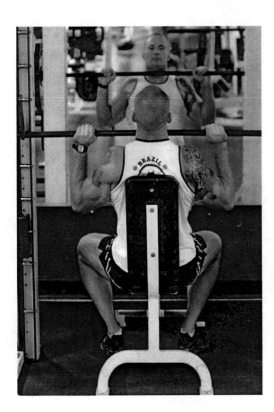 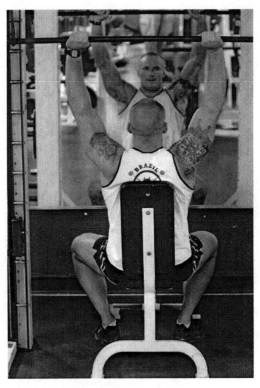

Front Straight Bar or Plate Loaded Military Press

Shoulders (side and rear deltoid)

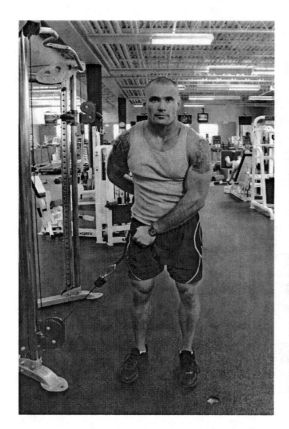 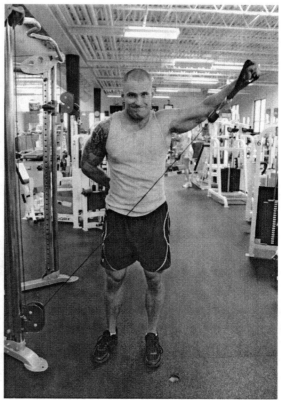

Cable Lateral Raise

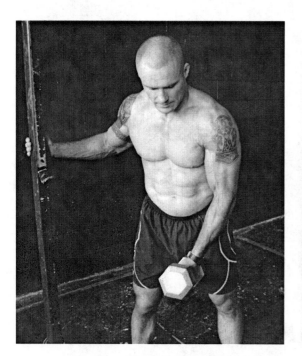 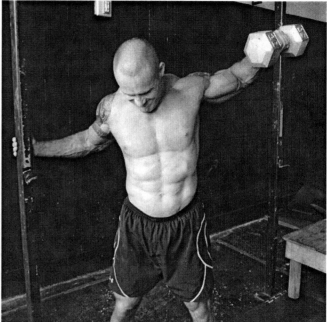

Standing Dumbbell Lateral Raise

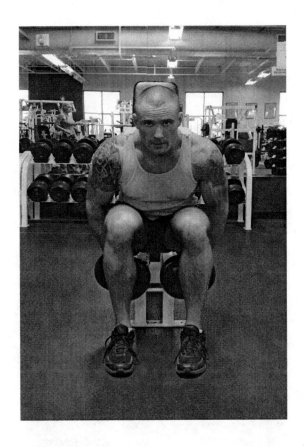

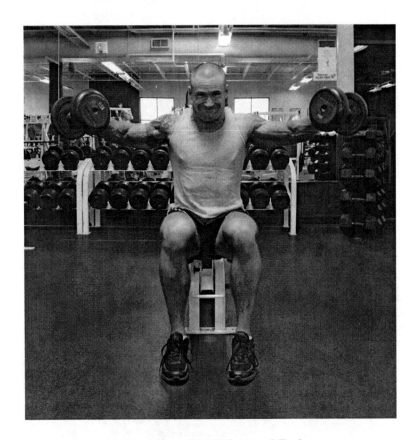

Seated Dumbbell Lateral Raise

Biceps

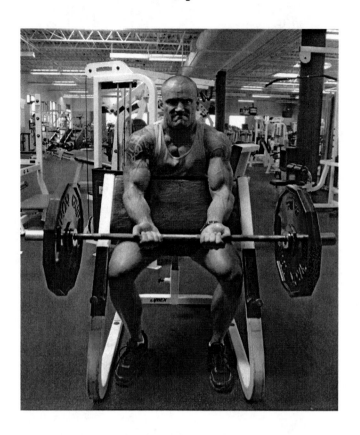

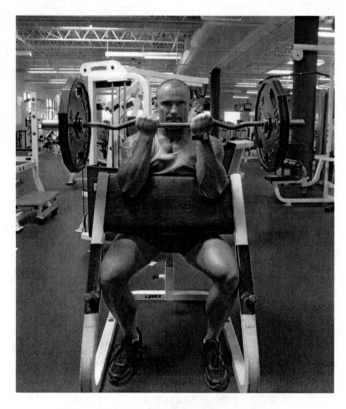

Preacher Curl with E-Z Curl Bar

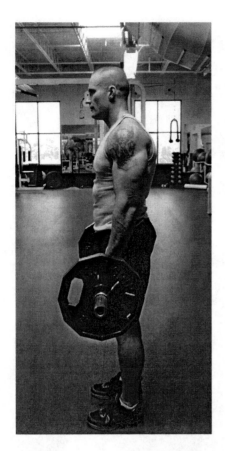 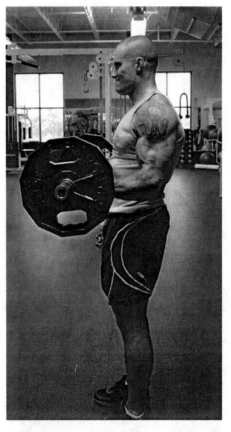

Standing Curl with E-Z Curl Bar

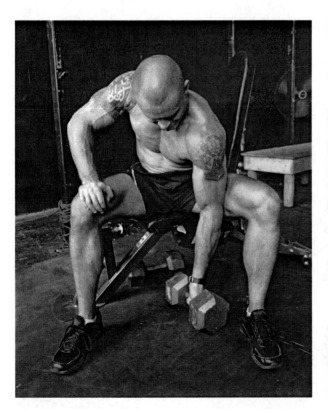 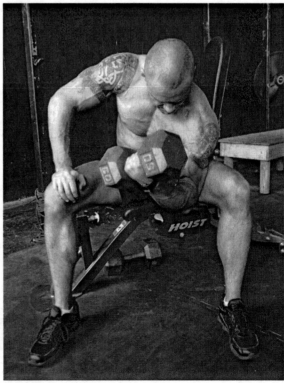

Concentration Dumbbell Curl

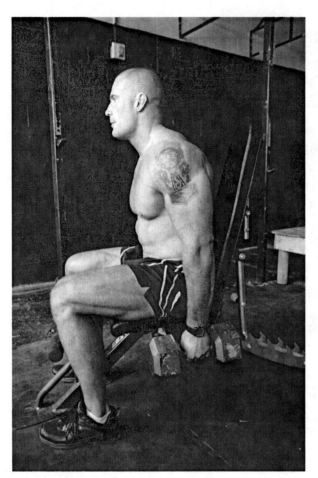
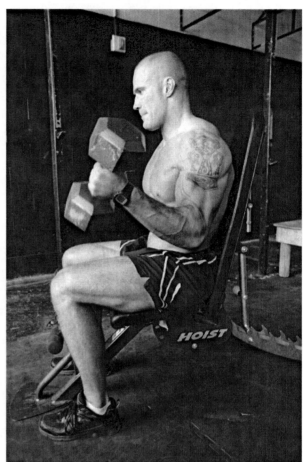

Seated Dumbbell Curl

Triceps

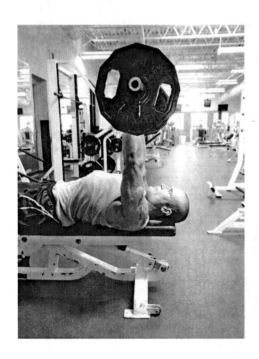
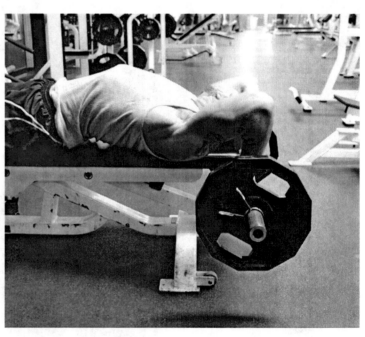

Skull Crushers/French Press

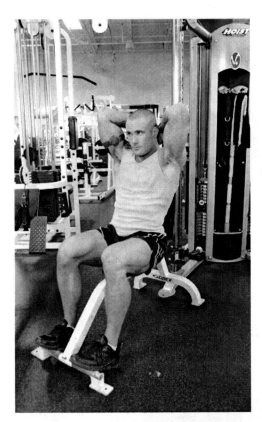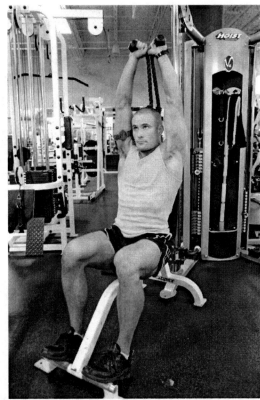

Overhead Triceps Extension with Rope or Bar Grip

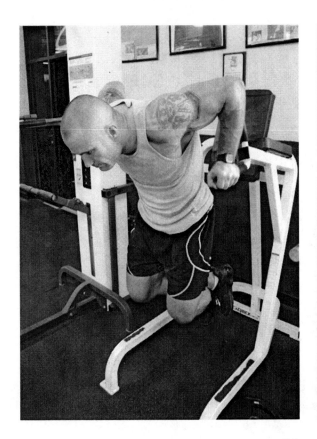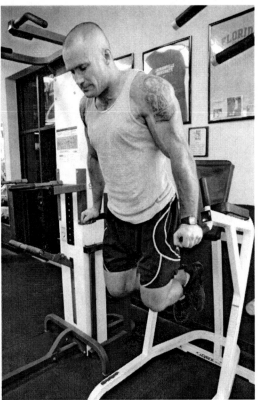

Dips

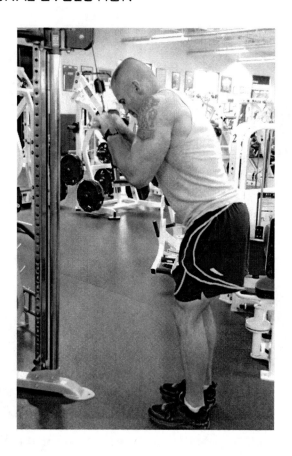

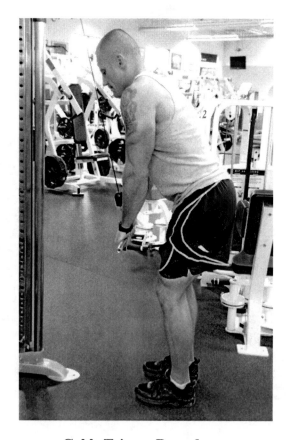

Cable Triceps Pressdown

Chest (Press)

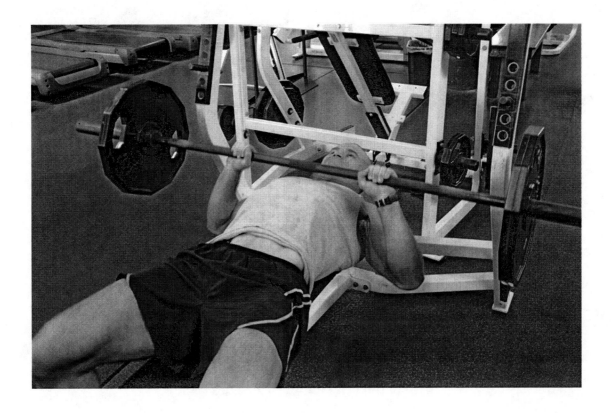

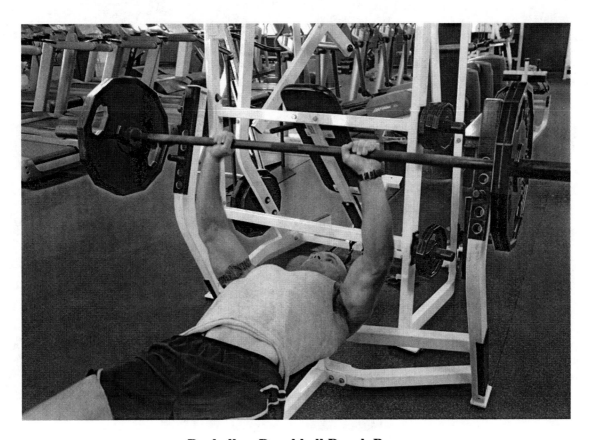

Barbell or Dumbbell Bench Press

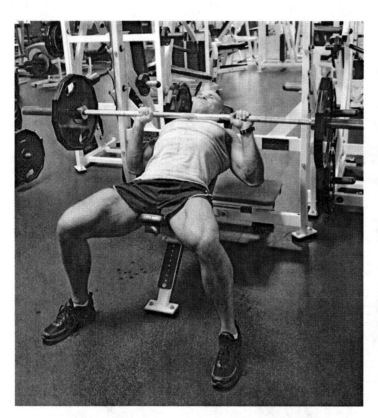
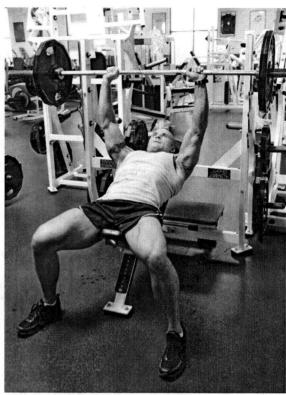

Incline Barbell Dumbbell Bench Press

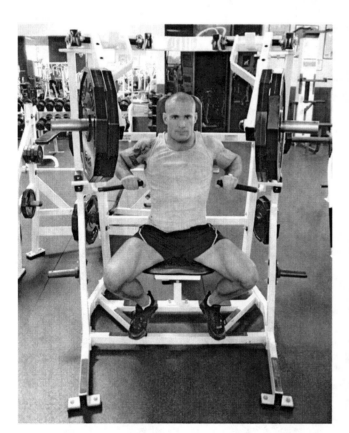
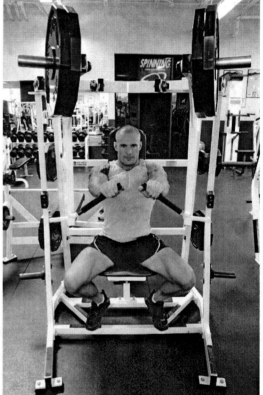

Plate Loaded Bench Press

Chest (Flyes)

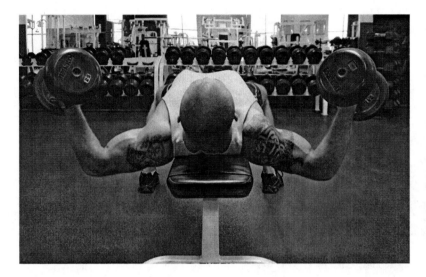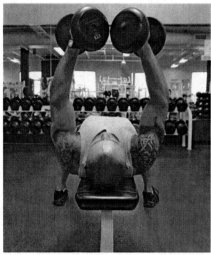

Flat Bench Dumbbell Flyes

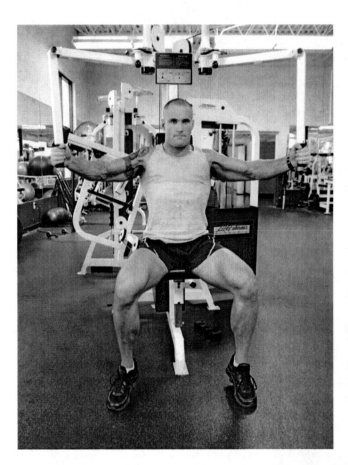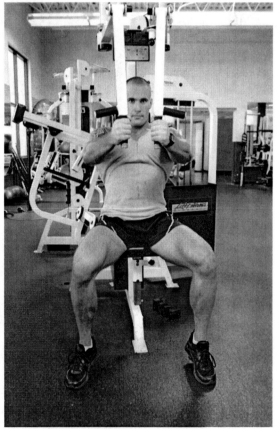

Machine Flyes

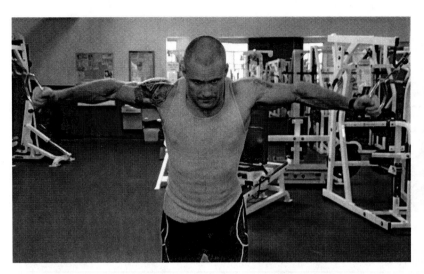 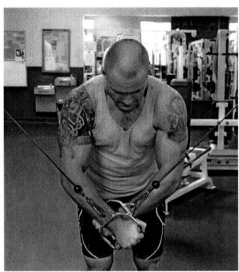

Standing Cable Cross-over

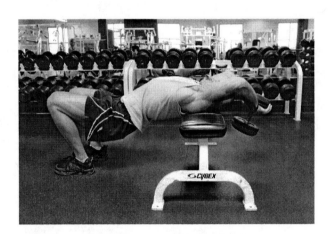

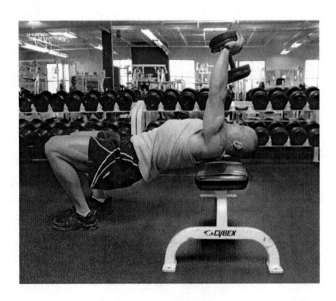

Cross Bench Pullover

Back (deadlift)

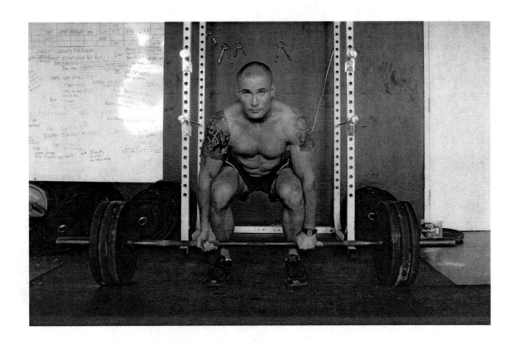

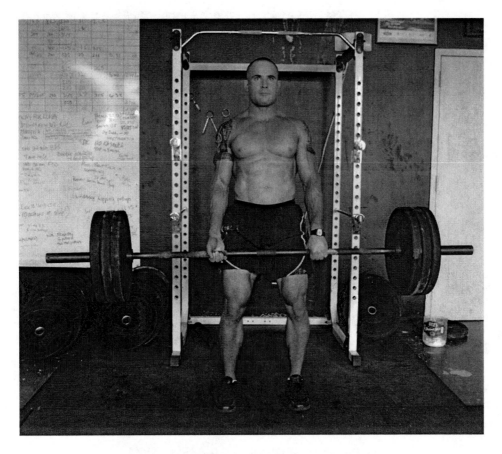

Conventional Deadlift (over-under grip)

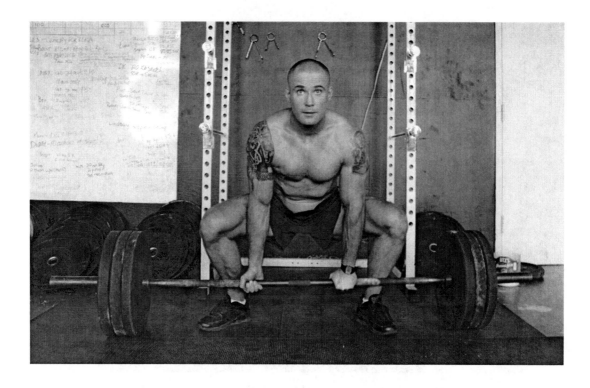

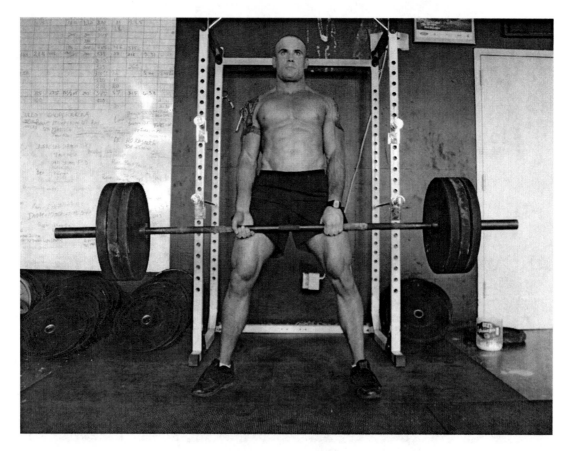

Sumo Deadlift (over-under grip)

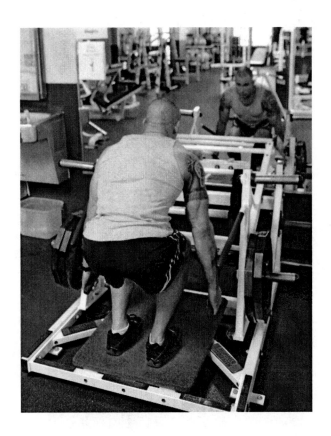

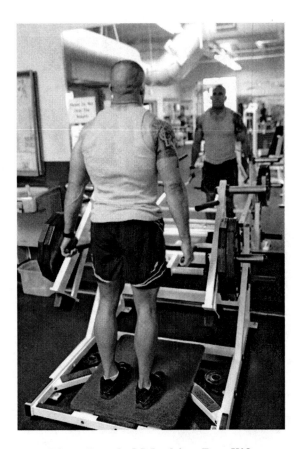

Plate Loaded Machine Deadlift

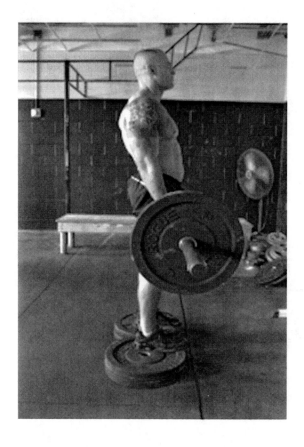

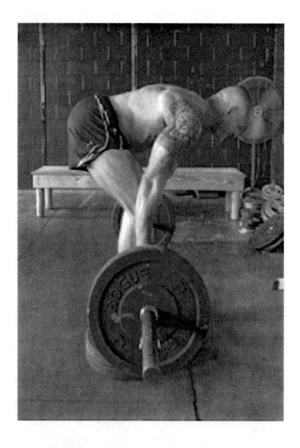

Stiff-leg Deadlifts (hamstring emphasis)

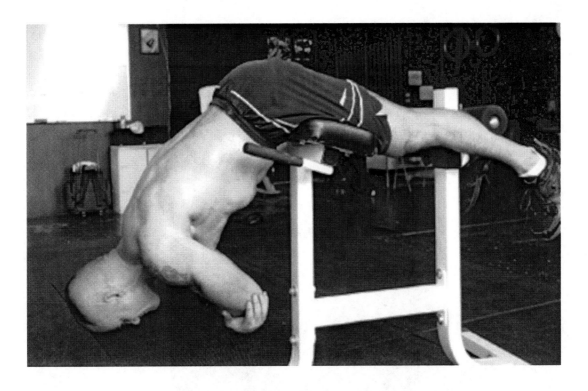

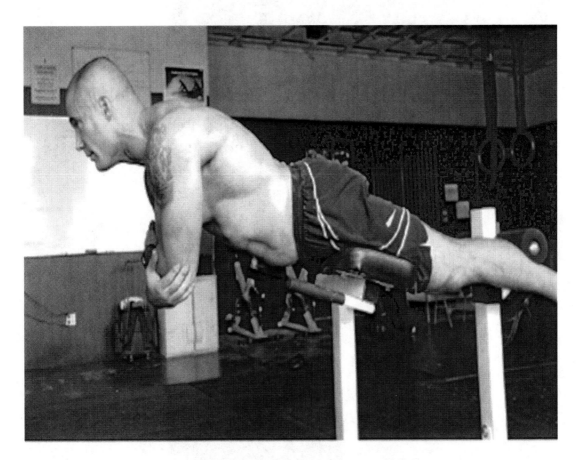

Hyperextensions (add weight as needed)

Back (wide grip)

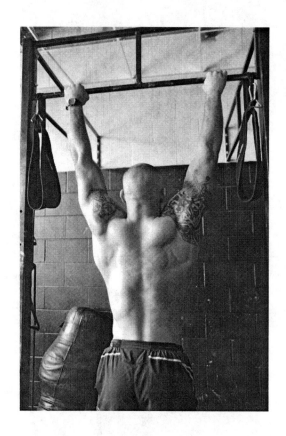

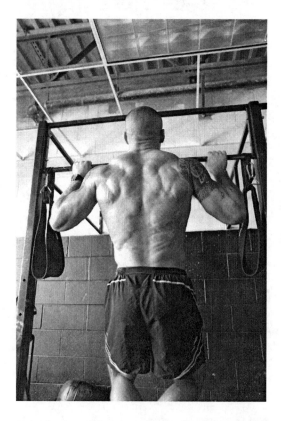

Wide Grip Pull up (add weight if needed)

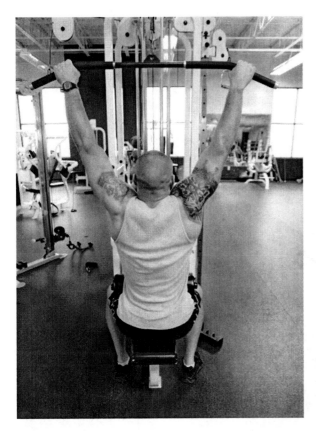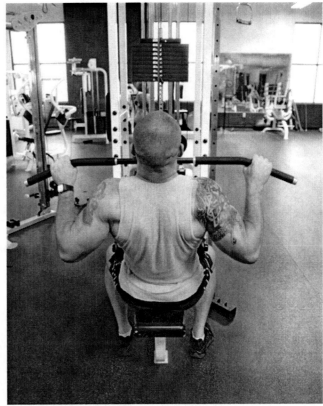

Wide Grip Pulldown

Back (Narrow Grip)

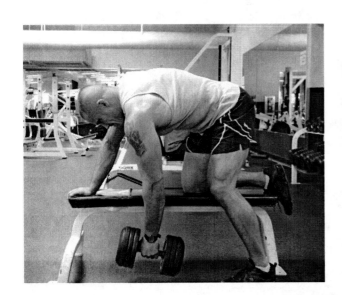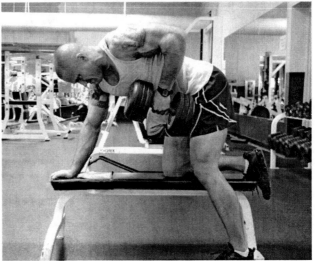

Dumbbell Bent Row

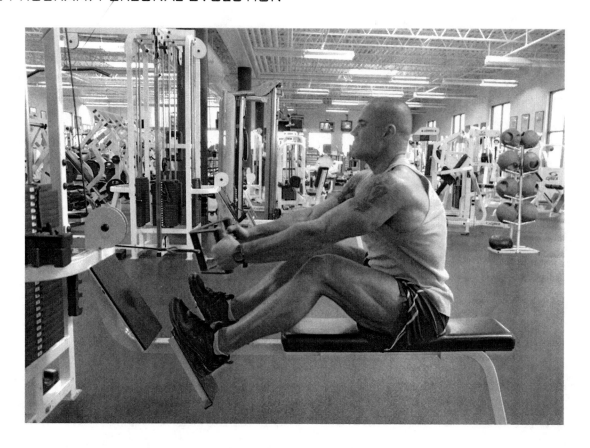

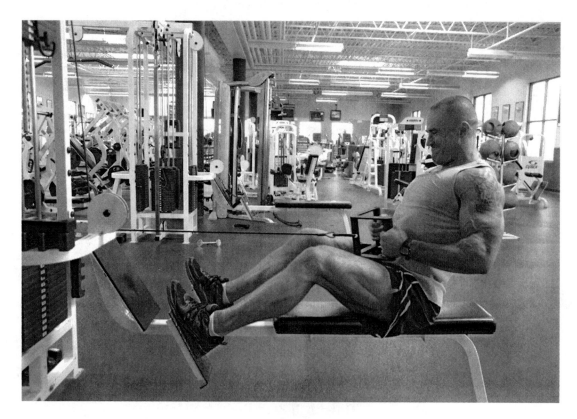

Seated Cable Row with Narrow Grip

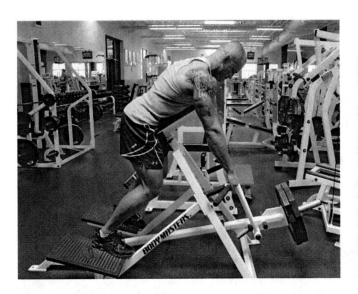
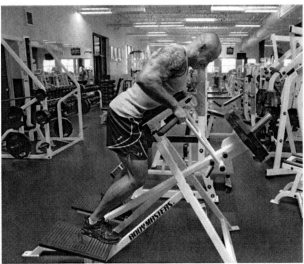

Plate Loaded T-Bar Row

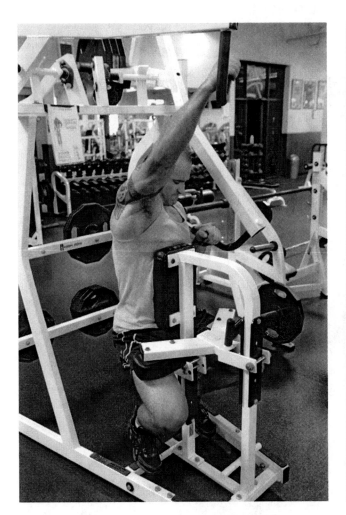
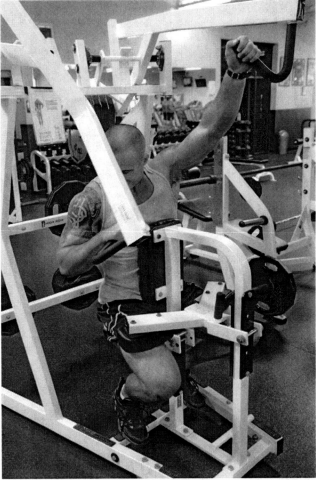

Plate Loaded Row (alternating technique)

Abdominals

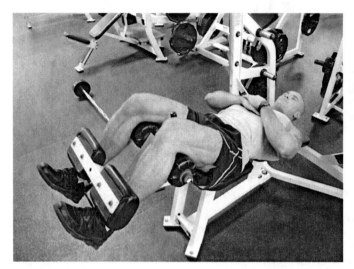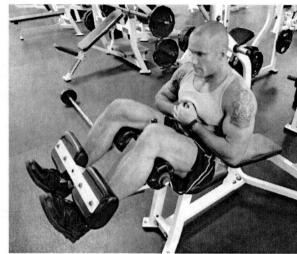

Incline Bench Sit-up/Crunches

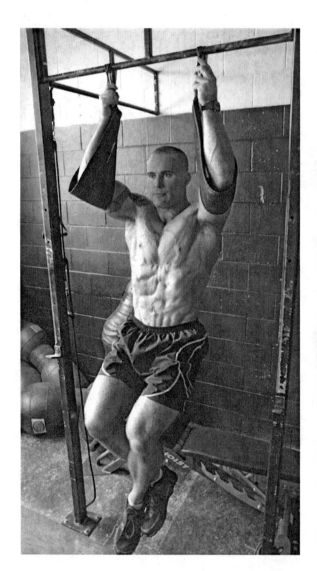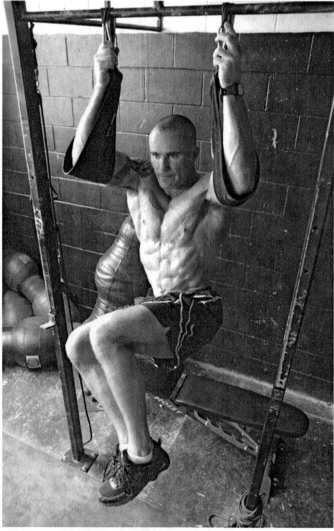

Hanging Vertical Knee Raise

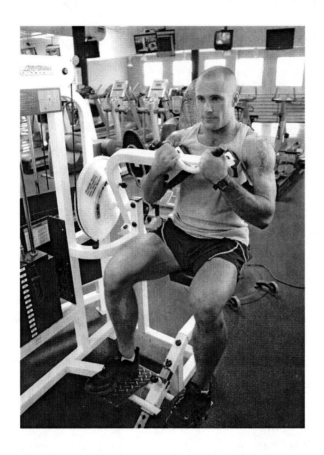

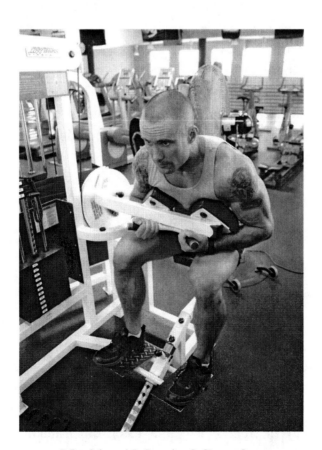

Machine Abdominal Crunches

Progress and Overcoming Sticking Points

Proper implementation of the core workout should lead to steady and continuous improvements every week as long as your nutritional needs are met and adequate time for recovery is provided. As your strength grows, you should notice an increase in either the amount of weight you can lift and/or the number of repetitions you can perform for a given exercise every single workout. Unfortunately, there will be times when you do not meet this goal. When this happens, do not become discouraged. Closely examining a few important factors will often provide a clue as to why you didn't improve from the previous week's performance. Look at your diet closely—have you consumed enough calories? Skipped meals or perhaps eaten a little too much junk food? Have you been getting adequate sleep and rest? Is there a source of extraneous stress (either mental or physical) that could be detracting from your workouts? There is a reason for everything, and careful investigation will often lead you to the correct answer.

Even with a perfectly planned training system, there will come a time when your progress in the gym slows down and eventually stops. Understanding a few basic principles will help you identify and avoid this problem before it occurs. As you grow stronger week to week and lift progressively heavier weights, the stresses placed on your physiology also increase. This inevitably leads to a state of overtraining if not compensated for. As a result, a longer recuperative period is needed between workouts. Additionally, as you become more accustomed to high-intensity training, higher intensity levels are required to stimulate the growth process. Whereas initially just performing a single set to positive failure was sufficient to stimulate maximal growth, you may need to utilize some of the advanced intensity techniques discussed here to sufficiently challenge your muscles.

When you notice that your progress is slowing down or stalled for more than two or three workouts in a row, you should perform the following analysis:

First, look for obvious changes in your lifestyle that could be contributing to the problem. Things like stress levels, sleep habits, diet, other sports, and travel can all have a negative impact on your progress. If possible, attempt to remedy any deficiencies in these areas.

Second, examine the intensity of your workouts. Are you putting out maximal effort in the gym or holding back? Are you taking every set to absolute failure or stopping short somewhere before that point? If you determine that the required intensity is lacking, consider including some of the special high-intensity techniques listed in the following section to take your workout intensity to the next level.

If you determine that you are performing your workouts to the highest possible intensity level, then the problem must lie elsewhere. Remember that as your strength increases and you lift progressively heavier weights, the stresses to your physiology also increase. Therefore, it follows logically this increased stress to your body's reserves requires a longer recovery period to replenish and eventually exceed what you started with. If this deeper inroad into your reserves is not compensated for with briefer workouts, longer rest intervals between workouts, or both, you can expect that your body will not have enough time to build new muscle tissue and your progress will at first slow down and then eventually cease.

To avoid this problem, first introduce an additional rest day to the Core Workout plan. For example, instead of training on Monday, Wednesday, and Friday, you would train Monday, take Tuesday and Wednesday off, and then train Thursday. Friday and Saturday are off and you would train again on Sunday, etc. This is the program that most trainees eventually end up on, and it seems to yield results for the longest period of time. There are some individuals who recover more slowly, however. If you notice that even with the addition of another rest day, you are still not gaining optimally, then consider adding an additional rest day so you would now be training one day and then taking seventy-two hours off before your second workout. This may seem like too long of a rest period, but remember, the higher your level of intensity, the longer your recovery period must be to compensate. Not everyone recovers at the same rate, so you must experiment somewhat and find the optimal training interval for you. And remember, the only objective criteria you should use to determine your optimal training interval is whether or not you are becoming stronger with every workout.

Finally, if you are on the Endomorphic Diet and losing strength to a significant degree, then it may be that you have cut your calories too severely and are beginning to lose muscle mass. While you are on the Endomorphic Diet, you should at least be maintaining your current strength levels. In most cases, you will make small but steady progress in your strength and muscle mass, but you really should not be losing strength from workout to workout. That is a red flag that you may be cutting calories too severely. Try increasing your calories just slightly, say by 10 percent, and see if that helps. The same rule applies if you are consuming below maintenance caloric levels on the Mesomorphic Diet.

Advanced High-Intensity Techniques

As discussed previously, the intensity level of exercise is the primary factor involved in the stimulation of muscle growth. When beginning The Program, you will be required to train with a very high intensity level. Each set is to be taken to the point of momentary muscular failure, meaning that despite your best efforts, you cannot perform another full-range repetition with good form. Many of you will be unaccustomed to this degree of effort. Don't worry. You will soon find that you will develop the proper mental focus and concentration needed to reach this point. As you progress, many of you will look for ways to increase the intensity of your workouts beyond simply training to momentary muscle failure. Indeed, as you become more advanced, you will need to increase the intensity of your workouts to continue stimulating growth.

There are a number of techniques available that you may incorporate into your workouts to achieve this goal. Those of you with weight-training experience may have used some of them before. In that case, you may want to begin incorporating them into the Core Workout from the beginning. For new lifters, I would recommend becoming comfortable with training to failure first before adding some of these techniques. Be aware that these tools can greatly increase the intensity of your workouts and therefore require a longer recovery period to compensate for their effects. If your progress slows down or you find that you are still very sore by the time your next workout is due, consider adding additional rest days to your workout.

1. Supersets

Supersets are a great way not only to increase the intensity of your workouts but also to greatly shorten their duration. A basic superset involves one exercise followed immediately by another (usually involving the same body part) with little or no rest between them. Supersets are easy to incorporate into the Core Workout. Any body part that has two exercises assigned to it is a potential candidate for a superset. For example, on day 2, you could superset dumbbell military presses with machine lateral raises for a very intense shoulder workout. Similarly on day 3, you could superset the conventional bench press with chest flies on a machine. Remember that you will be fatigued by the time you start the second exercise in the superset and will have to adjust the weight you are lifting accordingly. Don't expect to perform as many reps or lift as much as you can when you are fresh. Ideally, there should be no rest between the two exercises. So set up your weight for the second lift in advance so you don't waste time adjusting plates or pins. As soon as you complete the first exercise, move directly to the second.

2. Negatives

Incorporating negatives into your training can be an extremely effective way to add greater intensity to your workouts. The term *negative* refers to the portion of the lift where the muscle lengthens against the resistance of the weight you are using (an eccentric contraction). In contrast, the portion of the lift where the muscle contracts or shortens is referred to as the positive portion (a concentric contraction). For example, when performing a repetition of bicep curls, you initially grasp the weight and begin to curl the weight toward you. As you do this, your bicep muscle contracts and shortens. This is the "positive" portion of the lift. When you have reached the fully contracted position, you then begin to slowly lower the weight. This phase is referred to as the "negative" portion. As you lower the weight, your bicep is contracting very strongly to control the weights decent, but it is also lengthening. Every conventional set you perform is a repetitive cycle of positive and negative contractions.

The strongest portion of every lift is the negative phase. You typically can lower at least 20 to 30 percent more weight than you can lift. Additionally, you will still have the ability to lower a given amount of weight even after you have reached positive failure. Examination of muscle tissue after repetitive bouts of negative exercise shows a significantly greater amount of microtrauma to individual muscle fibers than does positive-only training. However, research to date has not shown that negative-only training is superior to conventional training in terms of developing muscle size. Training with negatives will greatly enhance your strength through the eccentric or lowering portion of the exercise, however. This is an area where clearly more research is needed. A certain degree of caution is warranted when incorporating negatives into your training. When using negatives, the forces placed upon your muscles and tendons are significantly greater. As a result, the potential for injury and the inroad into your body's recovery ability are increased. Be sure to compensate for this by using strict form and adding additional recovery time as needed.

Negatives can be used to enhance your training in several ways. First and most simply is to have your training partner assist you after you have reached positive failure. Have your partner help you lift the weight and then in a slow and controlled manner perform two to three additional negative-only repetitions. This is an excellent technique to fully stimulate the muscle group you are working and will leave you feeling completely exhausted. Obviously, certain exercises are more suited to this technique than others. It would be difficult and potentially dangerous to try this with squats and deadlifts, but most other free-weight and machine exercises are conducive to this technique.

The second way to incorporate negatives is to perform so-called "negative-only" training. This type of training involves using significantly heavier weights than you typically use and produces the greatest amount of muscle fiber trauma. A negative-only set involves using approximately 20 to 30 percent or more weight than you use for your conventional sets. Your training partner assists you in the positive portion of the lift until you reach the fully contracted position. At that point, you slowly lower the weight until you reach the fully extended position. This should take approximately three to five seconds and be performed in a very deliberate and controlled manner. As with your other sets, your goal should be eight to twelve repetitions. Again, be aware that this type of training is very intense and causes significantly more microtrauma to your muscles. As a result, expect to have sore muscles and require a longer recovery time before your muscles have fully compensated. There is insufficient research in humans to recommend that you make negative-only training the foundation of your training. It is not suitable when you are performing three workouts a week because (except for the most genetically gifted), there is usually not enough recovery time between workouts for adequate growth to occur. If you would like to incorporate some negative-only training into your workouts, I recommend choosing one workout or one body part per cycle as your negative-only day. The following cycle, pick a different workout or muscle group and so on. This way, you can reap the benefits of this very intense training style while avoiding overtraining.

3. Static Holds

Static holds involve maintaining the fully contracted position for as long as possible before lowering the weight to the fully extended position. This technique is best used in combination with negatives at the end of a set you have taken to positive muscular failure. This takes advantage of the fact that even after reaching positive failure (where you can no longer lift the weight you are using), you still have a sufficient reserve of muscle fibers that can hold the weight in the fully contracted position for a certain period of time before fatiguing. And even then, as mentioned above, you still have sufficient strength left to lower the weight in a controlled manner. An example of a set of pull-ups performed using this technique would look like this: you would perform as many pull-ups as possible; in this case, we'll say ten. At the end of your tenth repetition, your arms and lats are in the fully contracted position where you then hold yourself as long as possible. When you are shaking all over and feel like you are in danger of giving out and falling to the floor, slowly lower yourself to the ground in a controlled manner. If you are performing this technique with negatives, have your training partner help you back up into the fully contracted position and perform two to four additional reps in the same manner. Having your partner count out loud as you stay in the contracted position can quantify how long you are able to perform your static-hold and give you a reference point that you can try to exceed the next time you perform the same lift. A wide variety of exercises are amenable to static holds if you want to incorporate them in your training. Most free-weight and machine exercises are conducive to static hold training.

4. Rest-Pause

Rest-pause training is a personal favorite. This advanced intensity technique allows you to lift near maximal weights to fully stimulate your fast-twitch muscle fibers while still performing the desired repetition range of eight to twelve. A typical rest-pause set would look like this: Choose a weight that is as close to your one-repetition maximum as possible. Perform a single rep, and then rest three to five seconds. Perform another rep, and rest a similar amount of time. Continue this until you have reached eight to twelve reps. Obviously, you will need to lower the weight slightly after about the third or fourth rep and extend your rest interval a bit. This is perfectly okay. As long as you are performing what, at that moment, is as close to your one-rep maximum as possible, you will reap maximum benefit from this technique. In some cases, a complete set using the rest-pause technique may take as long as one to two minutes. As with negative-only training, you will be handling significantly heavier weights than you are accustomed to. Therefore, the risk of injury is increased, and the recovery time between workouts should be increased. Use strict form, and do your best not to cheat the weight up. Rest-pause training can be a fun and challenging way to up the intensity levels of your workouts. Use it sparingly, however, since regularly incorporating it into your workouts can lead to overtraining. Rest-pause training is best introduced at random or on days when you feel especially energized and want to really challenge yourself.

5. Strip Sets

Strip sets (or drop sets as they are sometimes called) are used to prolong a set beyond the point where you would ordinarily reach muscle failure. They involve selecting your usual weight for a given exercise and performing it to muscular failure. At that point, you or your training partner decreases the weight enough to allow you to continue. In general, aim for a weight reduction that allows you to perform about five more repetitions. If you lower the weight too much, you will end up performing a larger number of repetitions with very light weight and are more likely to stop for cardiovascular reasons than true muscle failure.

6. Heavy Partials

Heavy partials are a technique that I used during the off-season between power-lifting competitions. They involve using a much heavier weight than you are accustomed to and lifting it through a limited range of motion instead of the full range that you typically perform. For example, many power lifters have difficulty performing the last third of the bench press where the arms are fully extended and the weight is lifted the maximum distance from the chest. To remedy this, they perform bench presses using heavy partials on a power rack. This involves setting the safety bars on the rack so that the bar rests about six to eight inches above the chest. From here, the lifter loads up to 50 percent or more weight than he or she typically uses and proceeds to press the bar upward and then lower it back to rest on the safety bars. Many lifts are amenable to this technique, but the power lifts—the squat, bench press, and deadlift—are particularly well suited to heavy partials. The disadvantage of heavy partials is that the muscle is not worked through its entire range of motion. If you performed only heavy partials, you would quickly develop strength primarily in the range you trained; however, your strength through the remainder of the range of motion would be lacking. Heavy partials allow you to challenge your body with very heavy weights, which is particularly good for stimulating growth of fast-twitch muscle fibers. Perhaps, their best use is for those of you looking to improve a weak area in a particular lift, such as the lockout phase of the bench press or deadlift. I encourage you to try heavy partials only once you have become fully comfortable training in a more conventional manner.

Combining Techniques

There is no rule stating that you can only use one of these high-intensity techniques at a time. In fact, combining them during a single set can be an extremely effective way of greatly increasing your workout intensity. We already used the combination of static-holds and negatives as an example of how to combine techniques for added intensity. In reality, it is possible to combine any one of these techniques with another in order to take your workouts to the next level. Be creative and feel free to experiment to find what suits you and your training partner best. Just remember that as the intensity of exercise increases, you dig a deeper hole in your body's reserves, and as a result, it will take longer to recover. Be sure to increase your rest interval between workouts accordingly to compensate.

Rotating Exercises

The exercises listed in the exercise database are ranked in order of their effectiveness at stimulating growth in a given muscle or muscle group. When starting The Program, you should make every effort to include the recommended exercises in your routine. Having said that, realize that The Program is flexible. If you have a favorite exercise that has worked well in the past for you, you may substitute it for the recommended exercise. If you have an injury that precludes you from performing the recommended exercise for a given body part, certainly feel free to substitute one that suits you better. There may also come a time when you experience a certain amount of mental boredom with a particular exercise and want to try something different for a while. This is perfectly acceptable and, in fact, encouraged. Before you decide to change exercises, take stock of your progress to date. Has your strength in that particular lift increased steadily? Does your body seem to be responding well to that exercise? If so, following the "if it's not broke, don't fix it" philosophy may be best. Use your best judgment. If you are having success with a given lift but are becoming a little bored, you may try another for a while. You can always return to the original exercise later. Most of the time, trainees do extremely well with the recommended exercises but at some point begin to develop minor injuries like tendonitis, joint pains, or other nuisances. When this happens, listen to your body and take a break from that particular exercise just long enough to let those problems heal up. Then resume where you left off.

The following is how the basic Core Workout would look when placed into a training log:

	1	2	3	4	5	6	7	8
Day 1								
Thighs								
Calves								
Day 2								
Front Deltoid								
Side Deltoid								
Biceps								
Triceps								
Abs								
Day 3								
Chest (Press)								
Chest (Fly)								
Deadlift or								
Narrow-grip Back								
Wide-grip back								

What You Can Expect

Most trainees have come to expect that gaining muscle and losing fat is supposed to occur at an agonizingly slow pace. They have been disappointed over and over again so that now they believe progress, if it comes at all, only does so in small increments over months to years. Indeed, I have seen people who come to the gym every day year after year and have literally made no progress whatsoever. Most people give up long before that. If you have been exercising regularly and not making the kind of progress you want, then it's time to make a change. The system you are using is not working, and it's not going to magically start working anytime soon. It's time to step back and take an objective look at how you are approaching your workouts and make the necessary changes.

One of my favourite quotes from Mike Mentzer is: "if you are in possession of a truly valid theory, then success should be nothing short of spectacular." He couldn't be more correct. Nowhere is this truer than in modern medicine. Think about how diseases were treated during the Dark Ages. It was thought that disease was caused by "evil humors," demonic possession, and other nonsense. As a result, the physicians at the time were spectacular failures at curing disease. With techniques like bleeding and cupping (the placement of burning hot glass cups on the skin to draw out evil humors) being used regularly, you often had a better chance of recovery by staying away from physicians altogether. In those days, a simple ear infection or scratch could be fatal. It wasn't until the Enlightenment and through the first half of the twentieth century that scientists and doctors began to understand the underlying cause of infectious diseases. Now we take for granted the fact that antibiotics can cure most of the diseases that meant certain death to our not-so-distant ancestors. Surgery has progressed in much the same way. Appendicitis used to have an incredibly high death rate until the twentieth century. An inflamed appendix invariably would rupture, spilling pus into the abdomen and, unless you were lucky and your body could wall off the infection, lead to sepsis and death. Now, appendicitis is usually caught in its early stages and cured with a short, routine surgery, and the patient goes on to live out the rest of his or her life as if it never happened.

Exercise science has undergone a similar revolution in the last half-century, and progress continues to be made. The fundamental principles that induce the human body to develop muscle mass beyond baseline levels are well established. Unfortunately, there continues to be a great deal of misinformation and confusion on the subject. The arbitrary training systems espoused by most bodybuilders and fitness magazines are not rooted in science. As a result, the results gained from such systems are usually disappointing. The principles of high-intensity training are the fundamental tools that are used in The Program to help you meet your goals of a more muscular physique. As mentioned before, exercise designed to increase muscle strength must be intense, brief, and infrequent. The human body, any human body, will respond to a training system firmly based on these basic principles. Obviously, there is considerable variation among individuals in just how much progress can be made. Not everyone has the genetic predisposition to be Mr. Universe. However, regardless of what your ultimate genetic potential is, everyone has the ability to gain muscle and lose body fat when placed on a properly designed training program. The only way to discover the upper limit of your genetic potential is to achieve it.

When you are training correctly in accordance with the principles of the theory of high-intensity training, keeping your training sessions short, and allowing adequate time to recover and grow between workouts, then your progress should be continuous from the day you start training up until you near the upper limits of your genetic potential. If you are training correctly, you should be increasing in strength every single workout. Those of you following the dietary recommendations for increasing muscle size will see a corresponding steady increase in muscle size as well. It is not uncommon for those trying to get bigger on The Program to gain steadily one to two pounds of lean mass every seven to ten days. How much you gain and how quickly you gain it has a lot to do with your genetic makeup and your age, but the gains will come and they will do so faster and with less time spent in the gym than with any other training system you have tried before.

"Hastiness and superficiality are the psychic diseases of the twentieth century."

—Aleksandr Solzhenitsyn

THE PERSONAL EVOLUTION QUICK START GUIDE

Most trainees who begin a new training regimen are wildly enthusiastic. They want to get started right away. Many people, when first picking up a copy of *The Program*, can feel a little intimidated by the hundreds of pages and sheer volume of scientific information presented. And, of course, not everyone is interested in learning all the minute details of why they are doing what they are doing. They want to be told exactly what to do and how to do it and don't want to be bombarded with facts about insulin, glucose, metabolism, or any of the other minutiae that go into understanding the "why" of The Program. "Just tell me what to do, Doc, and I'll do it!" is something I hear quite often. I can certainly understand this perspective. That's why I've written this particular section of the book in such a way that it stands somewhat separate from the rest of the material. If you just purchased this book and want to get started *today*, then this section is for you.

As you move further into your training, however, I do encourage you to take the time to start from the beginning and read *The Program* cover to cover. Many of the ideas on both nutrition and training presented here are unconventional and need to be applied correctly for optimal results. Ultimately, I don't want you to adhere slavishly to this system unquestioningly for all time. I want you to be able to understand the underlying principles upon which The Program is built. When you grasp these fundamentals, you can then make intelligent adjustments in your training and nutritional program that fit your specific needs while still obtaining excellent results. Remember, The Program is the "thinking person's" training system. I wouldn't be doing you much good long term if I just told you what to do and didn't explain why you're doing it. I don't expect you to become a PhD exercise physiologist, but grasping a basic understanding of how your body responds to changes in nutrition and to specific training stresses will broaden your understanding and allow you not only to meet your own personal goals but assist others in doing the same.

Prelaunch Checklist

Before you start The Program, you should run through this prelaunch checklist:

1. Set goals:

   Write them down. Do you want to gain muscle, lose fat, or both? Be *specific*.

2. Before photos:

   Optional but strongly encouraged

3. Blood work:

   Ask your physician to order some basic screening tests:
   - a. Fasting glucose
   - b. Fasting lipid panel
   - c. Liver function tests
   - d. Vitamin D level
   - e. Testosterone, including bioavailable testosterone level
   - f. Any other tests specific to any particular medical problem you may have

4. Estimate your body-fat percentage:

   Use skin calipers, a bioelectrical impedance device, hydrostatic weighing, DEXA, or whatever equipment you have available.

5. Estimate how much total body fat you are carrying in kilograms:

   Weight in kg x body fat % expressed as a decimal= **kg of body fat**

   (Ex: 100 kg individual with 15% body fat has 100 x 0.15 = 15 kg of body fat)

6. Estimate your basal metabolic rate:

   Use either the Schofield equation or the Harris-Benedict equation:

The Schofield equation:
Men:
10–17 years BMR = 17.7 x W + 657 SEE = 105
18–29 years BMR = 15.1 x W + 692 SEE = 156
30–59 years BMR = 11.5 x W + 873 SEE = 167

Women:
10–17 years BMR = 13.4 x W + 692 SEE = 112
18–29 years BMR = 14.8 x W + 487 SEE = 120
30–59 years BMR = 8.3 x W + 846 SEE = 112

Key: W = body weight in kilograms (Convert body weight here!)
SEE = standard error of estimation

The SEE (standard error of estimation) is a built-in "fudge factor." It is the degree to which your calculated BMR may be off (either over- or underestimated).

If you are within three years of the young end of your age group, then add your SEE. If you are within three years of the older end of your age range, then subtract your SEE from your BMR.

If you already have a lot of muscle mass (>200 lbs), you should also add the SEE to your BMR. Obese individuals should subtract the SEE from their total.

As a general rule, if you are close to the young end of your age range, you should add the SEE to your total since younger people have higher BMRs. If you are toward the upper end of your age range, you should subtract your SEE from your BMR. Similarly, if you already have a lot of muscle, you should add the SEE to your total since you will naturally have a higher metabolic rate. Obese individuals (>25% body fat for men and >35% for women) should subtract the SEE from their total.

The Harris-Benedict Equation:

Men:

BEE = 66.5 + (13.75 x kg) + (5.003 x cm) – (6.775 x age)

Women:

BEE = 655.1 + (9.563 x kg) + (1.850 x cm) – (4.676 x age)

7. Calculate your maintenance calorie level:

Using your BMR (basal metabolic rate) calculated above:

Sedentary—none or very little exercise = BMR X 1.2
Program workout + no cardio = BMR X 1.4
Program workout + cardio 3/week = BMR X 1.6
Program workout + cardio 5–6 times/week = BMR X 1.7

8. Higher activity levels, i.e., program workout + cardio 5–6/week + other sporting activity = up to 2 x BMR

9. Choose a diet:

This will depend on your goals.

- The Ectomorphic Diet for those of you who want to gain as much muscle mass as possible.
- The Mesomorphic Diet for either maintenance or gradual weight loss/gain.
- The Endomorphic Diet for the fastest possible weight loss.

The Endomorphic Diet in a Nutshell

Total Calories:

Maintenance calorie level (as calculated above) – maximum calorie deficit

The maximum calorie deficit = Your total kg of body fat (as calculated above) x 70 x 0.75

Carbohydrates:
- Begin with a total of 30 grams per day
- Less than 10% of total calories from carbohydrates
- Keep carbohydrates low for breakfast
- Composition of carbohydrates should come, as much as possible, from high-fiber, leafy-green vegetables
- Optimal time for bulk of carbohydrate intake is prior to the daily workout.

Protein:
- Total protein intake should be 2.0 grams per kg of body weight divided roughly equally between 6 daily meal
- No more than 30% of total calories will come from protein
- Fast proteins should be consumed immediately before and immediately after the daily workout
- Slow proteins (egg, soy, or casein) should be consumed before bed
- Goal is for a minimum of 20 grams of leucine and 100 grams of BCAAs per day divided between 6 meals
- Protein should not exceed 40% of total calories

Fats:
- Approximately 60% of daily calories come from fat
- Approximately 60% of daily calories come from fat
- Goal is near equal omega-6 to omega-3 fat intake
- Omega-3 fatty acid supplementation with a goal of 2–3 grams of DHA+EPA total per day from fish oil or flax
- Zero trans fats

"Cheat Day"

Once a week, you may break from the diet and eat however you like. Attempt to consume the same amount of quality protein you would normally consume, but you may eat any carbohydrate or fat foods that you wish.

Do not consume carbohydrates after 10:00 p.m.

The Mesomorphic Diet in a Nutshell

Total Calories:

If your goal is to lose weight:

a. Estimate your maximal caloric deficit:

Your maximum allowable calorie deficit is 70 calories per kg of body fat per day.

As an added safety margin, this number is decreased by 25% to give you the initial number of calories you should subtract from your maintenance calorie level.

*Kg of body fat x 70 x 0.75 = **maximum caloric deficit***

(Ex: an individual with 15 kg of body fat could burn 15 x 70 = 1,050 calories of fat per day.)

b. Subtract this deficit from your maintenance caloric level calculated above to give you your daily caloric intake.

If your goal is to gain weight:

Add approximately 500 calories to your maintenance calorie level and monitor your progress. If you aren't gaining enough weight, add an additional 250 calories every two weeks until you are gaining weight at the rate you are happy with. If you are gaining too much fat, then cut back your calories by 250 and reevaluate your results in two weeks.

Carbohydrates:

- Approximately 35% of your total calories
- Less than 25% of total carbohydrate items from the "restricted" list
- Composition of carbohydrates should come, as much as possible, from high-fiber, leafy-green vegetables, fresh fruits, nuts, legumes, and whole grains.

Protein:

- Total protein intake should be 2.0 grams per kg of body weight divided roughly equally between 6 daily meals.
- Approximately 30% or less of total calories will come from protein
- Fast proteins should be consumed immediately before and immediately after the daily workout.
- Slow proteins (egg, soy, or casein) should be consumed before bed
- Goal is for a minimum of 20 grams of leucine and 100 grams of BCAAs per day divided between 6 meals.
- Protein should not exceed 40% of total calories.

Fats:

- Approximately 35% of daily calories come from fat
- Saturated fat no more than 10% of daily fat calories
- Goal is near equal omega-6 to omega-3 fat intake

- Omega-3 fatty acid supplementation with a goal of 2–3 grams of DHA+EPA total per day from fish oil or flax.
- Zero trans-fats.

"Cheat Meal":
Once a week, you may break from the diet and eat one meal containing whatever you like.

The Ectomorphic Diet in a Nutshell

Total Calories:

Add approximately 1000 calories to your maintenance calorie level, and monitor your progress.

If you aren't gaining enough weight, add an additional 250 calories every two weeks until you are gaining weight at the rate you are happy with.

If you are gaining too much fat, then cut back your calories by 250 and re-evaluate your results in two weeks.

Carbohydrate:

- Approximately 60% of your total calories
- Consume at least 50–100 grams of high-glycemic carbohydrate during three critical windows: after 11:00 p.m.; approximately 3 hours before breakfast; immediately after the day's workout.
- The remainder of the day's carbohydrate should be a mixture of moderate- and low-glycemic carbohydrates from fruits, vegetables, and grains

Protein:

- Total protein intake should be approximately 2.0 grams per kg of body weight divided roughly equally between 6 daily meals and a 7th early morning meal.
- Approximately 20% or less of total calories will come from protein.
- Fast proteins should be consumed immediately before and immediately after the daily workout and with the early morning meal
- Slow proteins (egg, soy, or casein) should be consumed before bedtime
- Goal is for a minimum of 20 grams of leucine and 100 grams of BCAAs per day divided between 7 meals

Fat:

- Remainder of total calories will come from fat, resulting in approximately 25% of daily calories coming from fat.
- Limit saturated fat to no more than 10% of daily fat calories.
- Goal is near equal omega-6 to omega-3 fat intake.
- Omega-3 fatty acid supplementation with a goal of 2–3 grams of DHA+EPA total per day from fish oil or flax.
- Zero trans-fats.

"Cheat Meal"

Sorry, no such thing!

Supplements for All Diets:

Add 5 grams of creatine twice a day

Minimum of 2 grams of DHA+EPA from fish oil or flaxseed oil per day

Training

All sets are between 8–12 repetitions and taken to momentary failure.

All exercises are performed for 1 set only unless otherwise specified.

Advanced high-intensity techniques may be included as needed.

Choose an appropriate exercise for each muscle group from the exercise database.

Beginners with no weight-training experience should start on the beginner's workout.

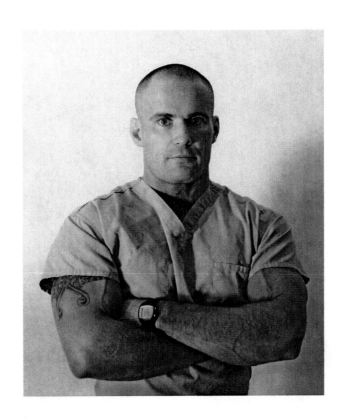

Andrew Winge, MD, graduated from the University of Oregon with a BS in Exercise and Movement Science. He obtained his medical degree from the Uniformed Services University and is board certified in Family Medicine and Emergency Medicine and a member of the American Society of Bariatric Physicians. Dr. Winge spent 17 years in the US Air Force practicing both Family Medicine and Emergency Medicine. He currently works full-time as an emergency room physician while also coaching, lecturing, and teaching about nutrition and high-intensity exercise. He runs an educational blog at www.personalevolution.net where he shares his thoughts on nutrition, training, and healthcare.

CPSIA information can be obtained
at www.ICGtesting.com
Printed in the USA
LVOW09s1020260617

539391LV00018B/432/P